APHASIA AND RELATED DISORDERS IN CHILDREN

Second Edition

Jon Eisenson

Professor Emeritus, Hearing and Speech Science
Stanford University

Former Distinguished Professor of Special Education
San Francisco State University

1817

HARPER & ROW, PUBLISHERS, New York
Cambridge, Philadelphia, San Francisco,
London, Mexico City, São Paulo, Sydney

Sponsoring Editor: Louise Waller
Project Coordinator: Total Concept Associates
Compositor: Jay's Publishers Services, Inc.
Printer and Binder: R. R. Donnelley & Sons Company

Aphasia and Related Disorders in Children, Second Edition

Library of Congress Cataloging in Publication Data

Eisenson, Jon, 1907–
  Aphasia and related disorders in children

  Rev. ed. of: Aphasia in children. c1972.
  Includes bibliographies and index.
  1. Aphasic children. 2. Language disorders in
children. I. Eisenson, Jon, 1907–   . Aphasia in
children. II. Title. [DNLM: 1. Aphasia—In infancy and
childhood. 2. Language development. 3. Perceptual
disorders—In infancy and childhood. WL 340.5 E36ab]
RJ496.A6E57   1984   618.92′8552   83–12740
ISBN 0–06–041889–3

Contents

Preface

Aphasia and Related Disorders in Children takes into account the scope and numbers of aphasic children and those with related problems. I wish it were possible to present firm figures—numbers and percentages—of the incidence of aphasia in the population of schoolage and younger children. Perhaps if the experts could decide on criteria (and here I offer my own), we could arrive at the necessary figures. Admittedly, the criteria I present in this text reflect my position. Fortunately, however, this position is shared with respected researchers in the field of child language. The first chapter discusses my approach, which is defined and explained at the outset—the better, I hope, to clarify my overall position.

This book is about children who are severely linguistically impaired and whose impairments permit the differential diagnosis of aphasia. It is also *for* these children, in the expectation that knowledge and clinical skill will help them overcome their impairments. In the first edition of this text, aphasic children were identified as a special population of the linguistically impaired. I provided evidence to support my position that these children had a congenital deficiency in perceptual functioning for those events that comprise the signals of oral language. Because of this underlying impairment, these children—the congenitally aphasic—are seriously delayed in acquiring and developing (or learning) language in the manner of the vast majority of children and of those who may be below the norm in intellectual capacity but have sufficient intelligence to learn to speak.

In this edition, we will cite other children who have perceptual impairments and who, to a lesser degree than aphasic children, also have language problems. Recent research strongly suggests that many children with reading problems—so-called hard-core dyslexics—also lack proficiency in their knowledge of language. This lack of proficiency is all the more significant because most of the indices of cognitive or intellectual potential for these children are well within normal range. I view these children as *brain different* and as a subtype of aphasic children. Support for this view will be found in the recent literature on dyslexia. In young children with *acquired aphasia,* the deficiencies, because they *are* acquired, become more apparent. These problems are considered in Chapter 1, in the section on acquired aphasia in children.

Aphasia and Related Disorders in Children includes expanded consideration of the perceptual dysfunctions that I firmly believe underlie the difficulties of some children in acquiring language through normal exposure and incidental teaching by parents and other key members of families. Classic and newer studies are reviewed to support this position in Chapter 3, "Perception and Perceptual Functioning Underlying Language Acquisition."

New chapters for this edition include Chapter 11, "Acquired Aphasia in Children," and Chapter 12 "Childhood Autism," by Adriana L. Schuler, an outstanding authority who has published widely in the area of childhood aphasia.

Chapter 2, an expanded chapter on normal language development, provides a basis for comparison with Chapter 5, "Congenital (Developmental) Aphasia." Chapter 6, on assessment, is also considerably expanded, with evaluations of tests and procedures that may be used with aphasic and other linguistically retarded children.

Some of my respected colleagues may continue to have reservations about the identification of a special population of children as aphasic or dysphasic. A line of argument offered by these colleagues is that even if there are aphasic children, therapeutic approaches for them would not be different from those employed with other linguistically retarded children. In Chapter 9, I present a counterposition: Aphasic children are a special population and so need specialized approaches. Such childen do improve with the approaches described and the materials presented in Chapters 8 and 9.

Chapter 10, "Congenital Motor Impairments for Speech Production," provides criteria for distinguishing the problem of articulatory apraxia from expressive aphasia.

For this and the first edition, I am grateful to my colleagues who participated in the clinical research that, for the most part, generated the data and my position on the nature of childhood aphasia. I am grateful also to the colleagues who shared their reservations with me, with the result that, from time to time, I had to review both theory and therapy with awarenesses that might otherwise have escaped me. Most of all, I am grateful to the parents and the children who were most active and involved in the many years of investigation on congenital aphasia, articulatory apraxia, and acquired aphasia in children.

Jon Eisenson

chapter 1

Introduction: Some Definitions and Defined Prejudices

This book will be concerned with three groups of children who are impaired in learning or producing an oral language system: the *congenitally aphasic,* the *oral (articulatory) apraxic,* and the *autistic.* It will also be concerned with a fourth group—children who acquired language normally but suffered from impairments in language proficiency as a result of brain damage incurred before age 12. These are children with *acquired childhood aphasia.*

Before defining or further characterizing these groups of children with aphasic or related disorders of language, this chapter will offer some definitions and explanations that may reveal some prejudices. It is hoped that these prejudices are not so personal that they cannot be shared.

THE DEFINITION OF LANGUAGE

Unless otherwise specified, the term *language* will be used to refer to a system that normally and primarily employs an aural/oral circuit for comprehension and production. This in no way implies that sign systems do not conform to the criteria and are not capable of serving the functions of an aural/oral language. Whatever the means of intake or output, language is a system that employs arbitrary symbols and rules relating to their use that permit human beings to express and exchange their thoughts and their feelings. A more elaborate definition is proposed for consideration by the Committee on Language of the American Speech-Language-Hearing Association:

> Language, one mode of human reasoning and communication, is an arbitrary or conventional symbol system which:
>
> 1. is perpetuated by a given linguistic community;

2. allows members of such a community to represent nonlinguistic and linguistic knowledge and share that knowledge with other members of the community through the comprehension and expression of an infinite number of novel productions;
3. can be shared through various modalities of transmission—listening, speaking, reading, writing, looking, and gesturing;
4. is acquired and used within variable biologic, psychologic, and environmental contexts resulting in multiple performance styles;
5. assumes, for full knowledge of and effective use of, a relatively intact central nervous system, a variety of cognitive processes, and a broad base of conceptual and social understanding; and,
6. appears to be comprised of multiple, interacting patterns of organization, i.e., phonologic (or analogous visual, tactile), morphologic, semantic, syntactic, and pragmatic. (ASHA, 1981, p. 143)

Language is actually a complex of subsystems, each of which has its own rules that somehow relate to the rules of the others. The subsystems are *phonology*—the sounds of spoken language and the rules governing their use; *morphology*—minimum units of meaning that are combined in "lawful" ways to form words; *syntax* (grammar)—the conventions that govern how we put words together to form sentences; *semantics*—the rules that determine the particular meaning of any given sentence; and *pragmatics* (situational semantics)—the system of practices and conventions that we must learn to increase the likelihood of achieving our purpose in speaking.[1]

Later discussions will elaborate on each of the subsystems of language and indicate how the groups of children with whom we are concerned are deficient in the use of the separate but overlapping systems. This chapter will present expanded explanations of the groups of children who, to varying degrees, are impaired in learning to comprehend and to express themselves in language, despite indicators that do not make such lack of proficiency readily apparent.

CONGENITAL APHASIA

Congenitally aphasic children have a primary impairment for processing (decoding and, in turn, encoding) oral language. This impairment, as indicated earlier, exists despite adequate intelligence, as assessed by clinical impression and nonlanguage measures of intelligence; despite hearing that, at least as measured by the usual audiometric procedures, is considered adequate for hearing spoken language; despite lack of evidence of a primary emotional (relating) problem; and despite membership in a family that provides normal opportunities and motivation for listening to interested and proficient speakers.

---

[1]Moskowitz (1978) defines *pragmatics* as rules that "describe how to participate in a conversation, how to sequence sentences, and how to anticipate the information needed by an interlocutor" (p. 92).

Other identifying terms for congenitally aphasic children, usually implying lesser degrees of impairment in language acquisition, are *congenital dysphasia* (Benton, 1978; Menyuk, 1978; Tallal and Piercy, 1978; Wyke, 1978) and *central auditory disorder* (Keith, 1981; Stark and Tallal, 1981). The position taken in this book is that the congenitally aphasic child is at the extreme negative end of a continuum that includes dysphasic children, those with central auditory deficiencies, those with learning problems, and perhaps a majority of children who have difficulty in learning to read and by age 9 or 10 may be identified as dyslexic.

Underlying the language problems of the congenitally aphasic child is an impairment in the auditory perception of contextual speech. This impairment is implied in the term *central auditory disorder*. (Chapter 3 will expand on this position.) Several investigators and theorists, however,—notably, Rees (1981) and Bloom and Lahey (1978)—take exception to this view. In a provocative article, "Saying More Than We Know," Rees states: "Auditory processing disturbances have become the iron bed into which all sorts of language and learning deficits are made to fit." Rees further argues that auditory processing approaches have not produced useful results in children classified as having central auditory dysfunctions. Even if this is so, it may well be a criticism of the particulars of the method rather than the diagnosis.

Bloom and Lahey (1978) do not object so much to the term *congenital aphasia* as to the value of the term as an indicator of determining appropriate therapeutic procedures. They argue: "To know that a particular child has been labeled aphasic does not tell the clinician or teacher what it is that the child needs to know about language, nor what the child's language development may have consisted of so far" (p. 512). The present author does not accept this assessment of the problem. Later chapters will discuss the approaches that have been found successful in the treatment of congenitally aphasic children.

Cromer (1978), who takes exception to the notion that congenitally dysphasic children have an impairment in their perception of sound per se, indicates that the underlying difficulty may be an impairment in the children's hierarchial structuring ability for language. This book assumes, however, that in aphasic children, both impairments—for speech perception at the outset and for syntactic structuring—are present.

ACQUIRED CHILDHOOD APHASIA

A second group of children with whom we will be concerned are those with *acquired aphasia*. These are children who have a normal history of learning to comprehend spoken language and to speak. Those above age 5 or 6 may have learned to read and write and may have established proficiencies in arithmetic and possibly in higher forms of mathematics. (In practice, age 14 is considered the upper limit for childhood aphasia.) Their language disorders and associated impairments followed brain damage from injury or disease that involved the language centers of the brain. Fortunately, the outlook for linguistic recovery is good for the vast majority of children with acquired aphasia, provided that one cerebral hemisphere is spared. (Chapter 11 will expand on this subject.) Nevertheless, there may be residual impairments that require therapy and that may have implications for continued language learning and educational achievement.

ORAL (ARTICULATORY) APRAXIA

A third group of children with whom we will be concerned in this book comprises those who can and usually do learn to understand spoken language but cannot make themselves understood orally. These are children whose articulatory problems are so severe that their speech is not intelligible. Their organs of articulation do not do their bidding. We identify these children as having *congenital oral* (*articulatory*) *apraxia*. Unless they are "turned off" and turned away from speakers and speaking because of their motor-productive impairment, congenitally apraxic children can continue to learn (decode) spoken language and to learn to read and write, provided that the teaching method used does not require articulatory behavior. These children will be considered in some detail in Chapter 10.

PRIMARY AUTISM

The fourth group of children with whom we shall be concerned are those with *primary autism*. This term implies that from the beginning of life, these children demonstrated behaviors or lack of behaviors that indicate normal ability to relate to caretakers. These children may well be a subgroup of the congenitally aphasic, with additional and complicating problems. Lovaas (1977, p. 30) considers language deficiency a salient feature for defining autism. Other features include apparent sensory deficit, severe affect isolation, and self-stimulatory behavior. Often, there is also "an absence of or minimal presence of social and self-help behaviors." Lovaas speculates that the problems autistic children show "may be the cause of their language deficiency or its effect. . . ." The autistic child will be considered in detail in Chapter 12.

BRAIN DIFFERENCE AND BRAIN DAMAGE

The four groups of children I have identified as those with whom we will be concerned in this book are considered *brain different*. The difference may be because of actual brain damage, because of maturational delay of the language centers of the brain, or because of "miss-wiring" within language centers or in conduction pathways between centers. The cause of the difference is clear for children with acquired aphasia, but it is not so evident in the other groups of linguistically impaired children. If we assume that behavior has neurological correlates, however, and that behavior is the result of how one nerve cell relates to another nerve cell in the nervous system and particularly in the brain, we must also assume that language deficits of a degree as severe as those in the children of special concern to us are a consequence of primary brain differences.

COGNITIVE DEVELOPMENT AND COGNITIVE CORRELATES WITH LANGUAGE

Cognition refers to those aspects of intellectual development that are usually correlated with physical and social maturity, and so enable us to make new and continuous differentiations and distinctions about our environment and experiences. On the basis of these differentiations and experiences, we organize and reorganize our thinking and our patterns of behavior, expressed and potential, for dealing with ourselves and with ongoing and anticipated events.

Cognitive processing refers to perceiving, conceptualizing, knowing, remembering, thinking, learning, and problem solving and usually to the way we codify the products of these processes. Language is, of course, the most frequent way most of us do the codifying. Through cognitive processing, we develop strategies to keep what we know in order so that we can continue in our pursuit of knowledge about our environments. Cognitive processing, in essence, is the way we as human beings learn to learn and, in the absence of abnormal influences, become increasingly proficient in attaining and using knowledge. We will accept Bruner's (1966) basic assumption: "Cognitive growth, whether divergent or uniform across cultures, is inconceivable without participation in a culture and its linguistic community" (p. 2). A corollary to this assumption is that different cultures may bring out different aspects of cognitive development that may be regular and ordered in development within a culture but may develop in a different order in a different culture or in a special subculture. This observation should be kept in mind when any cognitive or intellectual system of development is studied—Piaget's not excepted.

Cognitive development is related to intelligence, of course, but it is more closely related to what we prefer to think of as intellectual and social maturation. Cognitive development emphasizes thought processes, but little thought is completely devoid of feeling (affect), so feeling cannot be completely ignored. The assumption here is that cognitive development is essentially *maturational*—an expression of development—and so for most children we can project stages or levels associated with behavior and kinds of thinking. We are most concerned with the relationship between cognitive development and language. Therefore, we will briefly speculate on some necessary cognitive abilities that are normally associated with the comprehension and meaningful production of language. We shall not attempt to conjecture about the possibility or even probability that children have inner language and function cognitively before they begin to speak. Comprehension of languge implies cognitive functioning, and most children reveal abilities to modify their behavior based on comprehension that normally precedes production. Our emphasis, however, will be on the verbal stages rather than the preverbal (prelingual) production stage of language that is essentially the sensorimotor phase in Piaget's developmental psychophilosophy.

A necessary cognitive ability in the earliest verbal stage is to associate a name (label) with an object or event. This ability implies a capacity to hold something in memory—for example, an object, such as *ball* or *cookie,* that can somehow be recalled even when it is no longer present. In Piaget's terms (Piaget and Inhelder, 1969), the realization that an object continues to exist even when it is not in view—out of sight is not out of mind—is referred to as *object permanence.* Presumably, the achievement of object permanence is related to an ability to perceive size, shape, color, and possibly texture, so that one object may be differentiated from another and the objects may be associated with names. These are the first words for comprehension, usually followed by verbal productions (labeling or identification).

A related physical maturational stage is the awareness of control over the organs of speech. The associated anticipation of what the child has in mind to produce will, in effect, be produced. Note that here, too, reception precedes production, so that what the child produces is much simpler in construction than what that child might accept from another. Thus, at 15 to 18 months of age, and perhaps up to 2 years, a child who says *pasghetti* for *spaghetti* may appear almost resentful if an adult says *pasghetti.* The object is in mind, and the child will reach it in time. At that time, the child is able to produce what he or she perceives, and what is perceived is within the child's ability for articulatory planning and monitored production.

We will jump to an appreciably more advanced stage in terms of Piaget's theory, one that usually begins at about 18 months and continues, interestingly

Table 1.1   PIAGET'S COGNITIVE STATES, BIRTH TO 4 YEARS

Piaget developmental scale	Linguistic stage
Sensorimotor period (birth to approximately 18 months): Movements related to sensory intake (perceptions); toward end of period, children arrive at notion of object permanence (out of sight is *not* out of mind)	a. Prelinguistic sound production, crying, vocal play, babbling, lalling, echolalia, and first words; gesturing (mostly pointing and pulling), but also anticipatory movements in response to caretaker language b. Toward end of stage, single-word productions for labeling and commanding; for some children, two-word utterances
Early preconceptual period (18 months to 48 months): Beginnings of symbolic representations; at the outset of this period, most mental activity is about the ongoing present—the here and now; in the later months, the child can also appreciate (comprehend and deal with) the past and the future and will engage in considerable symbolic play	a. Two-word utterances, usually without grammatical features b. Gradual increase to three- and four-word or longer utterances that incorporate grammatical features of word order and syntax; verbal productions approximate those of older speakers and are likely to be well-constructed, simple sentences

and perhaps not purely coincidentally, up to about 11 years, when syntax is almost completely mastered. First, children have to decenter themselves from their worlds, to begin to know themselves as part of a world but not the core about which all else revolves. Second, children begin to categorize events into classes and subclasses, so that all men are not *daddies* and all four-legged creatures are not *doggies* or *kitties*. Third, children become able to combine units into related events and to recombine them in some order according to the needs of a situation. Such ordering and combining need not be performed but may be entertained in mind, with a *projected consequence*.

What has been described is a perception of some of the components of the early aspects of Piaget's *concrete operational period*. Intentionally selected were those aspects believed to be correlated with the acquisition of syntax by children, especially during the period between 18 and 36 months, between the end of the sensorimotor period and the beginning of the long period of concrete operations. Highlights of these stages are summarized in Table 1.1.

THE SUBSYSTEMS OF LANGUAGE

At the beginning of this chapter, oral language was described as a symbolic system that incorporates five subsystems: phonology, morphology, syntax, semantics, and pragmatics. Each of the subsystems has rules that are usually observed by proficient speakers. Intended meanings emerge from the individual's knowledge and use of the multifaceted linguistic system. These meanings— semantics—are expressed in how the speaker selects and combines words to produce sentences. This selecting and combining is done with due awareness of social settings or the context in which verbal communication takes place. This due awareness is referred to as pragmatics. The following sections expand the consideration of each of the identified subsystems of spoken language.

Phonology

The basic units of the sound system of a language are *phonemes*. These are the speech sound units that contrast with one another to indicate difference in meaning. Thus, *den* differs in meaning from *pen* and from *ten* because of the first sound of the word. If we substitute different final sounds for these words, we may get *deaf* (the middle sound is the same, though the spelling is different), *deck*, or *dell* (these last two words have only one final sound, or phoneme, despite the spelling). Changing the vowel may give us *din, pin,* or *tin* or, with other vowel changes, *done, pun,* or *tun*. In each example, lexical meaning has been changed by substituting a different phoneme in each position of the word. Except for single-phoneme words, such as the letter *a* pronounced as a/e/ or *I* pronounced with the diphthong i/aI/, phonemes are sounds without meaning that make for meaningful differences in words.

Allophones are the realistic variants of the basic and abstract constructs referred to as phonemes. In contextual speech, speech sounds are modified according to their phonetic environment. Thus, the *t* in *ten* is somewhat different from the *t* in *its, let, at, time,* and *Pat thinks*. Despite differences, we recognize the essential sameness of the sounds. A well-intentioned listener would not be overly concerned with whether all /t/ words were produced with the characteristics or features of the /t/ in *ten* or more naturally—as most of us would produce these words, in a natural rather than a self-conscious utterance.

There are rules that govern positions of sounds and blends (combinations) of sounds within a language system. In English, we do not begin words with the sound usually represented by the letters *ng*, but we have *ng* in *sing, youngster,* and *belonging*. We have no initial *dn* or *nd* combinations except in foreign words, but *nd* is a common *blend* in the middle (*candy*) and final (*stoned, found*) position in words. We have dropped the *k* and *g* in words of Anglo-Saxon origin (*know, gnostic*), but we retain them in *acknowledge* and *agnostic*. Similarly, we do not sound the *p* of *psychic* in initial position, but we do in other positions, as in *apes*. We do not begin words with *tl*, although we have final *tl*, as in *settle*. We have many *shr* words, such as *shrimp, shred,* and *shrug*, but we do not have initial *sr* blends, except as we pronounce some foreign words, such as *Srinagar* (the capital of Kashmir). We are prolific in other *s* blends, as in *spend, step, slip, scat, scrape, stride,* and *asks*. (The *-sks* blend is a difficult one for many children and for some adults.) These examples of speech sounds in word position and in accepted or unaccepted blends are part of the conventions children learn as they develop the sound system (phonology) of their language. It is interesting that most multilingual children have little trouble developing separate phonologies for each of the languages they acquire.

Morphology

A *morpheme* is a word or an element of a word that carries meaning. Morphology is the system of rules that governs how morphemes are used either as words or as inflections (prefixes or suffixes) that modify the meaning of the root word.

Let us examine the word *speakers* for its morphological structure. *Speakers*, a complex word, has three separate (minimal-meaning) morphemes: *speak, -er,* and *-s. Speak = talk,* the basic meaning of the word; *-er =* one who (the agent of/for the *speak*); *-s* indicates plural (more than one speaker). It is interesting that *-'s* (we do not hear the apostrophe but must arrive at it and its meaning from the context that incudes the word) changes the meaning from more than one speaker to *belonging* (possessive) to a single speaker. While children learn phonology, thay also manage to learn that they can produce compound and complex words by putting separate words together, such as the early, most important one for them, *caretakers*. They will also learn *busybody* and possibly *mudslinger* as well as *gunslinger*. They also learn that some morphemes may be used freely (separately) as words, such as *less*, and that others are used either at the beginnings or ends of words (prefixes or suffixes), such as *-re, -un* (*return, unless, unkind*) and *-er* or *-or* (*farmer, speaker, actor*). In the next chapter, we will consider fourteen "obligatory" morphemes that almost all children learn before they come to grips with syntax, the third subsystem of their language.

Syntax

Syntax is the way speakers of a language combine words to form sentences. The conventions or rules that govern how we combine words constitute the grammar of utterances (sentences). Children learn not only the most consistent (reliable and regular) rules of the speakers of their language but, in time, the irregular or exception-to-the-rules constructions. Oddly enough, these exceptions include the various forms of the verbs *to be* and *to have,* which are very high in frequency of usage.

Semantics

At the risk of sounding simplistic, *semantics* can be defined as the rules that determine how individual words and their meaning or meanings are combined to produce the intended meaning of a sentence. *Linguistic semantics* (verbal meanings) relates to the words selected and to syntactic structure. Meanings are also inseparable from pragmatics. Dale (1976) observes: "The semantic system of a language is the knowledge that a speaker must have to understand sentences and relate them to his knowledge of the World" and "Semantic development is the aspect of language development most directly tied to the broader cognitive development of the child" (p. 166). We will not discuss linguistic semantics beyond these statements, at least for the present. Later chapters will consider semantic relationships as expressed in the functions of language and in some basic syntactic structures that are learned by normal children in the ongoing process of language development.

Pragmatics

While children learn their language systems and become increasingly proficient in the application of the three subsystems, they also learn *pragmatics.* They learn how to say what they mean—to observe the conventions and the not-so-rigid rules of language usage that enhance if not entirely determine relational meanings. In essence, children learn how to be practical if they want others to know what they mean and what they expect others to do according to what they mean. Most children are on their w —having learned how to tell others what they mean—by 18 months of age. They are considerably more proficient by 36 months and much more so by age 10. This is what we mean by the assertion that language is a human species-specific function. To be human and normal, or relatively normal, is to have the potential for language, the most astonishing of all human creative achievements.[2]

---

[2]Recent successes in teaching a few chimpanzees and gorillas to use sign systems are impressive, but these achievements are still a far cry from the rich and complex language that most children can understand and use by 2 years of age.

The creative achievement may begin with a differential cry, develop into how long and how best to cry, and continue with selections of words and multiple word utterances. At almost all verbal stages, children will have to decide whether they can get what they want by asking questions, by imploring ("Please, pretty please."), by using imperatives (when and with whom), by saying things directly ("Would you close the window, please?") or indirectly ("Isn't it cold outside?" or "It's cold outside."). All of these processes, and much, much more, are part of learning how to mean. These kinds of learning are associated, of course, with social and intellectual maturity, with cognitive development, and, to some degree, with sex differences.

Pragmatics describes, if it does not prescribe, when and how to say what you need to say if you want your communication to be successful. The when and the how are specific to a given set of circumstances. Infants may begin pragmatic learning at a prelinguistic stage by modifying their crying so that needs, including social needs for some form of attention (action), can be achieved. Later in their linguistic, cognitive, and social development, children learn how to address persons who are important to them—how to address mother, father, or a grandparent in ways that are likely to bring about intended and desired results. In learning how to use language effectively, they also learn, or at least have the opportunity to learn, about the sensitivities of persons with whom they interact. As with the other aspects of language, we should not expect all children to be equally competent in the pragmatics of language. Neither, of course, are adults. In their observations of adults, children may note that "Darling, it's cold outside" may on some occasions be a comment about the weather, but it may also be an implied request for an action that a window be closed, or the heat turned up, or a log lighted in the fireplace. In brief, what children learn are the practices in language usage that are appropriate for a given situation. To some degree, they may learn that there are differences in what may be appropriate for a boy or for a girl, for a man or for a woman, as well as differences in what members of one sex say to members of the other. Rees (1980) sums up the current interest in studying the pragmatics of child language:

> The pragmatic turn has focused on the fact that children do not merely learn language but, from the very start, learn to do things with language. Investigators of child language using pragmatic approaches have sought to understand the processes by which language becomes functional for young children in social situations, and have looked to the social-communicative basis as the very source of language learning. . . . While earlier investigations sought to account for children's mastery of form and meaning in language, the pragmatic approach introduces an additional goal, that of explaining the child's development of communicative competence. (p. 25)

As suggested earlier, it is believed that meanings (linguistic semantics) are intimately related to if not inseparable from pragmatics. In his introduction to his book *Meaning in Child Language,* Leonard (1976) points out:

"Children do not only learn a set of relational meanings, but also contexts in which the meanings are expressed and the uses to which the expression of meanings may be put." Thus, children who learn *ball* concurrently learn a variety of meanings in a variety of contexts—some of the related uses for *ball.* Also learned are the children's own relational uses as well as those uses expressed in the actions of others who are related to them. The children learn that they or someone else can bounce a ball, throw it, roll it, squeeze it, or hold or withhold it. So also, even before the label for *mother* or *daddy* is learned, children, if fortunate, have also learned that *mother* and *daddy* are those who may hold you to their body, feed you, burp you, bathe you, dress and undress you, that they are someone to cry to or cry at, coo to (or coo with), and so on.

The implication of the relationship between semantics and pragmatics for children who are linguistically deficient is clear—whatever we teach them about language must be taught in contexts that are both meaningful and useful to them.

In addition to the writers and investigators already cited, references on pragmatics in child language include Bates (1976), Bruner (1975), Ervin-Tripp (1973), Halliday (1975), Hymes (1971), Moerk (1977), Prutting (1979), Prutting and Kirchner (1983), and Rees (1980).

CHILD LANGUAGE AND ADULT LANGUAGE

"When I was a child, I spake as a child, I understood as a child, I thought as a child; but when I became a man, I put away childish things" (1 Cor. 13:11). Child language is not adult language, nor is child language a garbled, diminutive, or token form of adult language. To be sure, child language uses a sound system that moves in the direction of the phonology of the adult. For a while, however, child language has its own phonology, with sounds that are present (selected?) from the speech of older members of the child's environment. The words produced are a selection that best meets the needs of the child. Child utterances—first words and early two-word utterances—begin by being asyntactic. Gradually, rules are acquired, so that the children not only speak in more aduult fashion but can express their wants, thoughts, and feelings more clearly. Presumably, such definition should also help in achieving success in communication. Why a child should give up speaking like a child is something about which we will not conjecture—at least not for the present. We will go on the assumption that except for a small percentage of children who come into this world ill equipped either neurophysiologically or intellectually, or for a very few with so negative an environment that they have no adults with whom to identify, continued progress to the use of adult forms, content, and structure of language is to be expected. A reasonable expectation and level of achievement is denied to very few children. Usually, this is accomplished with the help of adults, but it may sometimes be accomplished despite the lack of help from particular adults. Although most children acquire their language system by exposure—by being in an environment in which there are caretakers who really care—they do obtain an appreciable amount of indirect help and some direct teaching. Obviously, no child can acquire a language system unless there is a speaker or speakers who are ready and available to interact with behavior that includes language. Children are usually exposed to two adult language systems: the first, adult to adult, they overhear; the second is addressed directly to the child. It is likely that children first decode the second system before they can make much sense of adult-to-adult language. Moskowitz (1978) characterizes caretaker speech (usually mothers' and fathers') as follows:

> Caretaker speech is a distinct speech register that differs from others in its simplified vocabulary, the systematic phonological simplification of some words, higher pitch and exaggerated intonation, short, simple sentences, and a higher proportion of questions (among mothers) or imperatives (among fathers). Perhaps the most pervasive characteristic of caretaker speech is its syntactic simplification. While a child is still babbling, adults may address long, complex sentences to her, but as soon as she begins to utter meaningful, identifiable words they almost always speak to her in very simple sentences. Over the next few years of the child's language development the speech addressed to her by her caretakers may well be describable by a grammar only six months in advance of her own. (p. 94)

Perhaps the foregoing is an overgeneralization. There are mothers who insist that they never modified their language in speaking to their children and that the children survived and thrived, at least linguistically. Another caretaker, however—perhaps a grandparent—may have been more accommodating, indulging in "baby talk" if only to show affection for the child. Nevertheless, what these mothers say about the way they talked to their children may explain some behaviors that are otherwise inexplicable.

Adults usually talk to children about what is present and concrete—the here and now that can be seen and touched—and so referents and meanings are likely to be clear. Based on a review of parent-to-child language de Villiers and de Villiers (1979) observe:

> Mothers (and fathers too, although they have not been studied as much) tailor the length and complexity of their utterances to the linguistic ability of their children. Mothers' speech to one- and two-year-olds consists of simple, grammatically correct, short sentences that refer to concrete objects and events. There are few references to the past and almost none to the future. (p. 99)

Other observed characteristics that distinguish adult-to-young-child language from adult-to-adult language include the following:

1. There are distinct pauses between phrases and at the ends of sentences.
2. Sentences often include partial or complete repetitions, such as "Give me the big block. Not the small one. Give me the big one." de Villiers and de Villiers (1979, p. 99) note that up to 30 percent of utterances

are partial or complete repetitions of an earlier sentence spoken by the child or the adult.

3. Sentence intonation and stress on key words are likely to be exaggerated.

Perhaps the most important feature of adult-to-child language is an absence of incomplete, agrammatical, and "I mean, I mean" and "uh-uh" constructions that characterize much adult-to-adult spontaneous conversations. In effect, fortunate children who are addressed by caring caretakers are likely to hear a version of their language that is simpler, more slowly articulated, and more clearly marked by pitch and intonation changes than what they overhear in adult-to-adult talk. The form and structure of the adult-to-child utterances are not too far from their own—constructions that they can understand and soon will be able to produce, not in slavish imitation but as tokens of linguistic models. The structures and content are not so far above the child to be out of reach, yet they are far enough (or close enough) to make the reaching worth the effort.

As a result of these modifications, adults who are sensitive to children with whom they have frequent communicative contact are able to make themselves understood. In so doing, they provide models for how young children can in turn make themselves understood. Verbal models must also change, however, or the children would not progress in linguistic and related cognitive development. Clark and Clark (1977) observe: "As children show signs of understanding more, adults modify the way they talk less and less. The shortest sentences and the slowest rate are reserved for the youngest children; both sentence length and rate of speech increase when adults talk to older children" (p. 327).

THE CRITICAL PERIOD FOR LANGUAGE ACQUISITION

Is there a critical period for language acquisition? If a critical period is defined as the range of time in the life of a member of a species when a particular function (behavior) peculiar to the species can be established (learned and practiced) with least effort, the answer is positive. If, however, a critical period is considered a range of time during which a behavior must be established or thereafter be beyond the possibility of achievement, the answer for human beings is either negative or equivocal. On the basis of our information about cognitive development and its onset and acquisition during the first three years, it is apparent that this period, from about age 12 months to 48 months, is one that incorporates the largest amount of language acquisition. We should not forget, however, that for several months before first words are produced, normal children reveal considerable understanding of language addressed to them. Beyond age 4, there is still much that children have to learn about their language systems, but unless they are required to learn an additional language, they will never make the gains at the rate of learning a first system or, for a bilingual child, first systems. Even so, up to age 12, most children can learn an additional language system and can sound much like native speakers of the new language. A few adults can do so at any age. For these adults, there would not appear to be any critical period for learning a new language. For most of us, however, the critical period for learning a new language by exposure and some direct instruction seems to end at about age 12.

A correlate of the critical period for language acquisition that was not previously considered is cerebral laterilization. At about age 3, most children show clear evidence of cerebral lateralization for motor functions—for example, handedness and probably ear preference. (These will be considered further in Chapter 4.) Language will be disturbed if the dominant hemisphere for language, usually the left, is damaged. For most children, the reacquisition of language proceeds very quickly, but perhaps not completely if the nondominant hemisphere, usually the right, is also damaged. Such rapid reacquisition implies that, at least up to age 12, the half of the brain that is not normally the one that processes language has the potential capacity for taking over language functioning when there is such a need.

The groups of children who are of special concern in this book—those who are severely linguistically retarded—are all too often not identified and treated until age 3 or 4. Some are misdiagnosed and inappropriately treated considerably beyond age 4. Fortunately, we see most linguistically retarded children before the end of their critical period, so that language intervention probably has the silent help of biological maturational factors.

How late can a child learn to talk who, for physical or social reasons, has been deprived of normal stimulation and normal opportunity? Frankly, we do not know. Expositions of so-called feral or wolf children who somehow survived living in a forest from infancy are probably fiction disguised as documentaries. Just why wolves should have the early responsibility as caretakers is also a conjecture that might better be addressed to writers of fiction. In any event, there is little reliable evidence that feral children really existed and even less that they were able to learn the language of their later human caretakers.

There is one recent and thoroughly authentic account of a child called Genie, who was isolated and deprived of all but a minimum amount of human contact, presumably including little or no speech (Curtiss, 1977; Curtiss, Fromkin, Rigler, Rigler, and Krashen, 1975). Genie was not discovered until she was age 13 and 7 months. She was considered to be retarded by her parents and, probably because of the father's rejection, was confined to a small, curtained area in her home from the age of 20 months until she was discovered. The child had spent most of her waking hours, and probably some while asleep, either strapped or sitting in a potty chair or in an infant crib. For the most part, Genie was a silent child. If she made sounds, the result was a paternal beating and angry, barking noises directed at her. The mother shared in the neglect. Visits were for the purpose of feeding, mostly with baby food. Rarely did the mother speak to Genie during her limited caretaking efforts.

Genie was placed in a foster home that included two other children close to her chronological age. She was also treated by a speech specialist so that she had the advantage of exposure to speakers in a favorable environment and some direct instruction.

Genie became the subject of intensive and extensive study by psycholinguists, speech pathologists, and neurologists in the Los Angeles area and by consultants from other parts of the United States. The staff of the Institute for Childhood Aphasia at Stanford University, under my direction, were among the evaluators.

Four and a half years after Genie was discovered, a report on the child (chronologically an adolescent) includes the following notes on her social achievements:

> It is surprising that she survived at all. It is not surprising that she was malnourished, unable to stand erect, unable to speak or comprehend spoken language—a primitive and unsocialized victim of unprecedented deprivation and social isolation. Many things have taken place during these 4½ years. She now expresses love, pleasure, and anger: she laughs and cries. She has learned many social skills: she can eat with utensils, chew her food, dress herself, brush her teeth, wash her hair, and tie her shoe laces. She rides a bus to school and sews on a sewing machine. She runs and jumps and throws basketball. And she speaks and understands— imperfectly to be sure. (Curtiss et al., 1975)

Questions that remained unanswered concern Genie's intellectual potential. Was she "normal"? Did an isolation of almost 14 years reduce whatever potential she had for cognitive development and language? Our impression is that after four years of very special care, Genie at her best was at about a 24- to 30-month stage in overall language proficiency. Whether Genie will continue to learn language beyond the last reported evaluations is conjectural but important. If she does, then we can argue that, at least in one instance, even a poor start (Genie spoke a few single words at 20 months) is better than no start. Beyond this, we can take the position that although there is an optimal (critical) period for normal language acquisition, there is a much extended period for language learning. This is the position that we take; it permits optimism in our efforts with children who are severely retarded in language development.

REFERENCES AND SUGGESTED READINGS

American Speech-Hearing-Language Association (ASHA), Committee on Language. *ASHA*, 23(2), 1981, 143

Bates, E. "Pragmatics and Sociolinguistics in Child Language," in D. Morehead and A. Morehead, (eds.), *Normal and Deficient Language*. Baltimore: University Park Press, 1976.

Benton, A. "The Cognitive Functioning of Children with Developmental Dysphasia," in M. A. Wyke (ed.), *Developmental Dysphasia*. London: Academic Press, 1978.

Benton, A., and Pearl, D. *Dyslexia*. New York: Oxford University Press, 1978.

Bloom, L., and Lahey, M. *Language Development and Language Disorders*. New York: Wiley, 1978.

16   INTRODUCTION: SOME DEFINITIONS AND DEFINED PREJUDICES

Brown, R. *A First Language.* Cambridge, Mass.: Harvard University Press, 1973.
Bruner, J. S. "On Cognitive Growth," in J. S. Bruner, R. R. Oliver, and P. M. Greenfield, *Studies in Cognitive Growth.* New York: Wiley, 1966.
Bruner, J. S. "The Ontogenesis of Speech Acts," *Journal of Child Language,* 2, 1975, 1–19.
Clark, H. H., and Clark, E. V. *Psychology and Language.* New York: Harcourt Brace Jovanovich, 1977.
Cromer, R. F. "The Basis of Childhood Dysphasia: A Linguistsic Approach," in M. A. Wyke (ed.), *Developmental Dysphasia.* London: Academic Press, 1978.
Curtiss, S. *Genie: A Psycholinguistic Study of a Modern Day "Wild Child."* New York: Academic Press, 1977.
Curtiss, S., Fromkin, V., Rigler, D., Rigler, M., and Krashen, S. "An Update on the Linguistic Development of Genie," in O. P. Dato (ed.), *Georgetown University Round Table on Language and Linguistics.* Washington, D.C.: Georgetown University Press, 1975.
Dale, P. S. *Language Development: Structure and Function,* 2d ed. New York: Holt, Rinehart and Winston, 1976.
deVilliers, P. A., and deVilliers, J. G. *Early Language.* Cambridge, Mass.: Harvard University Press, 1979.
Donaldson, M. *Children's Minds.* New York: Norton, 1978.
Eisenson, J. *Is Your Child's Speech Normal?* Reading, Mass.: Addison-Wesley, 1976.
Ervin-Tripp. S. "Some Strategies for the First Two Years," in T. More (ed.), *Cognitive Development and the Acquisition of Language.* New York: Academic Press, 1973.
Greenfield, P. M., and Smith, J. H. *The Structure of Communication in Early Language.* New York: Academic Press, 1976.
Halliday, M. A. K. *Learning How to Mean.* London: Edward Arnold, 1975.
Hymes, D. "Competence and Performance in Linguistic Theory," in R. Huxley and E. Ingram (eds.), *Language Acquisition: Models and Methods.* New York: Academic Press, 1971.
Keith, R. W. (ed.). *Central Auditory and Language Disorders in Children.* Houston: College-Hill Press, 1981.
Lenneberg, E. *Biological Foundations of Language.* New York: Wiley, 1967.
Leonard, L. B. *Meaning in Child Language.* New York: Grune and Stratton, 1976.
Lovaas, O. I. *The Autistic Child.* New York: Irvington, 1977.
Menyuk, P. "Linguistic Problems in Children with Developmental Dysphasia," in M. A. Wyke (ed.), *Developmental Dysphasia.* London: Academic Press, 1978.
Moerk, E. L. *Pragmatic and Semantic Aspects of Early Language Development.* Baltimore: University Park Press, 1977.
Moskowitz, B. A. "The Acquisition of Language," *Scientific American,* 239(5), 1978, 92–108.
Olmstead, D. L. *Out of the Mouth of Babes.* The Hague: Mouton, 1971.
Piaget, J., and Inhelder, B. *The Psychology of the Child.* New York: Basic Books, 1969.
Prutting, C. A. "Process \prá|ses\: The Action of Moving Forward Progressively from One Point to Another on the Way to Completion," *Journal of Speech and Hearing Disorders,* 44, 1979, 3–30.
Prutting, C. A. and Kirchner, D. M. "Applied Pragmatics," in T. Gallagher and C. A. Prutting, (eds.), *Pragmatic Assessment and Intervention Issues.* Houston: College Hill Press, 1983.

Rees, N. S. "Learning to Talk and Understand," in T. J. Hixon, L. D. Shriberg, and J. H. Saxman (eds.), *Introduction to Communication Disorders*. Englewood Cliffs, New Jersey: Prentice-Hall, 1980.

Rees, N. S. "Saying More Than We Know," in R. W. Keith (ed.), *Central Auditory and Language Disorders in Children*. Houston: College-Hill Press, 1981.

Stark, R., and Tallal, P. "Perceptual and Motor Deficits in Language Impaired Children," in R. W. Keith (ed.), *Central Auditory Deficits and Language Disorders in Children,* Houston: College-Hill Press, 1981.

Tallal, P., and Piercy, M. "Defects of Auditory Perception in Children with Developmental Dysphasia," in M. A. Wyke (ed.), *Developmental Dysphasia*. London: Academic Press, 1978.

Wyke, M. A. (ed.). *Developmental Dysphasia*. London: Academic Press, 1978.

chapter 2

Normal Language Development

To appreciate the language acquisition problems of the severely linguistically retarded children with whom we are concerned, we need base lines for comparison. Accordingly, we will consider normal language acquisition and follow normal language development of children from their earliest crying and vocal play to their first sentences. As we proceed, we will make comparisons with the linguistically retarded at each stage of development.

The capacity to acquire some form of language—that is, to learn a linguistic code that normally employs distance reception, hearing or vision—is a human-species–specific ability that is denied to very few. These few include only the most severely mentally retarded, the severely perceptually impaired, and a very small percentage of nonrelating children (the nonverbal autistic). Almost all other human beings can acquire some form of language behavior, although the extent and complexity of this form of behavior varies considerably from individual to individual. The achievement is not denied to the blind, although they may be somewhat slower in language acquisition than are seeing children; it is not denied to the deaf if we accept the premise, as we should, that a visual sign system constitutes a symbol code with conventions and rules that may parallel and be equivalent to those of an oral linguistic code. Language as a potential human achievement is not indefinitely denied to congenitally aphasic children and may not be denied to autistic children, even if its onset is late and its development is retarded and deviates in some respects from that of normal children.

THE MANNER OF LANGUAGE ACQUISITION

Most children learn to speak by ear; that is, they acquire spoken language through aural-oral means and learn an aural-oral system. Almost all children begin their careers as speakers by producing single-word utterances. By age 3, most children have become sufficiently proficient as speakers to be able to meet the following criterion: they demonstrate through their productions that the utterances conform to the conventions of other speakers in their environment. These conventions include the acquisition of a speech sound (phonemic) system, a morphemic (sound-combining) system of words, and a syntactic or grammatical system (the combining of words into strings or formulations that approximate the utterances of important other members of the environment). The important other members may be siblings, parents, or family-related or unrelated regular caretakers. In most instances the mother is likely to be the most important early influence and so is also likely to be the most significant shaper of the child's initial language acquisitions. In some instances, the father may play the role and have the responsibilities and influences usually assumed by the mother.

Children normally neither duplicate nor slavishly replicate the language or languages to which they are exposed as spoken by key important others. Although children learn the form (the phonemic, morphemic, and syntactic structures of one or more languages) through which they express the content (what they have to say), they also manage to express themselves as individual selves in the ways they speak. These ways may include vocal differences, the selection of words, and, possibly, even such factors as the choice of passive or active mode for their linguistic productions.

Children also learn something about intended meanings, both as listeners and speakers, and about when and how one way of saying something may be more effective than another. Early in life, children may intuitively learn that there is an intended difference in meaning, however slight, between "Have a cookie," "Do you want a cookie?" and "You want a cookie, don't you?" Later, children may sense the intention in adult-to-adult talk of an observation, "Darling, it's cold outside," as really constituting a request from one adult to another to have the one close a window, or seek, find, and supply a shawl or a sweater to the other.

Children also learn when question forms are really disguised demands such as, "You want a ———, don't you?" Children also learn that it is not always what is said that is important, but how something is said, by whom, to whom, and with what accompanying vocal changes, facial expressions, or gestures—all of which may be unconscious additives to the selected words and the surface form of the words.

CRITERIA FOR LANGUAGE ACQUISITION

Sometime between 9 and 18 months of age, most children who will acquire speech produce their first true words. The first words are likely to be the designation-identification (labeling) of persons or things, spoken only when the persons or things are actually present. Shortly thereafter, however, most normal children will begin to announce by naming and designating what they wish to have present. Thus, "Mama" or "Dada" or "wawa" may be said to have mother come, or to be given an out-of-reach and perhaps out-of-sight doll or other play object. The child has discovered the magic of speech. Before these pronouncements are made, the child is likely to have learned to comprehend a considerable number of words, or sentences with key words, and she or he may point to the nose, place a hand on top of the head on command, or even play peek-a-boo with an admiring adult. Normally, comprehension, with or without overt reaction, both precedes and exceeds production of language throughout life.

Between 18 months and 3 years of age, or earlier for the linguistically precocious, most children become creative listeners and speakers. At this stage it becomes evident to discerning listeners that:

1. The child understands and derives meaning from a conventionalized system of audible and visible signs (symbols).
2. The child, without specific and direct teaching, understands verbal formulations to which there has been no previous exposure. Thus, a child trained to "Give me the dolly" but not to "Give me the block" nevertheless understands and behaves appropriately to the second utterance. When this is demonstrated, the child is listening creatively—showing an ability to understand new verbal formulations based on what has previously been learned.
3. The child produces new verbal formulations (new strings of utterances) that listeners can understand. Now the child is speaking creatively. The creations are the products of an inventory of intelligible words and word phrases now under the child's command.

The second and third criteria indicate that the child is capable of generalizing directly from specific words and utterances that have been learned (taught) to comprehension and production (generation) of an indefinite number of new formulations. In a very real and important sense, the child has become a self-generator of language. Somehow, mostly through indirect teaching (through interchanges with an important other and sometimes through direct teaching), the child learns the structure and rules for verbal expression. The normal child generalizes and frequently overgeneralizes some linguistic rules. (It is no fault of the child that adults use *sheep* for both singular and plural, or that *child's* is possessive and not plural, or that *children* is plural and *children's* is a possessive plural.) Later, the child may well generalize that adults or persons who commit so many exceptions to the rules they supposedly use are not to be trusted, or perhaps are just too full of exceptions. Ultimately, of course, children accept adult ways of talking and have their turn in imposing their rules on a new generation of creative and generally, but not consistently, rule-abiding listeners and speakers.

DEVELOPMENTAL LANGUAGE STAGES

Prelingual Stages

Before children utter their first words, which are usually intended to name or to bring about an event—to make something happen that they want to have happen—they normally go through a sequence of overlapping stages of vocalic and articulatory behaviors. In their early vocalizations, as well as in their responses to human sound making, normal infants demonstrate that they are compulsive communicators. They make eye contact and coo to attract attention, to evoke a response, and to maintain the attention of a respondent. If attention is lost, they may cry. If crying reinstates attention, visual flirtation and cooing may be resumed. Thus, very early in life, infants are able to express social behavior that is reinforced by the responses of others who are important to them (Bricker and Carlson, 1981, p. 480).

In all stages of language development, normal children are active participants in their acquisitions. To be sure, almost all children follow patterns and stages, but what is acquired—what is learned of language and what is produced—is an active and ongoing process. Nothing in the way of language or even prelanguage happens to the child without the child's assistance in having it happen.

The earliest stages—crying, cooing, and the beginning of babbling—appear to be universal and appear not to be directed toward the language or languages the child will later learn to speak. Beginning with later babbling, perhaps as early as 5 or 6 months, speech sounds and syllables the child will later be using in his or her first words are incorporated in vocal play. (Oller, Weiman, Doyle, and Ross, 1976). With very few exceptions, the prelingual stages that are identified with later babbling are precursors of true speech. (Carroll, 1961; Dale, 1976). The few exceptions are of children who do not engage in any sound play or who have reduced amounts of sound play, compared with their age peers. These exceptions may include a deaf child born into a family of hearing parents, the child born with a structural anomaly of the speech mechanism, the absence of a speaking caretaker, and the absence of a caring speaker. Otherwise, we believe that there is a continuity between early articulated sound play and later spoken language. Even the earliest stages have important general implications. Carroll (1961) suggests:

> Vocalizations, crying, cooing, and miscellaneous nondescript sounds of the first three or four months are probably most significant in that, in addition to exercising the maturing speech apparatus they make it possible for the infant to learn, through appropriate reinforcement, the instrumental, communicative character of vocal sounds, as when crying brings relief from hunger or pain.

Early Crying

Babies normally announce their entry into the postuterine world with a cry. Those who fail to do so spontaneously (reflexively) are usually helped to cry by the services of the attending physician in the form of a sharp slap on the tender backside. The cry, if appropriate in character, provides some assurance that all is well. It is likely that the birth cry is a reflexive expression of the pain or discomfort the baby experiences in having to breathe entirely through its own efforts. For the first few weeks of life, the baby is likely to cry in discomfort states and to sleep much of the rest of the time. The cryings are for the most part undifferentiated, in that the nature or characteristics of the cries, except for intensity, are not discernibly different in regard to the specific cause of the discomfort. Early infant crying includes sudden changes of pitch and levels of loudness and turbulence. Nevertheless, children vary greatly in their individual cries. In a sense, just as they will learn to speak as individual personalities, their first cries are expressions of themselves, and each is a highly individualized self.

Assuming that we are dealing with a normal, full-term baby, the cries in the first few weeks may be considered reflexive manifestations of physiological, internal changes. From the point of view of the oral (speech) mechanism, crying indicates that the respiratory, laryngeal, and oral mechanisms are functioning normally. The child is able to approximate (bring together) the vocal bands, and can set them in motion by inhaling and exhaling. Identifiable sounds produced during crying are likely to be nasalized vowels.

Some infants may vocalize in periods we would regard as comfortable—for example, after a bath or after a feeding and burping. Such noncrying vocalizations are infrequent in children younger than 1 month. Comfort vocalization increases in the normal child, beginning with the second month.

It may be noted at this point that deaf children are not different from hearing children in their early vocalizations. Differences in sound making begin to occur at about 6 weeks when normal-hearing infants may be heard to produce more speechlike sounds than the deaf do (Maskarinec, Cairns, Butterfield, and Weamer, 1981). Autistic children are likely to do very little crying and to be regarded as good babies. However, some autistic children cry excessively and are not likely to be comforted by caretakers. Moderate to severely mentally retarded children are usually delayed "shadows" of normal children in their early development, in both prelanguage and early language stages. Brain-damaged infants tend to respond differently from normal infants when crying is induced by a painful stimulus (e.g., the snapping of a rubber band on the sole of the foot). Karelitz and Fischelli (1962), and Fischelli and Karelitz (1963) found that infants identified as brain-damaged were slower in beginning to cry (latency after application of painful stimulus) when compared with normal infants. Furthermore, these investigators found that the abnormal infants required more stimulation than the normal ones to evoke the same amount of crying. In addition, the crying of the brain-damaged infants was found not to be so well sustained as that of the normal neonates. As with normal children, there is considerable range in the characteristics and patterns of early cries. Some brain-damaged children cry excessively (when compared with most normal children), and some brain-damaged children are not so readily comforted as normal children once their crying is under way. Bosma (1975) states that, in general:

... crying is a phenomenon that is greater than its respiratory manifestations. It is an arousal state of the organism with gestures of struggle in trunk
and limbs and with conspicuous vascular changes, including elevation of
blood pressure, tachycardia and vasodilation in the skin, particularly of face
and hands, and in the oral and pharyngeal mucosa. The surging motions of
the pharynx, mouth and face are grossly correlated with the expirations.

The cry of an infant at term is composed of stably balanced elements
that are characteristic of the individual infant. Appropriate to this interin-
dividual heterogeneity, the range of normal variation is great. (pp. 471–
472)

Bosma (1975) also notes:

Crying differs from developing speech in its occasion of stress and arousal,
in the associated exclusion responses to incidental stimuli, and in its
stability of performance pattern. In the young infant, crying may be recip-
rocal to the prologues and early speech. (p. 475)

It would appear, therefore, that despite considerable variation from
infant to infant, there are identifiable patterns that may serve to distinguish
most children who are potentially normal from most children who have brain
damage or are at high risk for abnormality associated with premature birth, or
from children who are different because of Down's syndrome, or from those
who will later be identified as suffering from Kanner's (primary) autism. Some
of these early cry differences are described by Karelitz and Fischelli (1962),
Truby, Bosma, and Lind (1966), and Wasz-Hockert, Lind, Vourenkoski,
Partanen, and Valanne (1968).

For the student of infant crying, the nature of the first cry may be both
informative and prognostic of later vocalizations to come. Truby, Bosma, and
Lind, in the introduction to *Newborn Infant Cry* (1965) tell us:

The cry of the newborn infant is a vivid manifestation. It is at once an
acoustically informative vocalization and a complex motor act sensitively
reflecting response to stimulus, beginning with the birth stimulation itself.
It demonstrates distinctive patterns of performance peculiar to the individual neonate. (p. 9)

Increasing Differentiation in Vocalization

Comfort vocalizations, as well as those associated with discomfort states,
become more expressive and differentiated as to quality and intensity as early
as the second month. Presumably, these differential productions, though
essentially reflexive, are indicators of a maturing neurophysiological system,
one that is becoming increasingly capable of responding in discernible and
various ways to different strokes and different pokes. A child may stop crying,
even if only for a moment, when the caretaker is present. An observant

caretaker may derive some meaning from the child's crying and may identify one cry as a likely call to be fed and another as a call for a change of linen. If this happens, the infant's cry has achieved a signal function. This, however, does not imply intention or voluntary production on the part of the infant. It does suggest that a mother, or any other caretaker (a significant other), is associating kinds of crying with several possible discomfort conditions and possibly with some comfort states. Cooing may then assume a possible broad intention, that of enjoining a caretaker in an interchange of vocalizations, a most important early noncontent dialogue.

By 5 to 6 months of age, most normal infants become competent differential vocalizers. At this age, children may well intend to bring about behaviors of caretakers that the caretakers infer from infant vocalizations. However, the caretakers may still be responding in keeping with expectations. For example, if it is about time for a feeding, a given vocalization may be interpreted as a hunger cry, as a postfeeding cry for a linen change, or as a cry for whatever else is supposed to happen because of the time and circumstances. Essentially, especially for infants under 6 months of age, the significance of a cry may be determined by contextual (circumstantial) cues.

After 6 months of age, there is little doubt that most parents of most normal infants are increasingly successful in correctly identifying the intention of their children's cries. These intentions include demands for feeding, for physical caretaking, and for play; they also include social greetings and expressions of surprise, pleasure, and displeasure (Ricks, 1975, pp. 75–80).

Cooing, Other Comfort Sounds, and First Articulation

During the second and third month, cooing, gurgling, squealing, and sounds that approximate consonants and a variety of vowellike sounds become part of the infant's inventory of vocalizations. At about 12 weeks, vowellike cooing may be sustained for 15 to 20 seconds (Lenneberg, 1967, p. 128). The infant is now becoming quite proficient in sound making, and at this period may show some sound preference but is not restricted to the speech sounds of the speakers in any particular environment or culture. Discerning adults may identify front vowels, those of *see* and *man,* as well as *oh, uh,* and *ooh.* Consonants that closely approximate *m, b, g,* and *k* may also be identified.

Babbling

By 5 months, many infants are proficient babblers and seem to show a preference for sounds produced at the front of the mouth (*b, m, t, d*). Earlier, many of the sounds (*g, k,* and even a uvular *r*) result from contacts between the middle or back of the tongue and the roof of the mouth. Occasionally, some of the sounds suggest consonant-vowel syllables such as *da, ba, ga, goo.* Whether these are the actual speech sounds produced or are perceived as such by listeners who try to fit what they hear into the categories of their own speech systems is a matter for conjecture. There is strong evidence, however, that in a few months children are actually producing identifiable speech sounds in their vocal play (Oller et al., 1976).

After the third or fourth month, children begin to spend an increasing amount of their waking time in vocal play—that is, in babbling for and to themselves as well as in the presence of and possibly to and for others. Children may squeal in what adults interpret as delight at the appearance of a caretaker or when removed from a confining crib to a playpen or from the playpen to the floor. Children also begin to show sensitivity to "no-no" sounds, a possible awareness that adults are not always accepting and approving. Sudden loud sounds, regardless of source (human included), are upsetting and are likely to produce crying. The absence of such behavior probably has negative implications for maturation and cognitive development. The normal child provides behavioral evidence that differentiation of response is a two-way affair.

Babbling is an important milestone in children's prelingual speech development and may serve as a predictor of language stages to follow. This does not imply that speech (oral language) emerges or develops in an ordered or lawful way from the infant's sound play identified as babbling; however, during the babbling stage—and, of course, at any other maturational developmental stage—innate drives for vocalization and sound play may be either reinforced or discouraged. The child's potential as a sound maker is now subject to external factors. The influences of the specific environment—how much, how, and when people respond—become determining factors in the child's future as a speaker. By 6 months of age, most children seem to be aware that vocal play is pleasurable as an accomplishment in itself and as a device, a form of behavior, that gives pleasure to others. If such pleasure is apparent, then the child has dual sources of reinforcement for vocal play. Thus, Lewis (1959) notes that although the forces that bring the child to babbling are innate, babbling is enhanced and sustained by the nature of the specific environment. A favorable environment, one that will sustain babbling and encourage further prelingual development, is one that includes attentive, responsive, but not overwhelming adults. It is likely that the same kind of environment and related dynamics will continue to influence the later language stages as the child matures and becomes capable of true speech.

DIFFERENCES IN VOCALIZATIONS IN CHILDREN LIKELY TO BE LANGUAGE-DELAYED

By the time an infant is 6 weeks of age, a discerning listener may be able to note differences in vocalizations between children who are developing normally and those who may be delayed. In comparing deaf and hearing children, it may be noted that the hearing produce more speechlike sounds than do the deaf (Maskarinec et al., 1981). Differences continue to increase with age. By the end of the fifth or sixth month, most of the differences will be in the responses the children make to other vocalizers. Although deaf children may engage in spontaneous, self-initiated vocal play, their repertoire of sounds is not as varied as that of hearing children. Lenneberg (1964) observes:

> The total amount of a deaf child's vocalization may not be different from that of a hearing child, but the hearing child at this age will constantly run through a larger repertoire of sounds whereas deaf children will be making the same sounds sometimes for weeks on end and then, suddenly change to some other set of sounds and "specialize" in these for a while. There is no consistent preference among deaf children for specific sounds.

In spontaneous vocalization, the voice of the deaf child is not different from that of the hearing child. Differences appear in the later stages of babbling, especially in the maintained play of sophisticated babbling that incorporates the intonation patterns of the language the child is acquiring or may already be experienced in using. In their later stages, usually beyond the sixth month, deaf children engage in less sound play than do the hearing. Autistic children (early or primary autism) seldom engage in sound play and rarely, if ever, in socialized vocal play. Retarded children as a total population are slower to begin vocal play and to continue babbling, and they are slower in other prelingual stages later in their lives, as compared with normal infants.

Lalling (Later Babbling)

The lalling stage is an extension of babbling. It is a stage characterized by self-imitation and less apparent random sound play. Lalling usually has its onset between 6 and 8 months. Syllable repetition such as "da-da-da," "ma-ma-ma," and "goo-goo-goo" may be produced, often with intonation patterns of the language they are in the process of acquiring. Such production-repetition of favorite sound combinations is likely to continue until children produce utterances with meanings apparent to adults. Lalling usually declines as true speech is produced; however, vocalizations that sound very much like lalling may be heard when children are at play, sometimes with one another.

During the early lalling stages, the intonations accompanying the articulated lalling may suggest that the child wants something to be done *now* or that the child is either pleased or displeased with what is being done. Utterances are no longer as random as they were in the earlier babbling stage. The child makes fewer sounds but seems to make them with some suggestion of intention. The child is now monitoring his or her own productions, is definitely listening to the speaker, and is apparently in control of his or her efforts. Some of the duplicated sound combinations, such as "ma-ma" and "da-da," resemble words and in some instances may actually be uttered as identification-designations of persons or things. However, very few children at 8 months have any actual intention of assigning meaning to their utterances. They may, however, begin to understand words and recognize such words as *baby*, the names of their playthings, and other labels that are important to them.

DeVilliers and deVilliers (1979) make an important observation about the babbling (and lalling) stage of prelingual development:

> Social and vocal rewards increase the amount of babbling, but they have little, if any, effect on the range of sounds babbled. Even when nine-month-old children are exposed to a concentrated input of syllables containing a wider variety of consonants than they themselves produce, they do not immediately broaden the range of consonants that they babble, although they babble more frequently. It is only at the very end of babbling that language input begins to influence the child's speech, and here the different languages begin to be distinguished. (p. 23)

The primary implication of the lalling stage for the normal child is the indication of a capacity for self-monitoring and control of production. Vocal play is no longer random. Recurrent sounds and syllables may indicate a choice (favorites) in sound production that may be increasingly influenced by adult speech. As with earlier babbling, autistic children are not likely to engage in lalling, although they may later repeat (echo) at length what they hear or overhear adults produce. Deaf children do not engage in lalling. Retarded children may continue in the lalling stage long after normal children have begun to say their first words.

Before considering the next stage—*echolalia*—in which hearing and listening (selective hearing) become paramount features, we will briefly review children's early responses to sounds.

EARLY RESPONSES TO SOUNDS

Normal children not only are persistent sound makers, but they are responsive to sounds and seem to show an early preference for human sounds. Normal children, we may speculate, are "prewired" to receive and differentiate human sounds (voices) from nonhuman and mechanical noises. In some respects, on a neurophysiological level, their systems show a remarkable capacity for identifying and differentiating human voices and the speech sounds that are produced by human beings. As early as 2 weeks, normal children begin to attend to a human voice and appear to be capable of distinguishing human voice from mechanical noisemakers such as whistles, rattles, and bells. If engaged in crying, they will stop at least momentarily if a human being vocalizes, but not if the sound is a bell ringing or a rattle shaking (Wolff, 1966, pp. 81–109). A generalized observation is that normal children have the capacity for distinguishing between human sounds and other, nonhuman, auditory events. Because normal infants can do this without training, they are expressing an innate capacity.

Charles Darwin (1877) explained the child's locking-in to the human voice as an "instinct of sympathy" and so an indication of the infant's dependency on an older human being. It is necessary for the infant to make the distinction between the human voice and other sounds in order to survive. Furthermore, from infancy on, voice is the primary way in which human beings perceive and express emotions. In this way—through the instinct of sympathy—a normal child responds to voice and uses voice to express feelings and emotions. Even when language is achieved, voice, unless controlled and concealed, expresses how human beings feel about what they wish to communicate.

Considerably more impressive, at least to students of infant speech, is the early ability of infants to respond differentially to syllables that are very close in sound (phonemic) structure—for example, distinguishing between the syllables *ba* and *pa*. Eimas, Siqueland, Jusczyk, and Vigorito (1971) demonstrated that 1-month old infants are able to perceive small speech sound (phonemic) differences by changes in behavior when the syllable *ba* is altered to become *pa*. This landmark experiment was conducted along the following lines: One-month-old infants were permitted to suck on pacifiers that were connected to an electric apparatus that monitored the sucking behavior and controlled a continuous recording of the syllable *pa* or *ba*. The level of loudness for the recorded syllable was maintained as long as the sucking behavior continued. When the sucking became weak (either because of fatigue or boredom—that is, adaptation) the syllable was changed either from *pa* to *ba* or from *ba* to *pa*, depending on which sound the infant was exposed to in the recordings. When this change happened, the infants began to suck with renewed vigor (interest?) in what is interpreted as an effort to keep the new (changed) syllable at an audible level. What the Eimas et al. study demonstrates is that on a neurophysiological basis, infants are "prewired" to respond differentially to syllables that are different only by the feature of vocalization (*ba* has an initial voiced consonant, and *pa* has an initial voiceless consonant). Older children and most adults would need contextual cues to make discriminative semantic judgments of sentences such as "*Ben* wrote with his *pen*" or "Three was *par* for Joe's drinking at the *bar*."

We may generalize the implications of the Eimas et al. study by observing that neurophysiological responses are not the same as cognitive judgments. What infants can do on one level (precognitively), they may not be able to do on another (cognitive) level. In fact, judgmental discriminations between voiced and voiceless consonants normally are not made by most children until they are at least 2 years of age. However, if they were not endowed with the necessary prewiring to make differential responses at as early as 1 month of age, they might have to wait longer than age 2 to make judgmental responses. Bloom and Lahey (1978) sum up this evaluation of this potential ability with the observation: "Thus, infants have such precursory capacities but need to learn how to use them for learning the relationship between form and content" (p. 91).

Children, even as infants, may reflexively (unconsciously) mimic a relationship between form and content, between how one says what one has to say and what is said, before there is any understanding of an utterance. Lieberman (1967) observes that the fundamental frequencies (basic pitch levels) in children's "babbled dialogues" with parents "transposed toward the fundamental frequency of the parent with whom they were talking, but the crying fundamental frequency remained high" (p. 46). Lieberman speculates: "The mimicry in speech perhaps represents a social use of speech, while the crying is egocentric since it still has an emotional reference."

Specifically, Lieberman observed that a 10-month-old boy, when alone in his crib, babbled to himself at a fundamental pitch level of 430 cps (Hz), cried at 550 cps, lowered the pitch to 340 cps in a dialogue with his father, but raised it to 390 cps when playing with his mother. Perhaps even more dramatic were the pitch changes of a 13-month-old girl, who cried at 450 cps, transposed fundamental pitch to 290 cps when playing with her father, and moved up to 390 cps when playing with her mother.

In summary, by 4 months of age, the child begins to make definite responses—by vocalization, cessation of vocalization, or change in body posture—to other human sounds and sound makers. On hearing a speaker, the child turns in the speaker's direction. If the speaker is not readily in view, the child's eyes scan the area in search for the sound maker. If the child is busy vocalizing, the initial reaction is to stop as he or she begins to search. If the search is successful and the speaker is located, the child may then respond by smiling or cooing. Vocal play may be maintained by continued interchange between the child and an adult. Infant vocalization may be encouraged and reinforced by the stimulating presence of a vocalizing adult. The evidence also indicates that children deprived of such stimulation (for example, children brought up in orphanages) do less vocalizing than children who are brought up and attended to at their own homes (Brodbeck and Irwin, 1946; Goldfarb, 1954).

ECHOLALIA

At about 8 or 9 months of age, most normal children enter the echolalic stage of their prelingual speech develoment. They do not, however, give up their lalling and occasionally may even revert to earlier babbling. The significant advance in the echolalic stage is that the child now begins to be an imitator of the speech-sound production that is heard. The early imitative efforts may seem, at first, to be somewhat wide of the mark, so that "ba-ba" may be the response to either "ma-ma" or "daddy," or both. Gradually, however, the approximations begin to be replications of what is presented. Imitative efforts may also be observed for what the child sees as accompaniments to the sounds. Thus, a child may wave and orally produce "bye-bye" without intended meaning. Vocal intonation may also be imitated, so that the child behaves as if actually speaking, in all but a change in postural set for doing what he or she seems to be saying.

If the child is not yet truly speaking as well as may be possible in another 2 or 3 months, he or she certainly is gaining in the comprehension of speech. The child shows increasing evidence of making differential and appropriate responses to some utterances addressed to him or her. For example, a child may reach or look for a ball on hearing "ball" and may reach for or hug a doll on direction or in answer to the question "Do you want your doll?" Echolalia may well continue into and overlap with the next stage, when children begin to name (assign verbal labels) some things and acts that are important to them in the worlds in which they live.

The persistence of echolalia is a feature of the speech of some children who show deviancies in earlier as well as later stages of speech. Autistic children—those who are not the silent, "good" ones—may be persistently echolalic. Their echolalic responses may be much more extensive than the single words or short phrases that are characteristic of normal echolalia. Thus, a pseudoverbal autistic child may respond to "Do you want a cookie, Jimmy?" with a replication of the very same words. Ross (1980) speculates that echolalia may "represent an early developmental stage of verbal behavior beyond which the autistic child has, for some reason, never been able to develop" (p. 207). This is possible, but we should keep in mind that the echo statements may represent one of many indicators of an underlying drive for sameness. Autistic children, whether silent or pseudoverbal, are also different in the prelingual stages that precede echolalia. Some of these aspects of early childhood autism will be discussed in more detail in our later consideration of autism (Chapter 12).

Table 2.1 summarizes the prelinguistic achievements of normal infants, from the first cries to possible first words. It is important to appreciate that all stages are approximate. Furthermore, there is likely to be much greater variation in production than there is in speech and voice reception—that is, the behavior appropriate to stimuli directed to the child.

IDENTIFICATION LANGUAGE (LABELING)

Sometime between the ages of 8 or 9 months and 18 months, most children utter their first words. The words may not necessarily sound like those of an adult, but they usually do approximate them sufficiently so that a moderately indulgent listener can recognize the target. Even if this is not so, a repeated articulated form that is consistently used in relation to a specific person, object, or situation meets the essential criterion for first words (deVilliers and deVilliers, 1979). Before the production of first words, most normal children indicate wishes and needs by pointing and grunting. The grunt may approximate "uh-uh," "guh-guh," or some other replicated syllable. Perhaps more important than the beginning of naming or labeling is the evidence that normal children provide of the comprehension of words addressed to them by older speakers. From the onset, normal children comprehend more language than they can produce.

Because echolalic utterances usually continue after the first true words are uttered, many children appear to have a much larger word inventory than they actually have. Operationally, we may now say that unless appropriate behavior accompanies an utterance (e.g., reaching for an object if an utterance resembling its name is produced) the child is not really speaking. On the positive side, we may say that any utterance, however wide the approximation

Table 2.1 MATURATIONAL MILESTONES, MOTOR CORRELATES, AND PRELINGUAL SPEECH STAGE

Approximate age	Speech stage (baby says)	Motor development (baby can do)
Birth to 4 weeks	Cries whenever uncomfortable, with little apparent difference related to the specific cause or irritant	Cries, eats, or mostly sleeps; most physical motor behavior involves the entire body; when crying there may be flailing movements of legs and arms
4 to 12 weeks	Crying becomes more differentiated and associated with the probable cause; cooing, laughing, and sound play (babbling) that may suggest some vowels and consonants; may engage in vocal dialogue with mother or other caretaker	Shows differential awareness of human voice; may turn head in direction of human sound maker; motorically, is usually able to support head when lying face down; may discover and inspect own hands
12 to 16 weeks	Coos and chuckles; overall increase in vocal play	Supports head in prone position; responds to human sounds by turning head in direction of sound source
20 weeks	Consonants modify vowellike cooing; nasals and labial fricatives frequently produced	Sits with support
6 months	Babbling, resembling one syllable utterances; identifiable combinations include "ma," "da," "di," "du"	Sits without props, using hands for support
8 months	Lalling and some echolalia (self-imitation and sound mimicry)	Stands by holding on to object; grasps with thumb apposition
10 months	Distinct echolalia that approximates sounds heard; responds differentially to verbal sounds and to some simple commands	Creeps efficiently; pulls to standing position; may take a side step while holding on to a fixed object
12 months	Reduplicated sounds in echolalia; possible first words for identification; responds appropriately to an increasing number of simple commands	Walks on hands and feet; may stand alone; may walk when held by one hand or may even take first steps alone

for the real thing, is true speech if appropriate behavior consistently accompanies it. Thus, "da-da" may refer to either parent or may be a general designation for an adult, if it is the utterance produced on the appearance of one of the parents or of any acceptable adult.

First words are usually reduplicated syllables such as "dada," "mama," or "baba." As we have indicated, they are produced as identifications or designations, as announcements for the presence of an event. The child at this stage, and when in the mood, may be able to obey verbal commands such as pointing to the nose when told "Show me your nose" or when asked "Where is baby's nose?'' The child may bang with a cup, a spoon, or a hand on the order to "go bang-bang." In this respect we should note that the child is identifying verbal events by appropriate behavior. The child who bangs a cup not on command but as a self-initiated act to get a game started or, better, to get some milk, or who says "cup" or something that approximates "milk" in order to get some, has entered into a significantly higher level (stage) of speech.

Most normal children, regardless of the age at which they start to speak, have an inventory of between 25 and 50 words that they use to label or identify objects or acts before they move on to the stage at which speech is truly magical. Now, merely by announcing an appropriate word, *they can make something happen*. At least, something will happen in keeping with anticipation if there is also an appropriate person available as an instrument to make the desired (anticipated) act possible.

If we accept that the major functions of language are *interaction, regulation,* and *personal control* (Halliday, 1975), then what are the functions served by the first words? Certainly, naming implies interaction, even if only to announce "See what I see!" Even this implication suggests that some other person should join in the seeing. However, when children are alone and name what is about them, the apparent interaction is between themselves and the things they nominate. Such language usage serves the function of expression of themselves, of their concerns, and of their needs. There is always the possibility of an imagined or wished-for other that extends the interaction beyond the child. In the next stage we need no longer guess about the possible presence of an important other. The other is there as an instrument to be controlled in the interest of the child.

TRUE SPEECH: ANTICIPATORY LANGUAGE

As was just indicated, by 18 months of age most children are able to employ a few words and some children many words to bring about an event, to make something happen that might not otherwise occur. We refer to this as *anticipatory language* for two reasons. First, the child, presumably on the basis of rudimentary inner language, appears to expect that something will happen as a result of an utterance. If the event does happen, the child will show satisfaction. If it does not happen, the child may repeat the utterance or may cry to show disappointment. Second, the child reveals by a postural change and by motor set that he or she expects something to happen and is prepared for it. If the child says "Mama," he or she looks for mother to come into view; if the child says "dolly," or "wawa," he or she acts ready for one or the other; and if the child says "up," he or she usually gets ready to be picked up. Words thus used have the power of magic. The child gets what is wanted, and usually the adult is happy to do the child's bidding.

Between 18 and 24 months, most children increase their productive vocabularies from a few words to vocabularies of from 3 to 50 or more words. Their comprehension vocabularies, of course, are considerably larger. Some children may have "collapsed" words that sound like two-word phrases—for example, "babyup." A small percentage of children in the 18- to 24-month age group may actually have several two-word phrase-sentences, such as "baby-nose" and "dolly-nose." The normal child under 2 shows rapid growth in linguistic competence and is now ready for the acquisition of much more complex verbal behavior. Comprehension continues indefinitely to be more extensive than production.

Functionally, the child's single-word utterances are sentences. The meaning of the individual utterance is determined by the word (lexical unit) and by the way it is intoned. Thus, "Mama," depending on accompanying intonation, may mean "Where is Mama?" "Mama, I want you here," or even "That's enough of you, Mama!" If we accept intonation as a form akin to syntax, then the child's variously intoned single-word utterances, if the intonation pattern follows the conventions (practices) of normal older speakers, functionally serve as complete sentences. In some ways this parallels what adults do with such single-word utterances as "yes," "no," and "uh-uh," or "tomorrow," as an answer to the question, "Are you going———?"

Although a strong majority of 2-year-olds are talking, and some are producing adult-type sentences, a few may not have uttered their first intelligible words. These children, if otherwise normal, do comprehend spoken langue, however, and may be able to carry out two-component commands. As a generalization, any child who does not understand language by the end of the first year is a child about whom we should be concerned. Such concern is not in order for a child who understands language but is not yet speaking, especially if the child is from a family with many late-starting speakers. There are children who are slow to start to speak, *but there are no normal children from normal families who are equally slow in their capacities and onset for the comprehension of speech.*

Children's early words may be used to communicate many things, sometimes beyond adult usage. Children often generalize the meaning of a word according to a dominant feature or function of what the word or act may designate. Thus, *dada* or *mama* may be used for any adult, for an adult who is a caretaker, or one who has a feature (height, weight, shape, a moustache or a beard) of a male (*dada*). Any four-legged domestic animal may be a *kitty* or a *doggy;* anything that is cuddly may be a *dolly* (*doddy*), and anything that can be held and then thrown may be a *ball*.

Any single word may be used as a label, as a demand, as a query, or even as a reflection of the "state of the nation" as children perceive it in their special environment. Actions usually accompany the early words. However, a child soon learns that it is not necessary to have accompanying action; it may not be convenient if the child's arms are occupied with a *doddy* but he or she needs a *cookie*. Intonation may then become the signifier of what the child intends by the word used. Thus, as indicated earlier, single words may carry full sentence meaning.

The single-word stage, except for the functional implications of intonation, is asyntactic. Beginning with the two-word stage, syntax—the rules governing the ways we combine words to form utterances (sentences)—

emerges. Syntax includes word order and the forms and structures we usually designate by the word *grammar*.

ACQUISITION OF SYNTAX

Syntax, as indicated, is the conventions (rules) that we somehow learn as young children regarding how to speak more than one word at a time. The conventions include word order, grammatical markers (word endings for expressing plurals, tenses, possessives), and the use of the little words of our language— the so-called function words (*to, of, in, on, for*) and the articles (*a, an, the*). The use of syntax is an indication that children are aware that the words of an utterance have a special relationship that is particular to what the child means to say and generalizable to other statements and other intended meanings.

A later chapter will consider the various constructions, the word order, and the syntactic forms normal children usually acquire and the usual order of these acquisitions. The information will be used in our programs for teaching severely linguistically retarded children basic comprehension and production of the American English language. For the present, however, we will review the now-famous longitudinal study by Roger Brown (1973) of three children whom he called Adam, Eve, and Sarah. Part of the study was concerned with the order of the acquisition of 14 English morphemes (suffixes and function words) by the three children.[1] The order of acquisition is summed up in Table 2.2, which is based on the Brown (1973) findings and adapted from Clark and Clark (1977). The generating subjects, Adam, Eve, and Sarah, acquired these morphemes over a period of 18, 9, and 21 months, respectively. Eve began using these obligatory morphemes—ones that are basic and essential to speaking the English language—at about 21 months, Adam and Sarah at 27 months. Eve acquired (used) all of the morphemes by 27 months, Adam at 42 months, and Sarah at 48 months. Despite differences in onset and individual time for acquisition, the order of acquisition shows high correlations. There are differences in the order in which each morpheme was acquired, but the similarity of order is more impressive than the differences.

Multiword Utterances: Factors That Motivate Acquisitions and Change

At this point it may be asked why any child who has learned to produce single words that have "magical" power should bother to get involved with multiple-word utterances. Presumably, almost all children are reinforced (rewarded) for their early utterances. Why risk involvement with complicated productions, with learning rules and conventions of syntax, with pronunciations that more and more approximate those of older speakers in their environment? Perhaps

[1]Although Brown and his associates considered only three children in this longitudinal study, the findings have been supported by other studies with a greater number of children (see Brown, 1973, pp. 273–281).

Table 2.2 FOURTEEN OBLIGATORY ENGLISH MORPHEMES (SUFFIXES AND FUNC-
TION WORDS) AND THEIR LIKELY ORDER OF ACQUISITION BY CHILDREN

Morpheme form	Likely intended meaning	Example
1. Present progressive: *-ing*	Ongoing action	Joe is eat*ing* lunch
2. Preposition: *in*	Containment	The cookie is *in* the box.
3. Preposition: *on*	Support	The cookie is *on* the box.
4. Plural: *-s*	Number (more than one)	The bird*s* flew away.
5. Past irregular: e.g., *went, ran*	The event took place earlier (before the time of the speaker's utterance)	The boy *went* away. The boy *ran* away.
6. Possessive: *-'s*	Possession	The girl*'s* dress is red.
7. Uncontracted form of the verb *to be* (copula): e.g., *are, was*	Plural number; past tense (earlier in time)	These *are* cookies. It *was* a cat. It *was* on the tree.
8. Articles: *the, a*	Definite and indefinite article	Bob has *the* stick. Bob has *a* stick.
9. Past regular: *-ed*	Event happened earlier in time	Tom jump*ed* (over) the fence.
10. Third person regular: *-s*	Third person, present action	He walk*s* fast.
11. Third person irregular: e.g., *has, does*	Present state (situation); ongoing action (third person)	He *has* a ball. She *does* the cooking.
12. Uncontracted auxiliary of *be:* e.g., *is, were*	Ongoing action; past action	Bob *is* eating. They *were* fishing.
13. Contracted form of *to be:* e.g., *-'s, -'re*	State of being (existence)	It*'s* a kitty. We*'re* at home.
14. Contracted auxiliary of *be:* e.g., *-s, -'re*	Time, ongoing action	He*'s* going. They*'re* eating lunch.

Source: Based on Brown (1973, p. 271) and adapted from Clark and Clark (1977, p. 345).

the question is as unreasonable (or as reasonable) as asking why songbirds sing or why so-called talking birds mimic the sounds—including those of human beings—that they hear. Essentially, the conjectural answer is that the potential for acquiring a language system is a form of behavior specific and peculiar to human beings. With few exceptions, this potential is achieved.

The exceptions are the children who are the major concern of this book. They include the congenitally aphasic, the autistic, and the orally apraxic, among whom are also found children with intake problems for language. These groups of children need to be taught directly to acquire, with considerable effort, the knowledge and ability to learn a mode of behavior that comes with relative ease for the vast majority of their age peers. Even for these exceptional groups, however, we may ask why they try. Again, the best conjecture is that perhaps they do not have much choice because they, too, are human, and the acquisition of language is part of their destiny.

One cannot achieve a destiny in a vacuum. Even if we accept Chomsky's (1972) abstract conceptual construction that a human being is born with a language acquisition device (LAD) by and through which what a child is exposed to is "filtered" and rules (order) somehow become generated, exposure to a speech (language) system is necessary. Beyond this, the child must be able to identify with and relate to speakers in order to be sensitive to the oral output perceived as language. Children may be preprogrammed (prewired) to be sensitive to language, but they must also be mature to be able to take in and decode what they hear and encode some of what they hear (listen to) in their own productions. If we accept this position, it is still necessary to ask whether the child can possibly acquire language by mere exposure, or whether the child must be an active participant in the evolving process.

To some degree, perhaps, the answer depends on the child and on the environment to which the child is exposed. Our position is that normal children are active participants in the language game. Children, if they are normal, are both inquisitive and acquisitive. Although most children need to pause from time to time to consolidate gains, and may be as reluctant to go from one construction to another as they sometimes are to accept new foods or new toys, the great majority of children seek some amount of variety in their lives. Language provides opportunity for variety of expression and variety of interaction. As Bloom and Lahey (1978, p. 367) point out, language allows the child to receive and send new information about the world in which he or she lives. Language permits the child, through verbal interchange, to learn about language, to learn what the most appropriate word is for an event and what the most appropriate construction is for the new word—the new and exciting piece of information. Of course, the child is likely to be reinforced for this active participation by parents, by older siblings, by peers, but perhaps mostly by himself with the realization, "I've learned to say (do it) the right way!" The right way, however, as will be seen later, is not a slavishly imitative way. The right way becomes increasingly individualized but manages to stay within the lawful boundaries determined by the language conventions of one or more environments in which a child interacts. Although words and syntactic constraints have their way with the maturing child, ultimately the child has his or her way with words. This achievement we refer to as the *idiolect* or, as we prefer, the *individuolect*.

Syntactic Speech

We have moved ahead of ourselves in our consideration of the stages in normal language acquisition. The implications of what we have already discussed will be applied in the discussion that follows.

By age 2, most children who have been speaking for 6 or more months have production vocabularies of from 50 to several hundred words. Their comprehension vocabularies are likely to be considerably larger. Some children will have names for all the objects and recurrent ongoing events in their environment, including words of their own invention. The most distinctive achievement, however, is not in vocabulary growth but in the ability to combine words into phrase-sentences. Although most of these early utterances may lack the conventional markers of syntax—the use of functional words (prepositions and conjunctions) and plural and tense endings—they nevertheless constitute functional sentences. The literal form of the words may comprise two nouns—for example, "Baby-milk" to mean "I want milk" or "Give me some milk," or an adverb and a noun, as in "More milk." Functionally, any words used by a 2-year-old may serve to indicate a variety of meanings. What matters is that the child is now using different words and is combining them to indicate different meanings. Frequently, one word may be used recurrently as part of a pivot utterance (Braine, 1963), so that the child may produce such phrase-sentences as "Here dolly" and "Here ball" as well as "Baby here" and "Cup here." There may also be such utterances as "More cup" and "More up" or the same words in reverse order. The significance of this achievement is that the child is developing awareness of sentence sense and word order. In time, usually within the next year, the word combinations will be modified by grammatical markers—the use of functional words to tie and relate to other words, and the conventions of word order according to the verbal practices (syntax) of older speakers.

By 2 years of age, half or more of the children's utterances are sufficiently intelligible to be understood by listeners, including those who may not be in regular and frequent contact with them. Presumably, this encourages continued efforts at word formulations. Of special significance at this stage is the child's ability to combine words in new formulations to which he or she has not been specifically exposed in the environment. Thus, from the inventory of known words, the child creates sentences that may parallel some that have been directly taught. If the child learned by imitation to say "Tommy up," for example, he or she may improvise "Dolly up," "Ball up," and "Mommy up," or, as indicated earlier, the same words in reverse order. The child now reveals an ability to generalize and to generate and has, in effect, become a creative speaker (an essential criterion for language acquisition).

Congenitally aphasic children at 2 years and beyond may be essentially nonverbal or at best at the one-word stage. They have fewer words in their lexicons than do their chronological and mental-age peers. Many of their verbal productions are unintelligible or show evidence of deviant phonology. Ingram (1976) emphasizes the apparently correct position that "deviant phonology may be not just a phonemic disorder, but a more global linguistic one" (p. 122). The more global aspects include deficits in the morphemic, syntactic, and semantic systems of language.

Echolalic autistic children are likely to be intelligible but noncreative in their productions; that is, they repeat what they hear, but usually without evidence of comprehension. There are variations, however, in kinds of echolalia. Their implications as possible communicative messages are considered in Chapter 12.

Children with congenital oral (articulatory) apraxia are often unintelligible in their verbal productions. Intonation, however, may be appropriate if the listener can guess what the child is trying to say. Unless the congenitally apraxic child is also aphasic, there will be a sharp contrast between aural comprehension, which may be normal or close to normal, and the deviant articulated productions.

Communicative Intent

Children show communicative intent in their early utterances, in the first words that are designated as *anticipatory language*. At a later stage, when they begin to use multiword utterances, they want more than an opportunity to say something that will result in making someone do something; they now want clear evidence that they have responding listeners and that, on occasion, the response that is wanted may be a verbal interchange. In responding to an infant's early utterances, the meaning and intention is essentially a responsibility assumed by the older listener. Increasingly, however, the responsibility shifts and is shared by the child and the listener. Between 18 months and 2 years of age, the child's intention to communicate is made increasingly clear in the very act of communicating. Bloom and Lahey (1978) sum up the change and progress in the young child's communicative behavior:

> Although still unable to use the conventions of language, infants come to know that their behavior can influence the behavior of others, and they behave with the intention of achieving that influence. Ultimately, in the second year, infants begin to learn the sounds and the signs in the context that are part of language, and communication becomes both intentional and *conventional.* An infant's progress, then, is from earliest communication (i.e., without intention and without convention) to intentional communication that is not conventional, to, eventually, communication that is intentional and uses conventional means. (p. 204)

When children learn to engage in behavior that is intentionally communicative, they may increasingly show evidence of frustration if their efforts are not understood. This behavior—frustration to express disapproval because an expectation has not been realized—is what parents exerience when their children are at the "terrible twos." Kagan (1980) states:

> We hazard the guess that the two central psychological victories of this period include the establishment of the first standards followed by the emergence of awareness of one's actions, intentions, states, and competencies. We call this function self awareness.

FUNCTIONS OF LANGUAGE: THE EMERGENCE OF SEMANTIC AND PRAGMATIC RELATIONSHIPS

The communicative efforts of young children may be classified into three broad categories: interaction, regulation, and personal control (Halliday, 1975). These functions begin to be expressed in infants' first words and continue as they mature and become linguistically competent. By age 2, or earlier in some children (Halliday found that all functions in his study were evident by 21 months), the three broad functions could be classified into seven, with their approximate order of appearance as follows:

1. Instrumental—language used to satisfy specific (material) needs; for example, "I want cookie," "I want doggy," "I want (something material)."
2. Regulatory—language used to exert control or direct the behavior of another; for example, "Mommy come," "Daddy throw ball."
3. Interactional—language used to establish or maintain contact with an important other (social-gesture languge); for example, "Hi mommy," "Please, daddy."
4. Heuristic—language used to investigate (explore) one's environment; for example, "There kitty," "What that?"
5. Personal—language used to speak of oneself, to announce and express individuality; for example, "I'm (me) a boy," "I (me) jump," "I (me) pretty."
6. Imaginative—language used in make-believe play, language used to create a pretended world; for example, "I'm a kitty," "I'm a birdie," or, even, according to need, "Me baby."
7. Informative—in contrast to heuristic, language used to provide information to someone who may not have it; may overlap the imaginative or be factual; for example, "I'm a big doggy" is informative and imaginative, but "Fido my doggy" may be factual.

Some of the purposes overlap, as indicated in the informative use of language. Some of the expressions of language function imply a need for a response, verbal or nonverbal; others more clearly call for an act (instrumental and regulatory). Often, caretakers will accompany action with oral language.

The regulatory function of language may also include *self-regulation*. A child who announces, "I throw ball" may be using self-expression (personal), may be asking for an audience (regulatory), or may be controlling his or her own behavior by specifically stating what he or she is doing or trying to do. The purpose or function of an utterance, whether simple or multiple, is determined, of course, by the circumstances as well as by the child's cognitive stage of development. Adults may project their own wishes onto what a child in a given situation is intending. This may account for the occasional confusion in the adult's response and, in turn, in the child's response to the adult for failure to be understood. Children, more unwittingly than adults, do not always make their intentions clear by the content of their utterances. Language usage is at best still a guessing game. As children mature, linguistically and intellectually, they become better guessers, but the possibility if not the probability for erroneous interpretation remains in almost all communicative efforts, even those by speakers of the same dialects of the same language system who are brought up in what may be considered the same environment.

Syntactic Stages

By age 2, the verbal constructions of most children indicate that they are aware of how words are strung together in an utterance. They show knowledge of syntax, and their sentences incorporate some of the grammatical features of older speakers in their environment. Some 2-year-olds may now be using three- and four-word utterances. By age 3, their sentences may include prepositions, articles, conjunctions, and other syntactic markers.

By age 3, many of the infantilisms, including those of pronunciation, give way to more grownup forms. The infantile "me want" is likely to be replaced by "I want" and "wawa" by "water" or something close to it. In general, phonemic proficiency is closer to that of the adult and is usually good enough that almost everything a child says is readily intelligible. Vocabulary growth is great, perhaps greater than at any other period in the child's life. Children at age 3 are also likely to understand the difference between the demonstrative pronouns *this* and *that* and between *here* and *there,* and some may even understand and appropriately use the forms for *come* and *go.* These unstable words, which have shifting meaning according to context and referents, have what linguists refer to as a *deictic function;* that is, the words have meanings in context that may not be determined by how they are defined in a dictionary. In a given context, the meanings are temporary and indicate a particular but temporary relationship that is determined by a given communicative interchange and by the persons participating in it. For example, knowledge of language usage and of speaker intention is required to appreciate that the *you* in the sentence "You should not cross without looking both ways" may be replaced by *one.* Furthermore, this sentence as a whole is usually not intended as a command but as a general observation about how one (you) should behave at a street crossing.

Age 3 to 4 Years: The Emergence of the Individuolect

Most children between 3 and 4 years of age are able to understand thousands of words and have a productive vocabulary that exceeds 1000 words. Almost all of their utterances are intelligible, so that a well-intentioned listener has little difficulty in understanding the child's message. This is not to suggest that all sounds in the child's language system are under control and are produced in a normal adult fashion. Many children still have difficulty with *s, z, ch, j,* and *l.* Their substitutions, however, are fairly regular, as are the tendencies to reduce sound blends such as *sp, sk, str, fr, br* to simple single sounds, depending on the sound under control. See Ingram (1976, Ch. 2) for a detailed consideration of normal sound (phonological) acquisition. Phonemic development will be considered later in this chapter.

There is considerable variation in articulation (phonemic proficiency) in 4-year-olds. Some speak with almost adult proficiency—happily, except for voice. Others sound quite infantile; yet most, as indicated, are intelligible because their messages can be understood. Most 4-year-olds have sufficient control of syntax to say what they need to say with few grammatical errors. Those that do occur may be a result of the children's generalizing what they will have to learn to consider as exceptions, such as the plural forms of *child, sheep*, and irregular verb forms. The majority of 4-year-olds, especially those who began to talk before 15 months of age, are probably more proficient in syntax than they are in articulation, but proficiency in one aspect of oral language is likely to be highly correlated with the other. Full syntactic proficiency, as indicated earlier, may not be achieved until age 10 or 11, and for some children not until early adolescence.

Four-year-olds are well on their way to becoming mature speakers with well-established language patterns, and they begin to show evidence of developing their own rhetorical styles. Each child may have favorite words and perhaps favorite ways of turning a phrase. Four-year-olds speak for themselves as individuals, and each speaks in a manner that expresses a self. Although they share a linguistic system with other speakers, some of whom they may indeed have imitated in their earlier language acquisitions, most 4-year-olds are adapting the system to themselves, to their needs and their personalities. In effect, 4-year-olds are developing their *individuolects*. Each has now become a speaker of a language, of a dialect of the language, and of an individualized adaptation of the dialect—an individuolect (idiolect).

Beyond Ages 3 and 4

Normal children beyond age 3 show continued growth in all aspects of language, for comprehension as well as production. For all of the subsystems of language, there are marked changes in the direction of adult forms and conventions. Nevertheless, even at age 4 and beyond, children have a way to go before they can understand and use irregular verbs and appreciate syntactic subtleties. Even at age 10, some children are not clear as to the meaning and appropriate use of word pairs such as *ask-tell, give-take, buy-spend* (Chomsky, 1969). In a sentence such as "Bill told Bob to catch the ball," there is little doubt that it is Bob who is to do the catching. However, in the sentence "Bill promised Bob to catch the ball," it is Bill rather than Bob who will be the catcher. Some 10-year-olds may not be certain or may be incorrect in applying the minimum-distance rule that is applicable to most verbs. If this rule is observed, the child will conclude that the verb closest to the noun indicates who does what. In time, most children beyond age 10 are able to comprehend such sentences despite the errant behavior of the verbs. They will also be able to understand the difference between "Ask Mary when to go" and "Tell Mary when to go" and between "Susan asked Mary to play" and "Susan told Mary to play."

ACQUISITION OF SOUNDS: PHONEMIC DEVELOPMENT

At about 6 months of age, the infant, in vocal play, produces some sounds and sound combinations that can be identified as belonging to the adult's language system. At about 8 months, the child begins to repeat syllables and word forms that closely resemble the adult's. The child's first words may sound like those spoken by adults or may be inventions of sounds that are easy to produce— "ma-ma" or "da-da." As the child learns to say more words, and even when he or she produces word-phrases or two- or three-word sentences, it becomes apparent that lexical (word) and syntactic proficiency are more advanced than articulatory (phonemic) proficiency. Between ages 2 and 5, children show great variability in phonemic development. Some children, especially girls, may be quite proficient by age 3 or 4, and may have adult-level proficiency by age 5. However, most girls do not level off in phonemic control until about age 6 or 7, and boys not until about age 7 or 8.

Children's errors in phonemic production and in phonemic control are not random or chance products. Children's first words are built of the sounds they can control—produced at will rather than as evocations in vocal play. These sounds are likely to include nasal consonants, labials (lip sounds), and vowels. Young children also engage in reduplication, possibly as an expression of normal perseverative behavior. Thus, with the sounds they are able to control, children build their inventories of first words. A word such as *mama,* which combines a nasal bilabial and a vowel, presents no problem. *Mama* is a "natural" in terms of phonemic proficiency and opportunity for reinforcement. *Mama* or a construction close to it is an almost universal designation for a mother. The word *dada* for daddy represents simplification through vowel reduplication. It is easier to say something twice than to say it once. *Dolly* may become "doddy" because of consonant and vowel duplication. The consonant /d/ is controlled before /l/. *Kitty* may be pronounced "kicky" because /k/ is usually controlled before /t/. "Kicky" may also be an expression of assimilation, the initial *k* influencing the change of the *t* to *k*. The pronunciation of "bummy" for *bunny* may be explained by the substitution of the bilabial /m/ for the tongue-tip nasal /n/; it is easier to produce two bilabials in a word. In fact, the pronunciation "bubby" for *bunny* is not unusual. Later, we shall consider in more detail the phonemic construction and the rules underlying such word forms in a discussion of the normal (usual) phonology of the first 25 to 50 words.

As children mature, first in auditory discrimination and then in articulatory control (here, too, comprehension or competence for intake precedes production or output), they begin to make distinctions between sounds that are phonetically close or similar.[2] As indicated earlier, by age 7 or 8, the great majority of children reach what is essentially an adult level of phonemic proficiency. In general, the process of phonemic development is characterized by progressive differentiation. Almost all children can detect fine shades of differences before they can produce them themselves. A child may persist in saying "kicky" for *kitty* but reject this pronunciation from an adult; he or she may still produce "wawipop" at age 5 but resent such an offering from an older person. What the child is demonstrating by this apparently inconsistent language behavior is that at age 4 or 5, he or she has better phonemic discrimination, and hence better expectations in regard to listening, than motor control over his or her own productions. In a year or two, motor control will be much improved, possibly because of a well-developed motor-kinesthetic auditory feedback loop. According to Liberman (1957, 1982) and Luria (1966), children may begin to perceive speech according to the way they produce speech sounds. Liberman (1957) states: "Speech is perceived by the articulatory stimulus and the events we call perception." Thus, children will perceive speech as they articulate the equivalents of what they hear. Whether or not this is indeed what takes place, an examination of the diagram of the brain will suggest that the proximity of the motor area for articulate speech to the temporal area for speech reception may well account for the establishment and interdependence of articulation and speech hearing (see Ch. 4, Fig. 4.1).

Normal phonological development will be reviewed in Chapter 7, "Phonological Deficiencies in Aphasic and Dysphasic Children."

PRAGMATICS: A STAGE ACQUISITION MODEL

As indicated earlier, in order to be successful in carrying out a communicative function, a child needs to know not only what to say but also how to construct and deliver the message according to the specific set of circumstances. Sentences are judged as appropriate and acceptable "under rules governing relations between scenes, participants, genres, channel, and the like—who can say what, in what way, where and when, by what means, and to whom?" (Hymes, 1971, p. 15). This kind of knowledge and performance is ongoing, beginning, as suggested earlier, in children's adjusted crying and cooing. Pragmatic proficiency, along with other linguistic achievements, normally continues into adult years. Prutting (1979) sees pragmatic competencies becoming clearly apparent after age 3; she provides a model that incorporates stages for acquisition of pragmatics.

Prutting (1979) considers her stage processes concept a model for research and study. She is aware that, despite the rich and extensive investigations into child language in recent years, there is considerably more to be

---

[2]It may be recalled that, as early as 4 weeks, infants respond differentially to speech sounds that are very close in phonetic features (Eimas et al., 1971). Reflex of innate neurophysiological responses are not, however, the equivalent of cognitive responses, and the implications of the early infant responses as possible precursors of later cognitive abilities cannot be ignored.

learned about the complex processes of early language acquisition, and she observes:

> There are obvious gaps and inconsistencies in the literature .The proposed stage process model should be viewed as reflecting a state of flux rather than reflecting a static state. With the research vitality in child language, additional evidence will be forthcoming. We will no doubt change aspects of our lexicon to describe the acquisition period, and add to, delete, and perhaps transpose information regarding the developmental stages as we learn more about the complex processes of language acquisition. (p. 21)

Prutting's proposed, but still tentative, stages for acquisition of pragmatics are presented in Table 2.3.

In a later writing Prutting and Kirchner (1983) provide principles and guidelines for the application of language to the understanding and treatment of language disordered children. They note:

> With regard to the use of various pragmatic abilities and certain cognitive precursors to language development, it may be erroneous to only assume that language disordered children are delayed compared to normals; although delay may be one of the profiles. (p. 57)

SPEECH READINESS

An examination of the speech stages in Tables 2.3 and 2.4 will reveal that the normal child appears to make great spurts in aspects of phonemic, morphemic, lexical, and syntactic acquisition at particular periods in his or her life. For example, we may note the large proportionate increase in vocabulary at about 30 months and the control of syntax at about 36 months. Consonant blends, which are not indicated on the tables, are usually established between 5 and 6 years. These acquisition times may be considered periods of readiness in which basic skills of previous stages are incorporated and the child is then ready and able for the next stage or level of development. Earlier, we also indicated that regardless of the language the child will speak, most children acquire their first words at the beginning of their second year. Periods of readiness are opportune times for potential abilities (capacities) to become manifest abilities, provided that opportunity and conditions are right. For most children, the essential right conditions are exposure to an older speaker and some reinforcement for their efforts. There is, of course, individual variation. For a given child, the rate of progress after onset of speech will be determined by a combination of innate factors—such as the integrity of the neurological mechanisms, sensory capacities, cognitive ability, and motor functioning—and cultural factors that, at least until age 3 or 4, are dominant within the child's own family. The factor of sex may give a girl a slight advantage over a boy, at least in the area of articulation, up to age 5 or 6. Bilingual exposure, especially for children from lower socioeconomic and disadvantaged groups, may be a negative factor.

Table 2.3 STAGES FOR ACQUISITION OF PRAGMATICS

Prelinguistic (birth–9 mo.)	Stage I (9–18 mo.)	Stage II (18–24 mo.)	Stage II (2–3 yrs.)	Stage IV (3+ yrs.)	Stage V (communicative competence, adult)
Perlocutionary acts: gazing, crying, touching, smiling, vocalizations, grasping, sucking, laughing (Bates, 1975)	Functions: instrumental, regulatory, interactional, personal, heuristic, imaginative, informative (Halliday, 1975)	Functions: pragmatic, mathetic, interpersonal, textual, ideational, (Halliday, 1975)	Responds to contingent queries, types of revisions, function of linguistic development (Gallagher, 1977)	Sustains topic (Bloom, Rocissano, and Hood, 1976)	Knowledge of who can say what, in what way, where and when, by what means, and to whom (Hymes, 1971)
Illocutionary acts: nonverbal and speechlike giving, pointing, showing (Bates, 1975)	Intentions: label, response, request, greeting, protesting, repeating, description, attention (Dore, 1974)		Rapid topic change (Keenan and Schiefflin, 1976)	Systematic changes in speech depending on listener (Shatz and Gelman, 1973; Gleason, 1973; Sachs and Devin, 1976)	Behavior speakers and listeners attend to; quality—informative but not too informative; quality—contribution should be true; relation—be relevant; manner—avoid obscurity, ambiguity, be brief and orderly (Grice, 1975)
Turn-taking (Bruner, 1975)	Verbal turn-taking procedures employed (Bloom, Rocissano and Hood, 1976)			Indirectives and hints (Ervin-Tripps and Mitchell-Kernan, 1977)	
	New information coded first (Greenfield and Smith, 1976)			Productive use of contingent queries to maintain the conversation (Garvey, 1975)	
				Role-playing, ability to temporarily assume another's perspective (Anderson, 1977)	
				Metalinguistic awareness, ability to think about language and comment on it (Gleitman, Gleitman, and Shipley, 1972; de Villiers and de Villiers, 1974)	

Source: Prutting, C. A. "Process \praͥses\: The Action of Moving Forward Progressively from One Point to Another on the Way to Completion," *Journal of Speech and Hearing Disorders,* 44 (1), 1979, 3–30.

Note: Plus or minus six months for all ages is considered normal. References for citations in this table are provided by Prutting (1979, pp. 27–30).

Table 2.4   MATURATIONAL MILESTONES, MOTOR CORRELATES, AND PRELINGUAL SPEECH STAGE

Approximate Age	Speech stage (child says)	Motor development (child can do)
18 months	Has repertoire of words (between 3 and 50); some two-word phrases; vocalizations reveal intonational patterns; great increase in understanding of language	Walks with ease; runs; can build two-block tower; begins to show hand preference
24 months	Vocabulary of 50 or more words for naming and for bringing about events; two-word phrases of own formulation	Walks with ease; runs; can walk up or down stairs, planting both feet on each step
30 months	Vocabulary growth proportionately greater than at any other period in life; speaks with clear communicative intent; conventional sentences (syntax) of three, four, and five words; articulation still includes many infantilisms; good comprehension of speakers in the surroundings	Can jump, stand on one foot; good hand and fingers coordination; can build six-block tower
36 months	Productive vocabulary may exceed 1000 words; syntax increasingly like that of older persons in child's environment; most utterances are intelligible to older listeners	Runs proficiently; alternates feet in walking steps; hand preference is established
48 months	Except for articulation, child's linguistic system much like that of the adults with whom child has most contact; may begin to develop an individual "rhetorical" style	Can hop on one foot (usually the right); can throw a ball to an intended receiver; can catch a ball in arms; can walk on a line

Source: Adapted from Lennenberg (1967, pp. 128–130).

Position in the family may give a first child an advantage over younger siblings. However, the most significant positive environmental factors are appropriate stimulation from good models (proficient and caring speakers) with whom the child can identify and relate.

REFERENCES AND SUGGESTED READINGS

Bloom, L., and Lahey, M. *Language Development and Language Disorders.* New York: Wiley, 1978.

Bosma, J. F. "Anatomic and Physiologic Development of the Speech Apparatus," in D. B. Tower (ed.), *The Nervous System:* (Vol. 3), *Human Communication and Its Disorders.* New York: Raven Press, 1975.

Braine, M. D. S. "The Ontogeny of English Phrase Structure," *Language,* 39, 1963, 1–13.

Bricker, D. D., and Carlson, L. "Issues in Early Language Intervention," in R. L. Schiefelbusch and D. D. Bricker (eds.), *Early Language: Acquisition and Intervention.* Baltimore: University Park Press, 1981.

Brodbeck, A. J., and Irwin, O. C. "The Speech Behavior of Infants Without Families," *Child Development,* 17, 1946, 145–156.

Brown, R. *A First Language: The Early Stages.* Cambridge, Mass.: Harvard University Press, 1973.

Carroll, John B. "Language Development in Children," in S. Saporta (ed.), *Psycholinguistics.* New York: Holt, Rinehart and Winston, 1961.

Chomsky, C. *The Acquisition of Syntax in Children from Five to Ten.* Cambridge, Mass.: M.I.T. Press, 1969.

Chomsky, N. "The Formal Nature of Language," in E. H. Lenneberg, *Biological Foundations of Language.* New York: Wiley, 1967.

Chomsky, N. *Language and Mind.* New York: Harcourt Brace Jovanovich, 1972.

Clark, H. H., and Clark, E. V. *Psychology and Language.* New York: Harcourt Brace Jovanovich, 1977.

Dale, P. *Language Development: Structure and Function.* New York: Holt, Rinehart and Winston, 1976.

Darwin, C. "A Bibliographic Sketch of an Infant," *Mind,* July 1877, 285–294.

deVilliers, P. A., and deVilliers, J. G. *Early Language.* Cambridge, Mass.: Harvard University Press, 1979.

Eimas, P., Siqueland, E. R., Jusczyk, P., and Vigorito, J. "Speech Perception in Infants," *Science,* 171, 1971, 305–306.

Fischelli, V. R., and Karelitz, K. "The Cry Latencies of Normal Infants and Those with Brain Damage," *Journal of Pediatrics,* 62(5), 1963, 724–734.

Furth, H. G. *Thinking Without Language.* New York: Free Press, 1966.

Goldfarb, W. "Effects of Psychological Deprivation in Infancy and Subsequent Stimulation," *American Journal of Psychiatry,* 12, 1954, 102–129.

Halliday, M. A. K. *Learning How to Mean—Explorations in the Development of Language.* London: Edward Arnold, 1975.

Hymes, D. "Competence and Performance in Linguistic Theory," in R. Huxley and E. Ingram, (eds.), *Language Acquisition: Models and Methods.* New York: Academic Press, 1971.

Ingram, D. *Phonological Disabililty in Children.* New York: Elsevier, 1976.

Irwin, O. C. "Speech Development in the Young Child," *Journal of Speech and Hearing Disorders,* 17(3), 1952, 269–279.

Kagan, J. *Psychological Growth in the Second Year.* Private communication; unpublished manuscript, 1980.

Karelitz, K., and Fischelli, V. R. "The Cry Thresholds of Normal Infants and Those with Brain Damage," *Journal of Pediatrics,* 61(5), 1962, 679–685.

Lenneberg, E. H. "Language Disorders in Childhood," *Harvard Educational Review,* 34(2), 1964, 152–177.

Lenneberg, E. H. *Biological Foundations of Language.* New York: Wiley, 1967.

Lewis, M. M. *How Children Learn to Speak.* New York: Basic Books, 1959.

Liberman, A. M. "Some Results of Research on Speech Perception," *Journal of the Acoustical Society of America,* 29, 1957, 117–123.

Liberman, A. M. "On Finding that Speech Is Special," *American Psychologist,* 37, 1982, 148–167.

Lieberman, P. *Intonation, Perception and Language.* Cambridge, Mass.: M.I.T. Press, 1967.

Luria, A. R. *The Higher Cortical Functions of Man.* New York: Basic Books, 1966.

Maskarinec, A. S., Cairns, G. F., Butterfield, E. C., and Weamer, L. K. "Longitudinal Observations of Individual Infant's Vocalizations," *Journal of Speech and Hearing Disorders,* 46, 1981, 267–273.

Oller, D. K., Weiman, L. A., Doyle, W. J., and Ross, C., "Infant Babbling and Speech," *Journal of Child Language,* 1976, 3, 1–11.

Prutting, C. A. "Process \prá|ses\: The Act of Moving Forward Progressively from One Point to Another on the Way to Completion," *Journal of Speech and Hearing Disorders,* 44(1), 1979, 3–30.

Prutting, C. A. and Kirchner, D. M. "Applied Pragmatics," in Gallagher, T. and Prutting, C. (eds.), *Pragmatic Assessment and Intervention Issues.* Houston: College-Hill Press, 1983.

Ricks, D. M. "Vocal Communication in Pre-verbal, Normal and Autistic Children," in N. O'Connor (ed.), *Language, Cognitive Deficits and Retardation.* London: Butterworth, 1975.

Ross, A. O., *Psychological Disorders of Children,* 2d ed. New York: McGraw-Hill, 1980.

Truby, H. M., Bosma, J. F., and Lind, J. *Newborn Infant Cry.* Upsala, Sweden: Almquist and Wiksells, 1965.

Wasz-Hockert, O., Lind, J., Vuorenkoski, V., Partanen, T., and Valanne, E., *The Infant Cry in Clinics in Developmental Medicine,* #29. London: Spastics International Medical Publications, Heinemann, 1968.

Wolff, P. H. "The Natural History of Crying and Other Vocalizations in Early Infancy," in B. M. Foss (ed.), *Determinants of Infant Behavior,* Vol. 4. London: Methuen, 1966.

chapter *3*

Perception and Perceptual Functioning Underlying Language Acquisition

The term *perception* will be used here to mean the cognitive process by which an individual organizes (establishes a pattern) and interprets received sensory data (events) on the basis of past experience or on the basis of a species-specific innate capacity for first experiences. If we did not invoke the concept of innate capacity, we would be at a loss to explain how any initial organization of sensory response could take place. Perception implies an act of categorization according to which stimuli (identified units or events) are sorted and given meaning.

Perception for language, whether spoken or written, necessarily deals with a series or sequence of events that have temporal order—that is, events that are extended in time or space. The discussion that follows will be concerned with the perception of those auditory events that constitute spoken language (speech). A primary and fundamental aspect of perception of speech is differentiating speech from other environmental auditory events that may simultaneously stimulate the potential respondent. Once again, we will invoke the notion of innate capacity, the capacity with which each normal newborn is endowed.

ATTENTION AND PERCEPTION

Normally, we are able to select voluntarily particular inputs for conscious intake and processing. Because at any given time we are bombarded by a multiplicity of stimuli, we must necessarily be selective regarding what we want to attend. Normally—that is, if we are not in a state of conflict of interest, or if the competing stimuli are not too intense or too persistent to be ignored, or if we are not suffering from excessive fatigue or from the effects of a drug—we succeed in attending, and so in perceiving, according to our situational wishes. How this is accomplished is in part explained in the passage that follows:

> We normally experience no difficulty with selection because the particular target we are interested in differs from all others on a large number of perceptual and cognitive dimensions. For example, it seems quite easy to have a conversation with one friend in the midst of a party. We do not consider it amazing that we are able to ignore a loud band and pick out a single person's speech from the 50 or 60 voices all around us. But the task seems so easy only because there are many cues to guide our selection. First, we know the person's location, and, for that matter, see the person's lips moving. We are also aware of the pitch, loudness, and speech style of the person's voice. In addition we are guided by the semantic content of the conversation, which helps us to know what the person is likely to say next. While our ability to focus attention on a single input is impressive, the effortlessness with which we can distinguish between such discriminable targets is largely a function of the natural diversity of the environment, and is misleading with regard to the extensiveness of the processing involved in the discrimination. This processing can be revealed by narrowing the differences between targets.
>
> As long as targets are conceptually distinct and differ on some perceptual dimension, one particular target can be processed in the presence of the others. For example, people can pick out visual targets of a particular color and auditory inputs of a particular pitch, location, or loudness. However, as the targets become more similar, it becomes extremely difficult to attend selectively to only one, even if they remain conceptually distinct. (Glass, Holyoak, and Santa, 1979, p. 201)

Some Assumptions about Perception

In the passage just quoted, the terms *perception* and *cognition* were used to indicate that there are perceptual and cognitive dimensions that facilitate attention. Do we perceive because we attend or attend because we perceive? We will not attempt to solve this chicken-and-egg sequence. Instead, we will consider some working assumptions relative to the *cognitive process of perception*.

Selectivity   As indicated earlier, perception is a selective process. We do not attend to and perceive everything that may come to us within a sensory field to which we are physically exposed. In most instances, we respond to those events that have some priority or importance for us at a given moment. Thus, it is possible to hear the voice and the words of the person for whom we are listening rather than the person who is talking to us, or to see only one face in a crowd though our sensory system may have taken in many.

Factors that determine selection include *set* (we perceive what we are prepared or set to perceive), *drive, motivation, training,* and *cultural values.*

The factors of drive and motivation need no explanation at this time, except to note that they may be negative; that is, there may be negative factors for us not to perceive. Training determines how we perceive cloud formation, automobile noises, or human noises. Bachelors because of either motivation or training, may not be adept at distinguishing a cat's crying in the darkness of the night from a baby's crying. Cultural values as well as training may determine the perceptions and both the covert and differential overt responses of parents to a baby's crying. Our knowledge (training) and our motivation determine whether we perceive or merely hear a foreign speaker when we are traveling abroad or at home when foreigners are present.

Discrimination   With the possible exception of figure–background discrimination, the discrimination of objects, or of any pattern of events, is established through learning. Our capacity for making discriminatory responses increases with experience and learning.

Categorization   In our definition of perception, we indicated that perception is a process of categorization. We may then ask where the first category that permits an individual to make additional categorizations came from. We accept, as a basic assumption, that a normal organism is born with some innate categories and develops some categories with maturation. Thus, specifically in regard to speech, the infant is born with a capacity for making broad categorical responses between speech and other auditory (nonspeech) environmental events. As infants mature and as their knowledge of language grows, their capacities for making finer discriminative responses enable them to establish categories for the components of the subsystems of the language or languages to which they are exposed and which they learn. Thus, we assume that normal infants and normal children have innate capacities for establishing categorical responses that, with experience, are refined and modified rather than rigidly set in keeping with first experiences.

PERCEPTION OF THE SPEECH CODE

Speech, as Liberman (1982) emphasizes, is special. As mentioned earlier, speech (oral language) is human-species–specific. We have no need, therefore, to explain why the infant normally is motivated to become a speaking member of a speaking culture; nor do we need to explain why the child gives up childish ways of speaking and, with normal physical and intellectual maturation, comes to assume grown-up ways of talking. Normally, the inner drive, the culture, and the opportunity are all present. A caring caretaker serves as a first teacher who, as was suggested in the first chapter, offers a model for speaking that does not exceed the child's emerging abilities. These abilities include making discriminative responses to components of the speech mode to permit categorizing with sufficient flexibility (events in essence the same but not necessarily identical) to allow meanings to emerge from verbal contexts and associated situations.

As we learn more about language and more about the speakers and the world in which we all live, what we listen to and how we listen and in turn comprehend come to determine the segments of the linguistic whole to which we are exposed. A sentence such as "They are sailing ships" means one thing when the speaker is pointing out to sea, where there are sailing ships, but means something else if the speaker had been asked, "Where are Tom and Bill?" The writings of Glass, Holyoak, and Santa (1979), Sanders (1977), and Liberman (1982) deal with the perception of speech by persons who are already able to speak. However, we are still looking for explanations and answers to related questions: Initially, how does an infant begin to derive meaning from the language to which he or she has been exposed? From where do the first perceptual responses come? In general terms, how does verbal utterance come to have meaning for a child who, at the outset, has only a potential for acquiring language but as yet no language?

How the beginnings begin and how first utterances are produced and understood are phenomena about which we can only conjecture. One explanation, identified with the linguist Noam Chomsky (1957, 1965), theorizes that human beings are born with a language acquisition device (LAD), an internal (hypothetical) structure that enables them to arrive at rules (grammar) after exposure to linguistic events. Accordingly, children acquire language because, through the use of the LAD, they are able to discover the underlying rules that govern the utterances to which they are exposed and to which they can respond. The rules or grammars are those that are concerned with the sound system (phonology), the morphemic system (morphology), and the verbal string system (syntax). While they are learning these rule systems, children also learn semantics and pragmatics. In learning all these aspects and rules of language, children learn what meanings utterances may have and how they themselves can express their meanings and feelings to others.

To some degree—probably to an important degree—the mystery of how an infant begins to decode spoken language may be explained by the way concerned adults talk directly to young children. What children hear in language that is directly addressed to them is likely to be shorter in total context, syntactically more correct and complete, and spoken more slowly, with key words emphasized. In addition, intonation contours are likely to be exaggerated and ends of phrases more clearly marked than in adult-to-adult talking. (See Chapter 2 references to Moskowitz and to deVilliers and deVilliers regarding caretaker-to-child language.) As a result of this kind of selected language exposure, and with the help of the LAD, the task of decoding is reduced in enormity. We assume that the modified utterances that infants hear in repeated situations provide the basis for the acquisition of verbal meanings.

DEVELOPMENTAL PRECURSORS TO SPEECH PERCEPTION

During the first month of life, probably as early as 2 weeks of age, a normal infant is capable of distinguishing a human voice from other sounds and noises in the environment. Thus, as Wolff (1966) has found, infants will stop crying, however momentarily, if a person speaks but will not do so at the sound of a rattle or the ringing of a bell. Not only is the human voice a selective stimulus for infants, but there seems also to be a very early capacity to discriminate differences in speech sounds long before children can make comparable distinctions in their own productions. Eimas, Siqueland, Jusczyk, and Vigorito (1971) were able to demonstrate that infants at 1 month of age could make differential responses (increase or decrease with habituation to nonnutritive sucking). The experimental task consisted of the presentation of two syllables, a voiced stop sound plus a vowel /ba/ in contrast with a voiceless stop plus a vowel /pa/. Infants showed an increase in sucking activity when initially exposed to /ba/, habituated to a normal level of sucking after several repetitions of /ba/, then increased sucking activity when the syllable was change to /pa/.

Sequencing

In our opening statements about perception we indicated that perception for language necessarily requires that the individual be able to deal with a series or sequences of events. The stimuli that constitute linguistic events, whether oral or written, occur in a temporal order. The order, as we shall see later, is not altogether random but, within limits, is predictable. To be able to deal with linguistic events, and so to acquire normal language behavior, the infant and young child must be able to keep in mind the order of stimulus presentation as the sequence is produced. Infants who succeed in repeating a sound complex, even if it is as brief as "da" or "ma," demonstrate that they have learned to sequence two sounds and to utter them as a single-syllabic combination. In learning to use a given linguistic system in acquiring a spoken language, young children somehow learn that some sequences or combinations of sounds are likely to occur while others just do not occur in a particular language. The mature adult who studies language systems will realize that some combinations do not occur in direct sequence because they are simply too difficult for the articulators to manage in a flow of utterance. A bilingual child may also learn (become aware of) some things about sound (phonemic) sequences that may have been long practiced; that is, some sound sequences are practiced in one linguistic system but not in another, or in some parts of an utterance but not in all parts. The child may learn that American and English speakers combine the sounds $k + l$, $g + l$, or $p + l$ at the beginning of a word or at the end, though not precisely with the same effect, as in *club, cycle, glad, single, play*, and *apple*. However, $d + l$ is not likely to occur at the beginning of a word, but often does at the end *(ladle, saddle)*. The sequences *dn* and *dv* will be reserved for foreign-looking words or names. By 2 years of age most children also learn, or at least begin to practice, word order according to the language or languages they speak. Thus, a child who speaks any of the standard varieties of English may, before 2 years of age, have uttered either "pretty girl" or "girl pretty," but it will not be long before he or she habitually says "pretty girl" if speaking English but reverses the order for saying the same thing in French. English–French bilingual children will learn both word orders as they acquire two linguistic codes. We assume that as a child acquires a language, he or she somehow acquires the rules for the language. By applying these rules for sound order and word order, the task of sequencing verbal content is facilitated. A rule, whether or not we are conscious or aware of its existence, permits us to anticipate or to guess what we may be responding to at a given moment in the light of a past response. The rule also permits us to anticipate the next event. The important effect is that it no longer is necessary to load or overload our minds with a greater number of events than we can easily process. We begin to "remember" even before the event has occurred. Of course, what we begin to remember is the anticipated event. Then we count on feedback to confirm or reject the impression.

Clark and Clark (1977) note that, by the fourth year, children show evidence of their knowledge of the acceptable phonetic sequences of the language or languages to which they are exposed and which they are learning to understand and speak. They generalize:

> Children apply the same procedures to intonation and stress as they do to sounds or phonetic segments. They build on what they learned to perceive at an earlier stage. They have to discriminate differences between intonation contours or stress patterns before they can learn to identify them. They learn the simplest intonations and stress patterns first and may take many years to master the more complex details of these suprasegmental properties of the sound system. (p. 376)

Sequencing is involved in memorization of content and in reproducing an order of events toward a particular objective. We memorize telephone numbers, addresses, social security numbers, and other numbers that our culture and economy make it convenient for us to reproduce readily. We memorize how to operate appliances that require an order of pushing buttons or twisting dials. To imitate or initiate a given action that calls for more than a single movement requires an ability for sequencing. Each step we take, each time we bring hand to mouth or to some other organ, calls for sequencing. Probably the most complex of all sequencing acts is articulation in speech. For articulation, we must assume that the unit for sequencing is an entire utterance. Normal persons, even allowing for normal hesitation phenomena or so-called disfluencies, speak in syllabic flows. We could not articulate in flows if utterance were controlled only by the preceding sound. Adults who suffer brain damage, with or without aphasic involvements, may have impairments in the control of a series or sequence of intended (nonreflexive) movements. Such impairments are known as dyspraxias. When they disturb spoken utterance, they are oral dyspraxias or, if severe, oral apraxias. We believe that most expressive or productive disturbances in severely linguistically retarded and developmentally or congenitally aphasic children are really oral dyspraxias and, as such, are impairments in motor sequencing for speech.

With experience, normal children come to learn relationships that permit them to anticipate the temporal order of events. To the degree that this critical language-learning function is achieved, children, and adults as well, no longer need to depend on sheer memory and recall to produce a series of events. The difference can be illustrated, perhaps simplistically, by trying to recall the digit series 3-7-1-9-5 compared with 1-3-5-7-9. Whenever a rule governing events can be discerned, it is no longer necessary to be restrained by the limit of how much can be recalled that is not rule-based.

Proximate and Distance Reception

Observations of the normal development of an infant reveal changes from proximate to distance reception, from an initial dependence on sensory intake of proximate (close to or in contact with the body) events to those at a distance. Our distance receptors—the eyes, ears, and nose—permit us to receive, perceive, and relate to the events of the world we cannot touch or taste. Some children, the autistic, seem to have difficulty in distance reception and so relate through direct body contact. Those who have visual or auditory impairments may need correction or assistance for distance reception. However, unless they also have central (brain) damage, they are able to integrate and perceive whatever they are able to receive.

The acquisition of speech is dependent on the capacity for distance reception. An impairment in distance reception, other than reduced sensory intake, and a related impairment in the ability to integrate and make differential responses to distant stimuli will prevent the child from learning to speak. This may in part underlie the nonverbal, autistic child's failure to acquire speech.

Perceptual Defense

Some stimuli (events) may have unpleasant or painful associations and may distress us or evoke anxiety when we are exposed to them. To avoid such distress or anxiety, at least unconsciously, we tend to raise our threshold of awareness and so establish perceptual defense. Bruner (1957) suggests another related basis for the development of perceptual defense. Perceptual defense may occur.

> ... first, through a failure to learn appropriate categories for sorting the environment and for following its sequences, and second, through a process of interference whereby more accessible categories with wide acceptance limits serve to mask or prevent the use of less accessible categories for the coding of stimulus inputs.

Bruner's notion has important implication for the brain-damaged and brain-different child. We conjecture that such a child may initially not have the capacity for making the discriminations between speech and nonspeech auditory events, and, when with maturation some basic categories are acquired, they may be so broad as to be essentially nonfunctional for speech perception.

However, the broad, crude categories, once established, may continue to interfere with further perceptual categories. So, because of perceptual defense, speech may be blocked out even though the cerebral system has matured enough to make the child capable of auditory perception for speech.

PERCEPTUAL FUNCTIONS THAT ARE BASIC TO LANGUAGE ACQUISITION

Earlier in this chapter, brief mention was made of normal developmental precursors for speech perception and reception. Now we shall make several general observations of what we consider the basic perceptual functions that must be established for normal speech perception. The statements made will be directly applicable to an aural-oral language code, although parallel statements could be made for a deaf child who is learning a linguistic sign system.

For a child to comprehend and produce and, in time, become a proficient user of an aural-oral language system, the following abilities must be established, initially by virtue of innate capacities and subsequently through experience and learning:

1. The ability to distinguish between speech and other auditory events.
2. The ability to receive stimuli that occur in a sequence or order.
3. The ability to hold the sequence in mind, to hold the sequential impression, so that its components may be integrated in some pattern. This may be achieved either through memory or by the application of a rule plus memory.
4. The ability to compare the pattern with other stored patterns or recalled impressions.
5. The ability to assign meaning on some level (to respond differentially) to the identified pattern or impression.
6. In order to speak, an articulatory system that makes it possible to produce a flow or sequence of movements that motorically encodes what the child means to produce.

SENSORY AND MOTOR INVOLVEMENTS AND PERCEPTION

As a general observation, we believe that limitations for the reception of sensory stimuli do not in themselves interfere with perception, provided that the stimuli are received. Thus, peripheral hearing loss or visual refractory defects do not impair perception once the stimuli have been received so that they can be processed by the central nervous system. Unless the limitations are corrected by an adjustment to the loss—getting closer to the source of sound, having an aid to amplify sounds, making distance adjustments to the visual stimuli, or having properly fitted glasses—intake will be difficult, and there may be problems related to such difficulty.

We believe that the combination of peripheral and central impairment certainly aggravates the problem. This combination is sometimes found in developmentally dysphasic or aphasic children who present evidence of mild-to-moderate peripheral hearing loss. It is also suspected that this may be an underlying problem for nonverbal infantile (primary) autistic children. To a lesser degree, the compounding effects also hold for moderately and severely linguistically retarded children who do not present the neurological and perceptual indices of aphasia (see Chapter 5).

PERCEPTUAL DYSFUNCTIONS

In determining possible perceptual dysfunctions in children who cannot report verbally whether or how they have received or organized stimuli presented for input (intake), we must resort either to conjecture or to the interpretation of experimental investigations. The first approach, conjecture, assumes that we know as fact what is accepted in theory. What we know as fact in regard to the brain-damaged comes, for the most part, from acquired impairments in adults. As a result of fairly recent investigations we have gathered a considerable amount of information about breakdown in auditory perceptual functioning in adults. For the most part, the observed data are well reconciled with theory. We even know something about distorted perception in adult schizophrenics. By analogy, we make assumptions for children. However, analogies may often be misleading. We need to be mindful of the differential effects of the time of onset of pathology on developmental processes. Thus, Eisenberg (1964) observes that injury before speech acquisition "is even more devastating than similar injury in the adult" (p. 68). According to Eisenberg (1964), an early injury to the brain, pre- or postnatal, might impair

> ... an elementary psychological function, the lack of which could then distort subsequent development. Thus, complex functions, the anatomical equipment for which might otherwise be intact, could have failed to evolve. Whenever the injury is such as to impair the development of the capacity to symbolize (language) all subordinate functions which are ordered by language will develop less optimally and all patterns of social interaction will be grossly impaired. (pp. 68–69)

If we resort to experimental investigations, we necessarily work on the assumption that the individual understands the task and the expected response to make. The child can be trained, of course, to make the responses and so reduce the margin of error in our interpretation of what the child actually does. However, we can by no means be certain that the child does indeed understand, and so the possibility for error must always be entertained. Earlier, it was indicated that dyspraxic involvements may make it difficult for a child—or for an adult, for that matter—to express intake in the form expected for a normal perceptual-motor activity. Thus, as Birch and Lefford (1964, p. 46) report, some brain-damaged (cerebral-palsied) children who make erroneous block-design reproductions are able, nevertheless, to choose a correct reproduction over their own product when directed to identify the one that most closely resembles the model. We have made a similar observation on aphasic children in regard to Bender-Gestalt figures.

Despite all these precautions, it is believed that some perceptual dysfunctions probably underlie the impairment for language acquisition in the developmentally aphasic and dysphasic child. For the present, let us consider these children to be *brain different* and, therefore, *perceptually different*. As a general and introductory observation, it can be stated that, as far as language acquisition is concerned, perceptual dysfunctions may occur as a result of an impairment of any of the input processes considered in the foregoing summary statement. Broadly stated, a perceptual disturbance for spoken language may be present because of the child's inability to organize sensory–auditory events even though received, to hold the events in mind, and to scan them and compare them with others stored by the central nervous system. Perceptual dysfunctions may also be a manifestation of categorical impairment. This may be based on an absence or inadequate number of basic or innate categories from which further categories may be developed. Categorical development for phonemes (the sound system of a language) may also be impaired if children do not modify their primary categories to permit the development of useful discriminations. If, for example, the primary category for sibilant sounds is so broad as to include all *s, sh, th,* and *f* sounds, the child will be unable to make the necessary discriminations from what is heard to respond differentially to contextual speech that includes these sounds. If this is indeed the case, the child will derive little meaning out of what is heard. At the other extreme is the possibility that the child's categories are too narrow, too restricted, and too rigidly set. Thus, the child may have too many categories for functional sound discrimination. The /s/ sounds in words such as *see, sue, its,* and *pest* are somewhat different in duration and somewhat different in lip position, each determined by its context within the verbal utterance. Even more so are the /t/ sounds in *too, let Tom, get that,* and *letter.* However different allophonically, by the age of two almost all children perceive the /s/ sounds and the /t/ sounds as categories that encompass each of the varieties. If the categories are discrete, the child necessarily has to overload his or her storage system with more individual sounds than can be recalled and matched while exposed to speech. If we bear in mind that no two persons articulate the same content in precisely the same manner and that no person articulates precisely the same way twice, even for the same content, we can appreciate the impairing implications of a precocious rigidity of sound categories. Children with such categorical involvement will be limited in perceptual development for speech and would, we conjecture, be considerably more impaired than those who can read only if the print type and size are the same as the first printed words to which they were first exposed.

AUDITORY DISCRIMINATION FOR SEQUENTIAL CONTENT

Spoken utterance, as indicated earlier, consists of sequences of sounds. The order in which they occur is in part determined by the phonemic rules of the given linguistic system (see the earlier discussion on sequencing). However unwittingly applied, unless we followed rules that permitted us to anticipate and to make correct guesses as to what we are hearing, it is extremely unlikely that any human being could literally hear (listen) and separately identify each sound in a flow of utterance. Nevertheless, it is necessary to be a fast listener to keep up with even a slow talker.[1] How fast must a child be able to listen, to resolve what sounds he or she is hearing, and to keep the order of sounds in mind in order to perceive the flow of sounds as speech? Unfortunately, this question çannot be answered directly. A later chapter will present some evidence on aphasic adults and on congenitally aphasic children indicating that auditory discrimination for sequential events is impaired and that there may in fact be a generalized impairment for dealing with (processing) sequential events.[2] This chapter will present some experimental evidence regarding how little time it takes for a normal perceiver to determine whether he or she is listening to two like events or two different events, and, if the latter, the order of presentation (reception and perception) of the events.

A rather common subjective response on first exposure to foreign-language speakers is that they seem to talk much more rapidly than we do. However, after increased opportunity for hearing the foreign speakers, even though we may not understand them, they seem to be speaking more slowly. This, of course, is not what takes place. It is much more likely that, with added exposure, we begin to tune in and, in effect, become faster listeners. Recent experimental evidence supports this subjective impression about the effect of experience on our auditory perception. Broadbent and Ladefoged (1959) report an experiment in which they themselves were involved as subjects. They report that the time required for them to discriminate *piss-hiss* from *hiss-pipp* was reduced from 150 milliseconds (msec) to 30 msec after repeated trials of the task. Hirsh and Sherrick (1961) report that an experienced subject required an interval of 20 msec to report correctly (75 percent of the time) the presented order when two events, a light and a sound signal, were presented repeatedly in the same order. In a later experiment, Hirsh and Fraisse (1965) report that naive subjects required about 60 msec for the same percentage of accuracy of performance when the discriminating decision had to be made on the basis of a single exposure of a light and a sound signal.

There have been relatively few investigations of the ability of persons

[1]Liberman, Cooper, Shankweiler, and Studdert-Kennedy (1967) point out that "speech can be followed, though with difficulty, at rates as high as 400 words per minute. If we assume an average of four to five phonemes for each English word, this rate yields about 30 phonemes per second. . . . Even 15 phonemes per second, which is not unusual in conversation, would seem more than the ear could cope with if phonemes were a string of discrete sounds" (p. 432). In essence, what these authors point out is that the ear can actually perceive more than it can possibly hear. This apparent inconsistency is related to the perceptual processing of speech sounds as part of a sound-decoding system which, as we indicated earlier, permits us to anticipate what we should be hearing, and in effect responding as if we did. For an expanded explanation, the provocative articles by Liberman et al. (1967) and Liberman (1982) are recommended.

[2]In a broad sense, aphasia (acquired) is a severe impairment in previously established language functions associated with brain damage. Dysphasia implies a lesser degree of impairment. Congenital (developmental) aphasia is a failure for normal language functioning to be established, presumably as a result of brain damage or brain difference associated with prenatal or congenital causes.

with verified brain damage in discriminating-sequence tasks. The evidence clearly indicates, however, that cerebral pathology markedly impairs this ability. Efron (1963) compared a group of aphasic adults who had incurred left temporal lobe lesions with neurologically normal adults in their ability to make correct judgments as to the order of two 10-msec sound pulses that were markedly different in frequency. Efron found that the neurologically normal subjects required approximately 50 to 60 msec to make correct judgments as to the presented order of the sound pulses. In marked contrast, most of the aphasic patients required significantly more time, a few as much as a full second between sound pulses, before they could make correct judgments.

It is necessary to be cautious about generalizing and applying the results of these studies to aphasic children. On the face of it, signals such as discrete sound pulses and light flashes would seem to present a much simpler task for discrimination and sequencing (time-order determination) than would speech signals. However, signals of this sort do not permit of anticipation and decoding, as spoken utterance might. The impairment for discrimination-sequencing, however—especially the appreciably longer time interval needed between signals for aphasic adults and children to make correct responses—is in keeping with clinical impressions. Aphasic children, as well as adults, seem to improve in comprehension of speech when the speaker reduces the rate of utterance. It is possible that this improvement is related to a reduction in quantity (bits of language to be processed) per unit of time. Investigations involving speech signals and spoken utterance are needed to give us the understanding we need about the perceptual functioning and impairments associated with severe linguistic retardation that are manifest in their most extreme form in dysphasic and aphasic children. Selected studies are reviewed in the chapters on the severely orally linguistically handicapped child (developmental aphasia).

PERCEPTION AND INTERSENSORY STIMULATION

In the earlier discussion of proximate and distance reception, it was mentioned that the perceptual development of the infant changes from initial dependence on proximate receptors to dependence on distance receptors. Birch and Lefford (1964) observe:

> In infants and young children, sensations deriving from the viscera and from stimuli applied to the skin surfaces appear to be predominant in directing behavior, whereas at these ages information presented visually or auditorily is relatively ineffective. As the child matures, the teloreceptive modalities assume an even more prominent position in the sensory hierarchy until, by school age, vision and audition appear to become the most important sensory modalities for directing behavior. Such hierarchial shifts are orderly and seem to be accompanied by increased intersensory liason in normal children. (p. 48)

The emphasis for this concluding part of the discussion on perceptual functioning for severely linguistically retarded children is on the development of intersensory reactions and perceptions. With a healthy degree of reservation, we will consider the findings and implications of studies conducted on frankly cerebral-palsied children.

Birch and Lefford (1964) report the results of an intersensory study on a group of neurologically damaged (cerebral-palsied) children. The sensory systems studied were vision, kinesthesis, and haptic (touch and active exploratory movement of the hand). The stimulus items were blocks cut out as geometric forms. The subjects were directed to judge whether simultaneously presented stimuli in pairs were the same or different. The same blocks were used as the visual and haptic stimuli. The findings for the brain-damaged children were compared with those for normal children. Birch and Lefford note that for normal children, errors decrease with age for all conditions of intersensory interaction. For the brain-damaged subjects, despite considerable variability, the overall finding was that "at the very least, the emergence of such relationships appears to be delayed in the 'brain-damaged' children, a factor which may seriously limit possibilities for the normal utilization and integration of environmental information" (pp. 48–58).

It cannot be assumed that linguistically retarded children who do not present the hard-sign evidence of the cerebral-palsied are equally impaired or delayed in their sensory-integrative functioning. Nevertheless, there is increasing evidence that many linguistically retarded children—especially those who are most severely delayed—when given a choice will tend to ignore auditory signals when they can respond to visual cues. Aphasic children in particular are likely to perform better on the visual association (nonlanguage) tasks than on the auditory (language) items of the Illinois Test of Psycholinguistic Abilities (Kirk and McCarthy, 1968). This finding is based on clinical observations and test data at the Institute of Childhood Aphasia at Stanford University (1962–1973) and at San Francisco State University (1973–1981). A related clinical observation is that moderately to severely linguistically impaired children were better able to accept and integrate training that employed a visual-plus-auditory input approach than training that began with emphasis on the auditory modality. In her discussion of neuropsychosocial substrates of oral language, Berry (1980) observes:

> The visual route for the majority of children (and adults) is superior. . . . With linguistically handicapped children it may indeed be the best way to teach—to teach language through oral reading. . . . What one hopes is that the language-retarded child will be able to use the multimodal input without disturbing his margin of safety, his homeostat. Can the limbic and reticular systems tolerate the bombardment of multimodal stimuli? (pp. 103–104)

Our observation is that a few children can handle multimodal stimuli, but most who are severely linguistically impaired—especially the dysphasic and aphasic—do better when responding to events one modality at a time. Obviously, spoken language requires intake through hearing. Perhaps the answer to Dr. Berry's concerned question is to reduce the quantity and rate of input, especially if it is necessarily multimodal. This is in keeping with the findings of Tallal in a series of investigations on the perceptual disabilities of dysphasic children. Essentially, Tallal and her associates report that dysphasic children have great difficulty in processing rapidly changing acoustic stimuli (Tallal and Piercy, 1978, Stark and Tallal, 1981). A therapeutic approach that considers the implications of this finding will be described later, in the discussion of speech sound processing.

REFERENCES AND SUGGESTED READINGS

Berry, M. F. *Teaching Linguistically Handicapped Children.* Englewood Cliffs, N.J.: Prentice-Hall, 1980.

Birch, H. G., and Lefford, A. "Two Strategies for Studying Perception in Brain Damaged Children," in H. G. Birch (ed.), *Brain Damage in Children.* Baltimore: Williams and Wilkins, 1964.

Broadent, D. E. and Ladefoged, P. "Auditory Perception in Temporal Order," *Journal of the Acoustical Society of America,* 31, 1959, 1539.

Bruner, J. S. "On Perceptual Readiness," *Psychological Review,* 64(2), 1957, 123–152.

Chomsky, N. *Syntactic Structures.* The Hague: Mouton, 1957.

Chomsky, N. *Aspects of the Theory of Syntax.* Cambridge, Mass.: M.I.T. Press, 1965.

Clark, H. H., and Clark, E. V. *Psychology and Language.* New York: Harcourt Brace Jovanovich, 1977.

Efron, R. "Temporal Perception, Aphasia, and Deja Vu," *Brain,* 86, 1963, 403–424.

Eimas, P. D., Siqueland, E. R., Jusczyk, P., and Vigorito, J. "Speech Perception in Infants," *Science,* 171, 1971, 303–306.

Eisenberg, L. "Behavioral Manifestations of Cerebral Damage in Childhood," in H. G. Birch (ed.), *Brain Damage in Children.* Baltimore: Williams and Wilkins, 1964.

Glass, A. L., Holyoak, K. J., and Santa, J. L. *Cognition.* Reading, Mass.: Addison-Wesley, 1979.

Hirsh, I. J., and Fraisse, P. Cited in *Central Institute for the Deaf Periodic Progress Reports,* 8(20), July 1964–June 1965.

Hirsh, E. J., and Sherrick, E. E. "Perceived Order in Different Sense Modalities," *Journal of Experimental Psychology,* 62, 1961, 423–432.

Kirk, S., and McCarthy, J., *The Illinois Test of Psycholinguistic Abilities.* Urbana: University of Illinois Press, 1968.

Liberman, A. M. "On Finding That Speech Is Special," *American Psychologist,* 37(2), 1982, 148–167.

Liberman, A. M., Cooper, F. S., Shankweiler, D. P., and Studdert-Kennedy, M. "Perception of the Speech Code," *Psychological Review,* 74(6), 1967, 431–461.

Sanders, D. A. *Auditory Perception of Speech.* Englewood Cliffs, N.J.: Prentice-Hall, 1977.

Stark, R. E. and Tallal, P. "Perceptual and Motor Deficits in Language-Impaired Children," in Keith, R. W. (ed.) *Central Auditory and Language Disorders in Children.* Houston: College-Hill Press, 1981.

Tallal, P. and Piercy, M. "Defects of Auditory Perception in Children with Developmental Dysphasia," in Wyke, M. A. (ed.), *Developmental Dysphasia*. New York: Academic Press, 1978.

Wolff, P. H. "The Natural History of Crying and Other Vocalizations in Early Infancy." in B. M. Foss (ed.), *Determinants in Infant Behavior,* Vol. 4. London: Methuen, 1966.

chapter 4

Brain Mechanisms and Language Functioning

The objective of this chapter is to present some basic information on the structures of the brain mechanisms that are related to and serve speech and language functions. We will consider such matters as the localization of functions that underlie verbal behavior, cerebral dominance (the functional differences between homologous areas of the two hemispheres of the brain), and the relationship of cerebral pathology to impairments of speech and language processes.

The contents of this chapter are not by any means to be considered a definitive treatment or a substitute for the available excellent and detailed considerations of brain functioning or of the brain and the mind. The materials here have been selected in the hope that they will provide the reader with a basis for understanding normal brain functioning and for understanding what brain mechanisms may be impaired in the special population of children who fail to acquire language or who are delayed or disordered in this acquisition. Extended considerations of brain mechanisms and language functioning may be found in the writings of Penfield and Roberts (1959), Luria (1966a, 1966b, 1970), Mountcastle (1962), Millikan and Darley (1967), Pribram (1971), Hecaen and Albert (1978), and Springer and Deutsch (1981). Briefer and more specialized, but not necessarily more technical, considerations of the relationship of the brain to language functioning are found in Lenneberg (1967), Masland (1970), Eisenson (1971), Gardner (1978), and Geschwind (1979).

PARTS OF THE BRAIN

Our consideration of the brain mechanisms that underlie the functions of language (the symbol-code system) and speech (the production mechanism) will begin with a brief description of the structures of the cerebrum. The brain with all its parts incorporates about 100 billion neurons (nerve cells).

The Cerebrum

The cerebrum, the largest part of the brain, consists of two apparently symmetrical, almost but not quite mirror-image hemispheres. These hemispheres, however much they look alike, have different and yet somewhat related functions. The functional differences are implied in the term *functional assymmetry of the brain*. The outer surface of the cerebrum is a thin layer of gray matter, which contains cell bodies. Beneath the gray surface is a thick layer of white matter consisting largely of fibers covered by myelin (white nerve sheathing). These fibers run to and from the cells of the cortex. The interior of the cerebrum consists of four cavities or ventricles.

The Cerebral Cortex   The cerebral cortex is the gray outer layer of the cerebrum. It is characterized by its many folds or indentations. The nature of this construction provides additional surface for the gray matter and for the 10 to 12 billion or more nerve cells to carry out their complex functions related to the reception, integration, and interpretation of stimuli and to the organization and expression of human behavior. Our special interest will be for that form of human-species–specific behavior we refer to as speech (spoken language).[1]

The shallow indentations or furrows of the cortex are known as *sulci* (singular, *sulcus*). The deeper indentations are known as *fissures*. The fissures permit us to consider the cortex as divided into major regions or lobes: the frontal (anterior), the temporal, the occipital (posterior), and the parietal. Another major area, the *insula,* or Island or Reil, is within the lateral fissure and is therefore not visible on the surface of the cortex.

Functional Areas   The cortex in broad plan may be considered to have two kinds of specialized centers or regions: projection and association areas. Those parts of the cortex that receive or send nerve fibers to or from the peripheral organs of the body are known as *projection areas*. These may be defined as regions of the cortex that communicate with lower centers of the central nervous system through specific nerve tracts. The cerebral cortex also contains association areas, which lie adjacent to the projection areas. Association areas make connections only with other regions of the cortex. Functionally, association areas may be considered as regions of the cortex that integrate nerve impulses, which are received from projection areas. Association areas are for the most part considerably larger than the projection areas. In the anterior and posterior parts of the cerebrum, the frontal and occipital lobes, the association

---

[1]Although we have made a distinction between language as the code system and speech as the productive mechanism, the term *speech* is also used to comprise the oral linguistic code and the production mechanism; hence the statement that speech is a human-species–specific function. Unless we wish to emphasize the distinction, the term *speech* may be used synonymously with *oral* or *spoken language*.

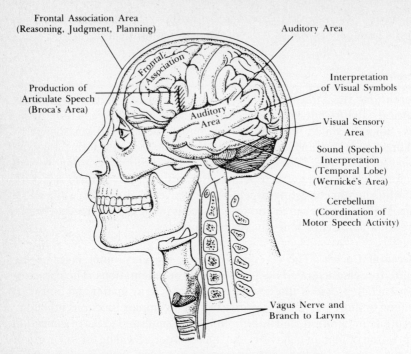

Frontal Association Area
(Reasoning, Judgment, Planning)

Auditory Area

Production of
Articulate Speech
(Broca's Area)

Interpretation
of Visual Symbols

Visual Sensory
Area

Sound (Speech)
Interpretation
(Temporal Lobe)
(Wernicke's Area)

Cerebellum
(Coordination of
Motor Speech Activity)

Vagus Nerve and
Branch to Larynx

Figure 4.1 Localization of brain function in relation to speech.

areas are particularly large. It is assumed that the interrelationships between
the activities of the sensory and motor areas take place in the association
cortex. Thus, presumably, complex functions such as listening and speaking
are able to be integrated and produced. Figure 4.1 features some of the
projection and association areas that have special significance for speech
(language) functions.

The Thalamus and Striate Bodies

The thalamus is a mass of cerebral tissue that is situated at the base of the
cerebrum and projects into the third ventricle of the brain. The thalamus is a
relay station for sensory (incoming) stimuli. All auditory, visual, visceral, and
somatic stimuli either terminate in the thalamus or make connections there that
continue on to the projection areas of the cerebral cortex.

The striate bodies are three gray nuclear masses that lie beneath the white
matter in the forepart of the cerebral cortex. The nerve pathways that go to and
from the cortex pass through the striate bodies. Functionally, in regard to
speech, the striate bodies may be considered a unit of the thalamus.

The Hypothalamus

The hypothalamus is located directly beneath the thalamus. Modifications in
the control of the visceral organs associated with emotional responses—for

example, changes in heart rate and blood pressure—are a result of activities of centers in the hypothalamus.

The Cerebellum

The cerebellum, or small brain, is situated directly below the cerebrum and is partly covered by it. The cerebellum has many complex connections through-out the entire nervous system. It has sensory connections with the nerve fibers that convey proprioceptive (muscle) sensitivity from the muscles of the body and from the balance mechanism of the inner ear. Coordination and control of voluntary movements are made possible by the elaborate connections between the cerebellum and the cerebrum. Presumably, precision of timing (synergy of movement) and the general character and tonus of muscular responses, both reflex and voluntary, take place as a result of the controls imposed by the cerebellum. Probably the best example of this function is the finely timed and coordinated motor activities involved in an act of speech.

The Brain Stem

The cerebrum and cerebellum are connected by large columns of neural tissue and central masses that are part of the brain stem. The lower (posterior) part of the brain stem is a flattened, cone-shaped mass known as the *medulla oblon-gata*. This part of the brain stem is continuous with the spinal cord by way of an opening in the base of the skull. The anterior part of the brain stem, which includes the thalamus, is continuous with the cerebrum. Later, we shall discuss the reticular formation, which for the most part consists of a neural network in the brain stem.

The Midbrain

The midbrain lies immediately below the thalamus. By means of connections with the cerebellum and the medulla, the midbrain has essential functions related to the regulation of muscle tone, body posture, and movement. By way of other centers, the midbrain is involved with functions that are integrated in the cerebral hemispheres. Of particular importance are reflexes controlling the eye.

The Pons

The pons is a unit of the central nervous system that lies just below the midbrain. This area, as the name suggests, serves as a bridge between the two sides of the cerebellum. Neural pathways to and from the cerebellum merge in the area of the pons.

The Medulla Oblongata

The medulla, or bulb, as indicated earlier, is a flattened, cone-shaped mass continuous with the brain stem and spinal cord. Nerve tracts (pyramidal tracts)

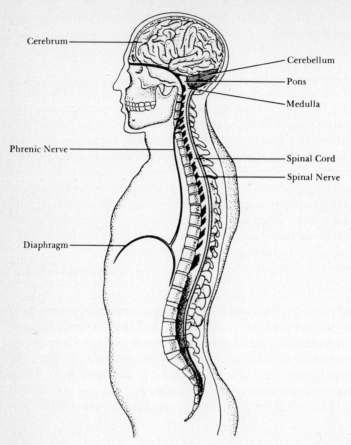

Figure 4.2 The central nervous system in relation to oral language production. (Reprinted with the permission of Macmillan Publishing Company from *Basic Speech,* 3d ed., by Jon Eisenson and Paul H. Boase. Copyright © 1975 by Macmillan Publishing Company.)

come to the medulla from the cerebral cortex. These tracts cross over (decussate) at the narrower, posterior end of the medulla. The medulla also has sensory tracts going toward the higher centers. In addition, the medulla has centers that are vital to biological functioning. These include the functions of respiration and circulation.

The spinal cord is continuous with the lower (posterior) portion of the medulla. Nerves emanating from the spinal cord go to the peripheral organs of the body.

Figure 4.2 is a diagrammatic representation of the central nervous system in relation to speech.

The Reticular Formation

The reticular formation is a rather vaguely defined organization or system of nerve cells in the brain stem. The cells of the reticular formation include fibers that extend (project) to the spinal cord, the cerebellum, and the cerebral hemispheres. In turn, the reticular formation also receives fibers from the same structures. Thus, the reticular formation may be functionally considered to have ascending and descending parts.

The *ascending* part of the reticular system seems, in effect, to constitute a central station where nerve impulses arrive from the receptor organs—the ears, eyes, nose, and the skin. Impulses from the reticular central station are conducted to various parts of the brain, including the projection centers of the cerebral cortex (see Figure 4.3).

The *descending* reticular formation receives impulses from the cerebral cortex and, in turn, sends impulses to the numerous fibers that come to it from the receptor organs. In this way, presumably, neural signals coming down from the cortex meet signals coming up from the receptors. As a result, a selection of responses may be made (perceptual selection). As an example, according to Krech and Crutchfield (1958):

> An impulse that comes down from the occipital lobe of the brain (the visual center) through the descending reticular formation can prevent impulses coming up from the ear from ever reaching the cortex. This can help us to understand the very common experience of not hearing someone speak to us when all our attention is directed at watching an object intently. (p. 172).

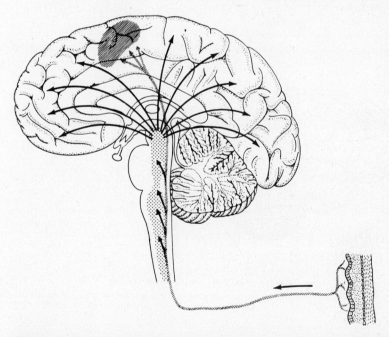

Figure 4.3 The reticular formation is the stippled area in this cross section of the brain. A sense organ (*lower right*) is connected to a sensory area in the brain (*upper left*) by a pathway extending up the spinal cord. This pathway branches into the reticular formation. When a stimulus travels along the pathway, the reticular formation may awaken the entire brain (*dark arrows*).(From J. D. French "The Reticular Formation." Copyright 1957 by Scientific American, Inc. All rights reserved.)

Although there is as yet no general agreement about all the possible functions of the reticular formation, there is agreement that one of its very important functions is to maintain a state of consciousness (awareness and alertness). Thus, we may generalize that nerve impulses from the ascending part of the reticular formation serve to arouse or alert the cortex so that normal perception may take place. According to Penfield and Roberts (1959, p. 16), the reticular system "provides neuronal mechanisms which seem to be essential to consciousness and the integration of function in the cerebral hemispheres" (see Figure 4.4). Lindsley (1961) indicates that in addition to serving as an arousal mechanism, the reticular formation may also serve as a specific

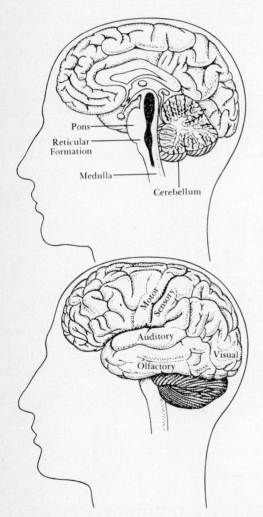

Figure 4.4 Relationship of the reticular formation (*black area*) to various parts of the brain is indicated at the top. The functional areas of the brain are outlined at bottom. (From J. D. French, "The Reticular Formation." Copyright 1957 by Scientific American, Inc. All rights reserved.)

attention mechanism, thus permitting the individual to make the appropriate differential responses (perceptual integration) to environmental stimuli. A third function served by the reticular formation is that of a feedback-control mechanism.

Some of the contributions of the reticular formation to cerebral functioning in particular and to human behavior in general may be summarized by this passage from French (1957):

> The reticular formation is a tiny nerve network in the central part of the brain stem. Investigators have discovered that this bit of nerve tissue, no bigger than your little finger, is a far more important structure than anyone has dreamed. It underlies our awareness of the world and our ability to think, to learn and to act. Without it an individual is reduced to a helpless, senseless, paralyzed blob of protoplasm.

> The actual seat of the power to think, to perceive, indeed to respond to a stimulus with anything more than a reflex reaction, lies in the cortex of the brain. But the cortex cannot perceive or think unless it is "awake." ... A sensory signal arriving at the cortex while it is asleep goes unrecognized. Experiments on anesthetized individuals have shown ... that stimulation of the cortex alone is not sufficient to awaken the brain. Something else must arouse the cortex: that something else is the reticular formation.

CONTRALATERALITY OF CEREBRAL CONTROL

In our discussion of the medulla, we indicated that nerve tracts come to the medulla from the cortex and cross over (decussate) in the lower portion. This is an example of the general plan of the nervous system, which results in

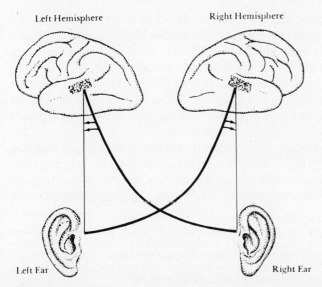

Figure 4.5 Neuroanatomical schema for auditory asymmetries indicating crossing of nerve fibers. (After D. Kimura, "Functional Asymmetry of the Brain in Dichotic Listening." *Cortex* 3(2), 1967, 174.)

contralateral control of motor and sensory functions. Thus, movements of the organs on the right side of the body are controlled by centers of the motor tract of the left cerebral hemisphere. Sensory function for paired receptors, the eyes and the ears, present a somewhat different arrangement. There are some fibers that do not cross. However, as may be noted in the diagrammatic representation of the ears (Figure 4.5), the greater number of fibers do cross, so that the basic scheme of contralaterality of the higher brain functions is maintained.

CEREBRAL DOMINANCE AND DIFFERENCES IN CEREBRAL FUNCTIONS

Our description of the cerebrum referred to it as consisting of two symmetrical, almost mirror-image hemispheres. Despite the physical similarity of the hemispheres, there are important functional differences (Eisenson, 1971).[2]

Some of the differences, based on clinical evidence following pathology, include the following:

1. The perception of spatial events (spatial perception, awareness of body scheme, and spatial relationships) is predominantly a function of centers in the right hemisphere (Masland, 1967; Geschwind, 1979).
2. The perception of auditory, nonspeech events (environmental noises, musical melody, tonal patterns, etc.) is processed (controlled) in the right hemisphere (Geschwind, 1979).
3. The perception of speech events is normally a function of the left hemisphere, and specifically of centers of the left temporal lobe.[3]

From what we have just indicated in regard to differences in cerebral functioning, the question of cerebral dominance or cerebral control is related to function. Some functions are dominated or controlled by the left hemisphere, others by the right. Language functions, the perception of the symbols of speech and of writing, and the production of spoken and written language are controlled (dominated) by centers of the left cerebral hemisphere for 95 percent or more of right-handed persons and for a majority of left-handed persons.

Figure 4.6 presents some of the differences in function for which each half of the cerebrum is normally dominant. As a generalization, we may infer that the left hemisphere is normally the dominant one for events that require analysis for understanding (decoding). In contrast, the right hemisphere is

[2]It is important to appreciate that the two hemispheres of the brain are not really as alike as they superficially appear to be. Geschwind and Levitsky (1968) "have found marked anatomical asymmetries between the upper surfaces of the human right and left temporal lobes." The area is significantly larger on the left side and "... the differences observed are easily of sufficient magnitude to be compatible with the known functional asymmetries."
[3]These observations and others about differences in cerebral functioning are considered in detail in Mountcastle (1962), Millikan and Darley (1967), Geschwind (1979), and Springer and Deutsch (1981).

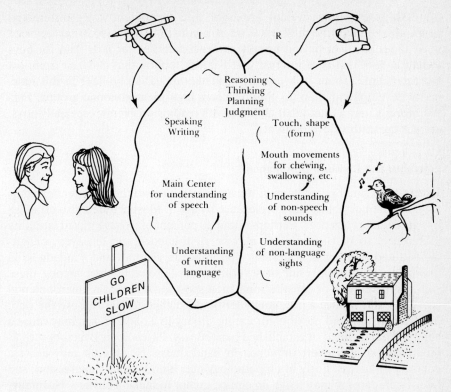

DIFFERENTIAL FUNCTIONS OF THE CEREBRAL
HEMISPHERES WITH SPECIAL ATTENTION TO LANGUAGE

Figure 4.6 The two hemispheres of the brain cortex showing special areas related to language (*left half*) and nonlanguage (*right half*). Although the hemispheres are virtually twins in superficial appearance, they have different functions. As may be noted from the diagram, many of the functions are related as to modality of intake. (Reprinted with the permission of Macmillan Publishing Company from *Communicative Disorders in Children*, 5th ed., by Jon Eisenson and Mardel Ogilvie. Copyright © 1983 by Macmillan Publishing Company.)

normally dominant for situations that can be taken in as a whole and do not require analysis to be appreciated and understood.

The Left Brain Is for Talking

As indicated earlier, recent findings on the differences between the two hemispheres permit us to generalize that normally the left brain is for talking. This is so primarily because the left cerebral hemisphere, particularly the left temporal lobe, is the processor of speech signals. Speech is normally established through listening. Thus, we accept the conclusions of Liberman et al. (1967) that "the conclusion that there is a speech mode, and that it is characterized by processes different from those underlying the perception of other sounds, is strengthened by recent indications that speech and non-speech sounds are processed primarily in different hemispheres of the brain."

Although human beings are born with the potential for differential hearing (listening), the differences do not seem to become clearly established until about age 4 or 5, and usually somewhat earlier for girls than for boys (Kimura, 1967). It is of interest that Kimura reports that children from low socioeconomic groups in Montreal, Canada, appear to be later in this functional development than do children from high socioeconomic groups. Furthermore, Kimura found that children with reading problems, especially boys, show a lag in this development.[4]

Laterality and Cerebral Dominance

Except for a small percentage of the ambidextrous and the ambinondextrous, most children establish hand preference by age 5. Most children also establish eye and foot preferences. Perhaps about 20 percent of us have mixed laterality preference, so that some of us may be right-handed and left-eyed, or left-handed and right-eyed. Laterality preference in general, and handedness in particular, may be a result of several factors. Probably chief among these factors is hereditary or constitutional predisposition. However, environmental pressures may induce a potentially left-handed child to learn to use the right hand for writing and possibly for eating. Injury to a hand or arm may cause a change from inclined or established handedness. Psychological factors such as identification may exert influence in handedness. Negativism may exert a contrary influence. Early brain pathology may limit laterality expression, and later brain damage may leave no choice except to make a change. Normally, however, once handedness is established, it tends to be maintained for life. Although, as has been indicated, handedness is only one form of laterality, it is probably the best single indicator of overall laterality preference.

Ear Preference

Unless there is a serious hearing impairment of one ear, a person listens with both ears. Normally, our ears listen together rather than competitively. Normally, also, if the occasion arises for listening with one ear, as we do in most telephone situations or when someone whispers into an ear, either ear can do alone what both ears usually do together. Suppose, however, that we were required to listen competitively—that is, to have different signals sent simultaneously, one signal or series of signals to one ear and a different signal or series of signals sent to the other. How would the signals be heard? Would there be an indication of ear preference, and, if so, would such preference be related to other aspects of laterality expression, especially to handedness? The answer, based on recent experimental investigations, seems to be positive. Some of the investigations, which are reviewed by Kimura (1967), employed the technique of dichotic (competitive) listening devised by Broadbent (1954). The basic

---

[4]Kimura's (1967) investigations were based on the expression of ear preference, which is believed to be related to cerebral dominance. We shall discuss ear preference later.

technique sets up competition between the two ears for the reception of auditory signals. In the initial Broadbent study, different digits were presented simultaneously to a listener's ears by means of a dual-channel tape recorder with stereophonic earphones. One sequence of digits was presented to one ear while another sequence was simultaneously (competitively) presented to the other ear. The subject was asked to report all the digits he could recall in whatever order he could recall them. Because the investigator knew the ear to which the digit sequences were sent, the report of the subject provided separate scores for the recall ability of each ear. The usual finding for normal right-handed persons is a statistically significant greater recall for digits that were sent to the right ear than for those sent to the left. Investigations using speech signals other than digits, such as words or short verbal utterances (Dirks, 1964), show results along the same lines as those found by Broadbent. In interesting contrast are findings when melodies rather than speech signals are presented to subjects dichotically. In such a study, Kimura (1967) found that nonverbal, melodic material is recognized more accurately by the left ear than by the right. Thus, we may conclude that ear preferences are part of overall laterality preference. The dichotic listening investigations provide support for the observation made earlier that there is a speech mode, and that the processing of speech is different from the processing of nonspeech auditory events. We emphasize this point because it sheds light on the clinical observation that most congenitally aphasic children can respond appropriately to environmental noises other than speech long before they can understand and respond to speech.

Ear preference and hand preference are both normally established by age 4 or 5, but this does not suggest that the two are in any way ca˙ sally related; neither should it suggest in any way that left-handed persons have left ear preference. In fact, most left-handed persons show the same preference for speech and nonspeech, though not to the same degree, as right-handed persons. To return to an earlier statement, the left hemisphere is for speaking—for the perception, control, and production of speech—for almost all right-handed persons as well as for a majority of those who are left-handed. Similarly, the right cerebral hemisphere, regardless of handedness, seems to be dominant for environmental, nonspeech auditory events. An excellent review of studies on the relationship of handedness, ear preference, and cerebral dominance for language may be found in Krashen (1975).

LOCALIZATION OF LANGUAGE FUNCTIONS

As was suggested earlier, most of what we know about the brain mechanisms that serve or control language functions is based on information from the pathology of impairment. Human brains have been mapped for lesions that are associated with disruptions of language functions that were established before the pathology was incurred. Based on such knowledge, it is assumed that certain areas of the cerebral cortex are normally in control of particular language functions; that is, the areas make special contributions to cerebral functioning as a whole in regard to language (speech).[5]

Based on data from several sources (Penfield and Roberts, 1959; Russell and Espir, 1961; Luria, 1965), from Masland's (1967, 1968) research review articles, and from the evidence presented in our earlier discussion, the following general observations may be made:

1. The left cerebral hemisphere serves overall language functions for a vast majority of persons, regardless of individual handedness.
2. Productive language functions are served by the anterior portions of the cerebral cortex.
3. Receptive or intake functions (the decoding of language) are served by the posterior portions. Auditory decoding is carried on in the left temporal area, and visual decoding primarily in the left occipital lobe.

The Auditory Cortex

We have made several references to the left temporal lobe and its functions, which are related to the perception of spoken language. We also cited the article by Geschwind and Levitsky (1968), who report anatomical differences between the left and right temporal areas "of sufficient magnitude to be compatible with the known functional asymmetries." We will now expand on the particular functions of the temporal lobe that are fundamental for the perception of the speech code.

Speech, as was pointed out in our discussion of perception, is a sequential or time-bound function. We also pointed out that temporal-order resolution is impaired in aphasic adults and seems to be impaired or slow in development in aphasic children. Hearing and language, as Masland notes (see Millikan and Darley, 1967, p. 234), require a preoccupation with time or temporal order. In listening to speech the hearer must make continuous and very rapid decisions about sequential auditory events. Thus, Masland says, "I have been intrigued with the possibility that maybe it is the integration of time bound activities which centers in the left hemisphere. . . ." We believe this to be so. Further, it appears that time-bound activities are impaired in the event of damage to the left temporal lobe.

Speech-sound (phonemic) discrimination is also served by the left temporal area. The effect of lesion on phonemic perception may be appreciated from the data in Figure 4.7.

On the positive side, Luria (1966a) indicates that the essential function of the left temporal lobe (the secondary divisions of the auditory cortex of the left hemisphere) is in

> *. . . the analysis and integration of the sound flow by identification of the phonemic signs of the objective system of the language.* This work must be

---

[5]The evidence of the investigations of dichotic listening referred to earlier permits us to make observations regarding auditory functioning of normal persons as well as the effects of pathology. The findings on normal persons support the evidence coming from those following pathology.

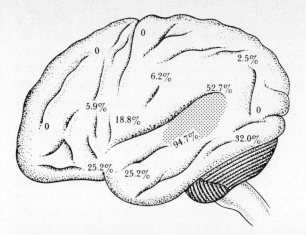

Figure 4.7 Percentage distribution of cases with impaired phonemic perception related to site of cerebral lesion. Stipple region includes the auditory projection and association areas considered to be essential for normal phonemic perception. Note the relatively high incidence of impaired phonemic perception related to lesions in areas immediately adjacent to the stippled region. (After R. L. Masland, "Some Neurological Processes Underlying Language." *Annals of Otology, Rhinology and Laryngology,* 77(4), 1968, 787; based on data from A. R. Luria, "Brain Disorders and Language Analysis." *Language and Speech* 1(1), 1958, 14–34.)

carried out with the very close participation of articulatory acts which ... constitute the efferent link for the perception of the sounds of speech. It consists of differentiating the significant, phonemic signs of the spoken sounds, inhibiting the unessential signs, and comparing the perceived sound complexes on this phonemic basis. (p. 101)

An inspection of the diagram for localization of function in relationship to speech (Figure 4.1) will reveal the close proximity of the area for the control of articulate speech to the auditory cortex. We also suggest a review of our basic definition of perception in relationship to Luria's emphasis that the auditory cortex differentiates the significant phonemic signs of speech signals and compares "the perceived sound complexes on this phonemic basis."

EXCEPTIONS TO LEFT CEREBRAL CONTROL

Although the left cerebral hemisphere is normally dominant for language function, there are some important exceptions. These exceptions include a very small minority of right-handed persons and perhaps a bare majority of naturally left-handed persons. The latter group, based on their ability to spontaneously recover language following acquired damage to the left hemisphere, seem to have either (a) bilateral cerebral control for language or (b), in the event of damage to the left hemisphere, a capacity for the right hemisphere to assume controls normally served by the left. Another important exceptional group is young persons below age 12, who also make excellent recovery of language function in the event of acquired damage to the left hemisphere. In this group we may assume that the plasticity of the young brain is such as to make a shift in cerebral dominance for language, which is not ordinarily the case in older persons (Penfield and Roberts, 1959, p. 102; Penfield, 1971).

From our brief review of cerebral dominance and language function, it is evident that although the left cerebral cortex is normally dominant (normally subserves language), the right hemisphere has the capability or potential for subserving language under certain conditions. One of these conditions, pointed out by Masland (1967), is found in children who incur serious injury to the brain and in children whose entire left hemispheres are removed prior to approximately 8 years of age. Most of these children, after recovery from the physical effects of the operation, resume language functions and seem to be able to talk normally. The assumption is that these children reestablished language function under the control of the right cerebral hemisphere. Masland (1967) asks: "If that is the case, what is the basis of the language disability of those children who *do* have language disabilities?" He then offers several possible explanations:

1. These children suffer from bilateral lesions involving both hemi-spheres.
2. The defect (lesion) lies in lower centers (the brain stem or basal ganglia) through which information is relayed to the higher brain structures.
3. "There are genetically or constitutionally determined organizational defects or peculiarities of the brain of such individuals which cause it to be difficult or impossible for them to form the associations or correlations essential to the establishment of language" (Masland, 1967).

A fourth possibility, which we consider in our discussion of perceptual dysfunction, is the position of Eisenberg (1964), who notes:

The psychological deficits we observe in the patient who has suffered early cerebral injury cannot be taken to imply that the tissue destroyed is in itself the sole cause of the entire pattern. The injury might have impaired an elementary psychological function, the lack of which could then distort subsequent development. Thus, complex functions, the anatomical equipment for which might otherwise be intact, could have failed to evolve. (pp. 68–69)

We believe that the same effects of psychological dysfunction, which Eisenberg suggests may come from brain lesion, might also be a result of maturational delay.

BRAIN DIFFERENCES

The general plan for the organization of the two halves of the brain for language and nonlanguage functions follows along the lines described in the preceding pages of this chapter. Disturbances in the event of acquired pathologies also follow along lines that may be anticipated from the general plan. There are differences, however, and it is important to appreciate that no two brains are precisely the same. Deviations from the general plan may be slight and minor, but sometimes they may be appreciable. The result may well be an individual organization that is functionally different from normal expectations. However, except in the event of acquired pathology or failure to establish an expected function within an expected time range, the difference may never be suspected.

Some children's difficulties in learning may be explained by interarea (associational) integration failures, which may be caused by individual maturational differences or may follow a genetic plan shared by other members of the family. Such children may have difficulty in multisensory intake, especially if they are taught by persons who assume that children learn the way the teachers themselves learned and accordingly so teach.

Familial left-handed and truly ambidextrous persons constitute a fairly large exceptional portion of the population—probably 10 percent. For this population, the two cerebral hemispheres have less functional asymmetry than is found in more than 95 percent of right-handed persons. They are brain different when compared with right-handed persons, but these differences are usually a plus, except in cultures where left-handedness is socially undesirable.

A study of Figure 4.7 also points out differences. The vast majority of cases of acquired impairments of phonemic (speech sound) perception have the lesions (damage) in the auditory area of the cerebrum, consistent with expectations. Phonemic impairments are also found, however, in association with lesions incurred in other areas of the brain. We cannot be sure of the cause or causes for these apparent exceptions. For the time being, we will accept the truism that human beings are themselves and each is a special self. They are individuals because of genetic differences, acquired differences, teaching, and other dynamics, singly or in combination. We can only conjecture how these individual variations account for what we are and what our brains are, and how they influence, predetermine, or ultimately determine our linguistic behavior and, of course, our other human behaviors.

REFERENCES AND SUGGESTED READINGS

Broadbent, D. E. "The Role of Auditory Localization in Attention and Memory Span," *Journal of Experimental Psychology,* 47, 1954, 191–196.

Dirks, D. "Perception of Dichotic and Monaural Verbal Material and Cerebral Dominance for Speech," *Acta Otolaryngologia,* 58, 1964, 73–80.

Eisenberg, L. "Behavioral Manifestations of Cerebral Damage in Childhood," in H. G. Birch (ed.), *Brain Damage in Children.* Baltimore: Williams and Wilkins, 1964.

Eisenson, J. "The Left Brain Is for Talking," *Acta Symbolica,* 2(1), 1971, 33–36.

French, J. D. "The Reticular Formation," *Scientific America,* 196(5), 1957, 54–60.

Gardner, H. "What We Know (and Don't Know) About the Two Halves of the Brain," *Harvard Magazine,* 80, 1978, 24–27.

Geschwind, N. "Specializations of the Human Brain," *Scientific American*, 421(3), 1979, 180–199 (also in *The Brain*, San Francisco: Freeman, 1979).

Geschwind, A. N., and Levitsky W. "Human Brain: Left-Right Asymmetries in Temporal Speech Region," *Science*, 161, 1968, 186–187.

Hecaen, H., and Albert, M. *Human Neuropsychology*. New York: Wiley, 1978.

Kimura, D. "Functional Asymmetry of the Brain in Dichotic Listening," *Cortex*, 3, 1967, 163–178.

Krashen, S. D. "The Development of Cerebral Dominance and Language Learning: More New Evidence" in D. P. Dato (Ed.), *Developmental Psycholinguistics: Theory and Application*. Washington, D.C.: Georgetown University Press, 1975.

Krech, D., and Crutchfield, R. S. *Elements of Psychology*. New York: Knopf, 1958.

Lennenberg, E. H. *Biological Foundations of Language*. New York: Wiley, 1967.

Liberman, A. M., Cooper, F. S., Shankweiler, D. P., and Studdert-Kennedy, M. "Perception of the Speech Code," *Psychological Review*, 74(6), 1967, 431–461.

Lindsley, D. B. "The Reticular Activation System and Perceptual Integration," in D. E. Sheer (ed.), *Electrical Stimulation of the Brain*. Austin: University of Texas Press, 1961.

Luria, A. R. "Aspects of Aphasia," *Journal of the Neurological Sciences*, 2(3), 1965, 278–287.

Luria, A. R. *Higher Cortical Functions in Man*. New York: Basic Books, 1966.

Luria, A. R. *Human Brain and Psychological Processes*. New York: Harper and Row, 1966b.

Luria, A. R. *Traumatic Aphasia*. The Hague: Mouton, 1970.

Masland, R. L. "Brain Mechanisms Underlying the Language Function," *Bulletin of the Orton Society*, 17(1), 1967, 1–31.

Masland, R. L. "Some Neurological Processes Underlying Language," *Annals of Otology, Rhinology and Laryngology*, 77(4), 1968, 787.

Masland, R. L. "Brain Mechanisms Underlying the Language Function," in *Human Communication and Its Disorders*. Washington, D.C.: National Institute of Neurological Diseases and Stroke, U.S. Department of Health, Education and Welfare.

Millikan, C. H., and Darley, F. L. (eds.). *Brain Mechanisms Underlying Speech and Language*. New York: Grune and Stratton, 1967.

Mountcastle, V. B. (ed.). *Interhemispheric Relations and Cerebral Dominance*. Baltimore: Johns Hopkins Press, 1962.

Penfield, W. "Language Learning and the 'Switch Mechanism,'" *Acta Symbolica*, 2(1), 1971, 22–32.

Penfield, W., and Roberts, L. *Speech and Brain Mechanisms*. Princeton, N.J.: Princeton University Press, 1959.

Pribram, K. *Languages of the Brain*. Englewood Cliffs, N.J.: Prentice-Hall, 1971.

Russell, W. R., and Espir, M. L. E. *Traumatic Aphasia*. London: Oxford University Press, 1961.

Springer, S. P., and Deutsch, G. *Left Brain, Right Brain*. San Francisco: Freeman, 1981.

chapter *5*

Congenital (Developmental) Aphasia

In the opening chapter it was indicated that a major concern in this text will be with the congenitally (developmentally) aphasic child. Such severely linguistically impaired children suffer from having too many names and too many opportunities for being misdiagnosed. *Dysphasic* and *Aphasoid* are other terms that, although they usually imply a less-than-severe degree of impairment, are sometimes used as synonyms for congenital aphasia. Still another term is *severely orally linguistically handicapped,* viewed here as a concession to medical colleagues, who believe that the term *aphasia* should be limited to acquired impairments and not applied to congenital or developmental disabilities.

IDENTIFICATION

Congenital aphasia will be used to designate the child who, despite evidence of adequate intelligence based on nonverbal assessment, despite an absence of abnormalities of the oral mechanism, despite a lack of evidence of early emotional (relating) problems, and despite a lack of evidence of hearing impairment—except for spoken language—fails to acquire language. This failure is present despite caretakers who are available and presumably eager to provide normal opportunities for language learning. The terms *aphasoid, dysphasic,* and *severely orally linguistically handicapped* will be used only when cited directly from the literature; the evidence indicates that each of these terms is essentially synonymous with *congenital* or *developmental aphasia,* as used here.

As mentioned earlier, some neurologists and speech pathologists take exception to the designation of congenital aphasia for the severely linguistically retarded child, who will be described in detail in this chapter. Critchley (1967), a neurologist, takes the position that the term *aphasia,* which literally means "without speech," should be reserved for acquired linguistic impairments associated with identified brain damage. Rees (1981) is not convinced that the perceptual deficiencies we will describe here are really relevant or have been proved to underlie the language difficulties of such children. Bloom and Lahey (1978) share Rees's lack of conviction. They also share the reservation that the use of the terms and related concepts of congenital or developmental aphasia make a contribution to determining the appropriate (differential) treatment of the child. It is hoped that this chapter will establish that *congenital or developmental aphasia* is an appropriate, differential diagnostic term and that corresponding differential treatment is available as well as productive.

In a separate chapter we will consider the child with *acquired aphasia.* The term *childhood-acquired aphasia* will be limited to designating a child who has acquired language normally and has subsequently suffered impairment as a result of cerebral pathology through accident or disease. If the child improves and has only residual language and cognitive deficits, as is usually the case when the damage is limited to one cerebral hemisphere, then the appropriate term should be *acquired dysphasia.*

Beyond early adolescence, usually beyond age 15, the recovery process increasingly resembles that of the adult with acquired aphasia. Fortunately for preadolescents, "regardless of the cognitive and academic sequelae that ensue, one cannot help but be struck by the rapid recovery from aphasia in a majority of the children" (Satz and Bullard-Bates, 1981, p. 421). The implications of these observations will be considered in Chapter 11.

THE SYNDROME OF CONGENITAL (DEVELOPMENTAL) APHASIA

Children who are born with brain damage because of prenatal (congenital) conditions, who are markedly delayed in cerebral maturation, or who incurred brain damage before the onset of speech are frequently severely retarded in language development. Some of these children are frankly cerebral-palsied—with obvious motor impairments—as well as being aphasic. Others, especially those with bilateral brain damage, may also be severely mentally retarded. A few may have severe hearing impairment. Our discussion here will be limited to the children who (a) are not mentally retarded, insofar as they have adequate intelligence as judged by other cognitive indices that are correlated with language acquisition; (b) are not deaf or even moderately hard-of-hearing, but in some ways suggest that they might be so (some do have mild hearing losses—15 to 25 decibels—that seldom cause problems in language acquisition in most children, but when hearing losses are present, they are likely to be in the middle and upper speech ranges); and (c) are not primarily autistic (nonrelating to human beings and so possibly nonspeaking) but all too often withdraw from speakers because of their inability to make sense of human oral language.

Some children who initially may be congenitally aphasic on the basis of slow maturation of their central nervous systems may have delayed onset and slower-than-normal speech development. At age 4 or 5, they may present a profile in language development that may be comparable in many ways to a 1½- to 2-year-old. We found this to be so in our investigations at the Institute for Childhood Aphasia at Stanford University during the period 1963–1972. Some children are conspicuously slow in their phonemic (articulatory) development, have a limited vocabulary suggestive of a child who is just beginning to speak, and have retarded syntactic proficiency. Their overall profile tends to shadow but does not quite parallel that of younger, normally speaking children. Other children present diverse and scattered profiles in their language acquisitions. For the most part, congenitally aphasic children are not retarded shadows of their age peers.

Hardy (1978) reviews the pros and cons of the concept of congenital aphasia. With some reluctance, Hardy concludes that there are two kinds of children with developmental disorders of communication: the congenitally aphasic and the congenitally apraxic. Hardy presents a case of a 6-year-old boy with developmental auditory aphasia. The child had "normal hearing sensitivity when given a pure tone hearing test, but his hearing could not be tested with speech stimuli because he seemed to have a complete inability to understand speech." The boy was able to respond appropriately to gesture. Hardy suggests that "difficulty in analysis of the sequencing of the language code" may be a partial explanation of the child's difficulty. Having seen many such children, we are inclined to agree.

DIFFERENTIAL DIAGNOSTIC FEATURES

As indicated earlier, the congenitally aphasic child often behaves as if mentally retarded, as if suffering from a profound hearing loss, or as if autistic. A differential diagnosis must therefore distinguish this child from other language-delayed and nonverbal children. Differential features include the following.

1. *Perceptual dysfunctions* are likely to be found in one or more sensory modalities, but not in all modalities. Auditory perception is almost invariably impaired. (See Chapter 3 for a review of perception, particularly the perceptual functions that underlie speech.)

2. *Perceptual auditory dysfunction* includes difficulty in speech-sound (phonemic) discrimination and phonemic sequencing (temporal order). By sequencing, we mean the capacity to hold a series of events in mind and to respond to an ongoing event in the light of immediate past events. Because spoken language is a flow of articulated sounds, a child who can discriminate but cannot sequence a flow or stream of auditory events at the rate at which such events are normally presented will not be able to understand what is heard. In effect, the child may be able to hear but is not able to decode speech.

This is the kind of child described by Hardy. Earlier, another Hardy (1965) referred to this disability as "auding."

Eisenberg (1976), in her chapter "Organization of Hearing Functions," reminds us of the need to distinguish between deafness and the inability to deal normally with acoustic information. Referring to a child who is not obviously deaf but is not yet old enough to talk, she says: "We can say that he responds at normal levels, but *we cannot* say that he *hears normally*." On the other hand, Eisenberg points out that if the child is not deaf but is old enough to be expected to talk and nevertheless is not able to deal normally with acoustic information, we cannot say that he or she hears normally. Eisenberg (1976) emphasizes the need to develop assessment procedures for children who show evidence of developmental disorders of communication: "These are disorders for which there are no adequate diagnostic labels, no adequate techniques for measurement, testing, or intervention" (pp. 151–152).

3. *Temporal order difficulties,* though most severe for auditory events and especially for speech, may be present for visual events. Except for signing, however, what we ordinarily take in visually is relatively static. We can usually look again—often for as long as we wish—at a visual display. Impairments in sequencing in the visual modality are seldom evident. In deaf adults, there are impairments for signing that parallel those for an oral spoken language (Albert, Goodglass, Helm, Rubens, and Alexander, 1981, pp. 125–127).

4. *Intellectual inefficiency* is characteristically over and above any objectively (psychometrically) determined mental limitation. Because it is assumed that we are dealing with children who are not basically mentally retarded, it is implied that their functional intelligence may not be consistent with expectations based on their cognitive indices and their obtained mental ages and intelligence quotients. Observations indicate that developmentally aphasic children require optimal conditions in order to function close to their cognitive potential. In clinical settings, such conditions include an absence of distraction and of noise of any variety, making certain that the child is not unduly fatigued or emotionally upset and is not hungry. A little bit of distraction, of fatigue, or of frustration generated by awareness of error may go a long way toward impairing the intellectual functioning of an aphasic child who is involved in an assessment procedure. In this sense aphasic children are regarded as having a strong inclination to function as if intellectually inefficient.

An aphasic child's test performance or performance in a learning situation will show considerable variability on the same type of task or test from time to time during a day, as well as from day to day. If the best performance is accepted as indicative of the child's intellectual potential, then developmentally aphasic children tend to approximate the norm in intellectual functioning, at least when the assessment is made on the basis of nonverbal standardized test inventories administered under optimum conditions.

Dr. Joel Stark (Stark, Poppen, and May, 1967), while a member of the Institute for Childhood Aphasia at Stanford University, studied the test performance of 75 aphasic children ranging from 3 through 8 years of age. He employed two scales, the Leiter International Performance Scale (Arthur

Table 5.1   TEST SCORES OF 75 APHASIC CHILDREN

Age group	N	Columbia mental maturity scale (CMMS)		Leiter international performance scale (LIPS)	
		Mean IQ	SD	Mean IQ	SD
3–4.11	16	99.5	17.95	93.8	22.18
5–6.11	35	87.0	12.59	89.3	21.06
7–8.11	24	73.1	16.56	79.4	12.62

adaptation) and the Columbia Mental Maturity Scale, both of which can be administered without verbal directions and require no verbal responses. The final diagnosis for the children in the Stark study was severe language impairment associated with established or likely CNS involvement. The results are summarized in Table 5.1.

It may be noted that the mean IQ for the 3-and 4-year-old children is within normal range. Also to be noted is the lower-than-average IQ for the older children. We interpret this difference in scores to be a reflection of the difference in task requirements related to form, color, and size. At the upper age level, correct performance requires an ability to categorize and abstract and either to select an item (on the Columbia scale) or to arrange materials (on the Leiter scale) according to some principle. An additional factor in the upper-level items is that in each test situation, the child has to deal with considerably more stimulus events than at the lower levels.

Observations of the behavior of the children when they are confronted with difficult items reveal a marked tendency toward perseveration, displays of frustration and hostility directed either at the materials or at the test administrator, and often considerable hyperactivity. Some children, however, simply withdraw from further involvement with the testing situation. Another clinical observation of the test performance of these children is their inclination to lose sight of the principle necessary for the completion of a task. For example, if a test task calls for the alternation of figures, such as a circle and a square, a child may arrange half of the figures in the appropriate order and then place the others in a completely random order. Another characteristic performance error is the failure to carry over a principle from one test task to another. Thus, if, as on the Columbia scale, a child succeeds in pointing to the appropriate (different) figure, we still cannot assume that he or she will remember the principle of this task for succeeding items. The performance may improve if the child is reminded of the nature of the task for each succeeding item. This is ordinarily not required for normal children. Failure to keep a principle in mind is another indication of intellectual inefficiency.

This is not meant to suggest that, by definition, all aphasic children are intellectually normal in potential or in functional intelligence when language is not directly involved. Earlier, we indicated that most aphasics have adequate intelligence when judged by nonverbal behavior and therefore, unless there were some other involvement, should be expected to learn to speak. We are mindful that moderately retarded children do learn to speak, and that even some moderately severely retarded persons understand uncomplicated oral language and can be taught some functional speech. The disparity between intelligence and language comprehension and production is considerably greater among congenitally aphasic children than among the mentally retarded. We have also noted that in regard to auditory processing, aphasic children show greater impairment than most children who have mild-to-moderate hearing losses.

Aphasic children may, in fact, also be mildly and perhaps moderately intellectually retarded. If intellectual retardation is judged to be severe, then we prefer to consider the degree of retardation as the basic cause for the language impairment. Benton (1978) suggests a possible relationship between intellectual level, cerebral abnormality, and language function:

> One possibility is that the variability in intelligence level is related to a corresponding variability underlying the specific language disability. In the case of some children the cerebral abnormality may be limited in extent and thus affect only those functions involved in speech and language learning. In the case of other children, the cerebral abnormality may be sufficiently extensive to retard their general intellectual development as well as have a specific effect on the acquisition of language skills. (p. 47)

Benton shares the frequently made observation that retarded children as a general population have a higher incidence of speech defects than their age-peer population as a whole. Moreover, Benton (1978) states: "There is also evidence that many retardates show pronounced impairment in the development of linguistic function that cannot be accounted for by their low mental age" (p. 48). Presumably, although these retarded children have a low intellectual level, their linguistic dysfunctions go beyond what we often find in "familial" retarded persons. These children may be considered dysphasic-retarded.

Language development in nonretarded aphasic children may be so delayed that at age 4 or 5 they may still be essentially nonverbal, both for comprehension and production of speech. In other instances, as indicated earlier, the child may have had a delayed onset of speech, perhaps with first words coming as late as 36 months. At age 4 or older, the child may be at a two-word phrase level when most age peers are using conventional syntax in multiword utterances. In general, the productive language of the less severely impaired developmentally aphasic child may be described as sparse in vocabulary and lacking in syntactic competence.

A-PHASIC DEVELOPMENT
OF THE CONGENITALLY APHASIC CHILD

Hyphenation of *a-phasic* directs attention to the out-of-phase developmental background of many congenitally aphasic children. Clinical histories reveal that these children often do not present the anticipated patterns and correlations of their age peers in regard to general sensory, motor, and perceptual functions as well as intellectual abilities. Even when brain dysfunction cannot be established on a hard-sign basis, congenitally aphasic children indicate by clinical history that they are *brain different*. Morley (1960) reported similar findings in a longitudinal study of aphasic children. Aphasic children are slow to develop laterality for handedness and, we believe, for ear preference. Both of these expressions of laterality are recognized as related to cerebral dominance for language.

NEUROLOGICAL FINDINGS

Except for severe language impairment, many developmentally aphasic children do not present clear-cut or hard-sign evidence of central nervous pathology. Hard-sign evidence includes motor disabilities, sensory dysfunctions, and perceptual-motor integrative impairments or delays. Perhaps about one child in two or three who is designated an aphasic child on the basis of psychological and psycholinguistic assessment also shows clear evidence of neuropathology. Many more, at least another third, show evidence of "at least minimal brain damage" (Brown, 1967, p. 357) or minimal brain dysfunction. Perhaps it is more accurate to suggest that these children show evidence of maximum brain dysfunction despite minimal hard-sign evidence of brain damage.

Kenny and Clemmens (1975) emphasize: "Uniquivocal or 'hard' neurologic signs are abnormal at any age. Borderline or soft neurologic signs indicate abnormality at a particular age only, suggesting a relative delay in some aspects of neurologic maturation" (p. 54).

Ferry, (1981), a pediatric neurologist, states as a basic premise:

1. Delay or deviation in language development is due to disordered brain function. Normal speech and language development is a reflection of an intact, functioning brain.
2. Speech and language delay or impairment may be the only symptom or sign of neurological impairment. This is a reflection of functional localization in which severe damage to a circumscribed area may occur while other areas of the brain remain perfectly intact. Thus, although a child with delayed speech development may have a perfectly normal general neurological examination, this should not rule out the possibility that his delayed speech development is due to a neurological problem. (pp. 5–6)

Electroencephalographic (EEG) and Related Findings

Several investigations indicate that the incidence of abnormal EEG findings is higher among congenitally aphasic children than would be expected from children in their age range who are not aphasic. Goldstein, Landau, and Kleffner (1958) report that about 40 percent of 69 aphasic children showed abnormal EEG findings. The percentage was about the same for the 114 deaf children with whom the aphasic children were compared. However, the aphasic children had a higher incidence of focal abnormalities (14.5 percent compared with 6.1 percent for the deaf). In a study at the Institute for Childhood Aphasia at Stanford University (Forrest, Eisenson, and Stark, 1967), about half (36 of 73) of the aphasic children had abnormal EEG findings. Twenty-two of the abnormalities were localized, with 19 of them in the left cerebral hemisphere. This is perhaps the most significant part of the observations because, as indicated earlier, the left cerebral hemisphere is the one normally assumed to be dominant for speech (language functioning).

Rapin and Wilson (1978) report on radiographic studies of children who were severely retarded in language development. Their findings on 87 children who were suspected of structural brain damage revealed that 26 showed enlargement of the left temporal horn, 6 of the right, and 14 of both left and right. Rapin and Wilson, (1978) remind us: "The lateral temporal cortex is concerned with auditory, and in the left hemisphere, with linguistic processing" (pp. 23–24).

It is important to note that Rapin and Wilson were investigating children with delayed language who were suspected of having structural brain pathology on the basis of other neurological observations. This may account for the higher incidence of positive radiographic findings than in the Stanford study.

Related Observations Regarding Cerebral Dominance

After a review of several studies on the prevalence of left-handedness or lack of strong indications of lateral preference among children who are delayed in language development, Zangwill (1978) notes: "In general, weak, mixed or inconsistent lateral preference are the most frequent findings" (p. 10) Incidentally, a comparable observation is made for children with dyslexia (severe reading difficulty) who are otherwise normal. Zangwill (1978) generalizes that "the developmental lag which in the absence of gross brain damage is generally held to underlie developmental aphasia, has its neural correlates in slow, faulty, or incomplete lateralisation of language processes" (p. 10).

PHONEMIC OR SPEECH-SOUND IMPERCEPTION

Some of the neurological findings discussed here have implications for the understanding of the developmentally aphasic child's difficulty with normal speech perception and, therefore, with the acquisition of oral language. With only rare exceptions, the aphasic child's basic perceptual impairment is considered an impairment for auditory perception for speech at the rate at which speech is normally presented. Even though some aphasic children may have a mild hearing loss and a few a moderate loss based on audiometric results, the typical pure-tone audiogram could be described as adequate for speech. For the developmentally aphasic child, the correlation between audiometric findings and hearing (really *listening*) for speech does not pertain. Even if a speech threshold is established to suggest that the child hears speech at a given level—

that is, presumably low enough so that the child should be able to learn to speak—other factors prevent or delay this acquisition. The most important of these factors is difficulty in speech-sound or phonemic discrimination and sequencing in contextual utterance.

Luria (1966), the Russian neuropsychologist, holds that an area of the left temporal cortex, which he designates the *auditory cortex,* has a special capacity for phonemic (speech-sound) discrimination. Thus, delayed maturation or damage to this area is likely to result in impairment for speech-sound discrimination and perception. However, it should be noted that appropriate perception of nonspeech environmental sounds may not be impaired. This probably accounts for the apparent inconsistency of the developmentally aphasic child's responses to sounds that are appropriate to animal, mechanical, and other environmental noises but inappropriate to speech. Perhaps the developmentally aphasic child is not really as inconsistent a listener as he or she superficially appears to be. Those of us who logically expect that a child who is able to hear and understand environmental sounds should also be able to hear and understand all sounds, including speech, may well be the ones who are in "consistent error."

Luria's findings are supported by investigations at the Haskins Laboratories in the United States. One of the laboratories' reports (Liberman, Cooper, Shankweiler, and Studdert-Kennedy, 1967) sums up their observations as follows:

> The conclusion that there is a speech mode, and that it is characterized by processes different from those underlying the perception of other sounds, is strengthened by recent indications that speech and nonspeech sounds are processed primarily in different hemispheres of the brain.[1]

PERCEPTUAL DYSFUNCTIONS

From the mid-1960s to 1973, the research staff of the Institute for Childhood Aphasia at Stanford University investigated the perceptual functioning of aphasic children as compared with their age peers. The findings indicated several differences that have implications for and explain some of the difficulties of these children in processing language.

Defective Storage (Memory)

One of the Stanford studies (McReynolds, 1966) indicated that aphasic children had difficulty in discriminating between speech sounds but could be taught through a reinforcement approach to make appropriate discriminations. The aphasic children needed considerably more time and trials to learn

---

[1]See also Liberman (1982). In Chapter 4, we reviewed the evidence for the differential functioning of the two cerebral hemispheres and the normal dominance of the left hemisphere for speech and language.

what most normal age peers could achieve in a few trials. Moreover, forgetting from trial to trial what they had learned to discriminate appeared to be characteristic. It is assumed that defective short-term memory accounted for the poor learning.

Defective Discrimination and Temporal Order

Rosenthal and Eisenson (1970) found that aphasic children have difficulty in making appropriate discriminative judgments for speech sound and have even more difficulty in making correct temporal order (sequential) judgments. The interstimulus interval (ISI) between signals and number of trials to arrive at correct judgments was used as a measure of difficulty. Some of the aphasic children required as much as a ten times greater ISI than the normal controls.

The results of the Rosenthal and Eisenson investigation are in keeping with an earlier study by Lowe and Campbell (1965) on a population designated *aphasoid*. In the Lowe and Campbell study, the aphasoid children made correct temporal order judgments within a range of 55 to 700 msec (mean, 357 msec), compared with a range of 15 to 80 msec (mean, 36.1 msec) for normal controls. An interesting note in the Rosenthal-Eisenson study is that their subjects included several children who had established a considerable amount of language, after a year or more of direct language instruction. Nevertheless, in a novel experimental situation, what we assume to be underlying difficulties again tend to be manifest. As a group, the language-delayed children and the children with a history of severe language delay performed poorly when ISIs were less than 200 msec.

INEFFICIENT DETECTION STRATEGIES

Rosenthal and Wohlert (1974) found that aphasic children showed less benefit from the release of a masking noise than did normal controls in a masking-level difference study in which signal intensity (pure tones) was varied. The investigators interpreted their findings to mean that language-delayed children have poor detection strategies for auditory task performances. Specifically, Rosenthal and Wohlert suggest that the delayed-language children—aphasic and postaphasic[2]—do not appear to anticipate and adequately tune their auditory systems "to expected signal parameters such as frequency, phase, duration, and intensity." As a consequence, the attempts of aphasic children result in higher-than-normal error thresholds and error rates. Another study (Springer and Eisenson, 1977) suggesting perceptual inefficiency used a dichotic listening procedure with 10 children aged 8.7 to 12.9 who had a history of severe language delay and controls matched for age, sex, and handedness. All the children, both experimental and control, showed a clear right-ear advantage in reporting consonant-vowel (CV) syllables such as *ka-ga* or *ba-da*. This finding implies left (contralateral) dominance for speech sounds, a normal expecta-

---

[2]*Postaphasic* is used to identify the children who had received a year or more of direct language instruction and were functioning adequately in school settings.

tion. However, the experimental (language-delayed) group made significantly more errors than did the control group. Specifically, the language-delayed group, much more frequently than the control group, reported hearing syllables that were not sent to either ear.

This study tends to confirm the findings of the Rosenthal-Wohlert investigation regarding the lability and inefficiency of the auditory system in aphasic children, at least for speech sounds. Their systems do well enough when tuned in, so that they can be taught language. For reasons that are not clear, however, the auditory systems do not stay tuned in long enough to acquire all the information they need to be successful in sustained tasks, at least when the tasks are novel, as in an experimental situation. It is also possible that the aphasic and postaphasic children performed poorly because they were slow to learn what it was to which they should have been listening.

Tallal and several associates have reported on a series of investigations on the perceptual abilities of dysphasic children for auditory events, both speech and nonspeech, and for visual events (Tallal and Piercy, 1978). Among the findings of the reported studies are the following:

1. An apparent perceptual problem of dysphasic children is in sequencing (processing the order) of auditory events at interstimulus intervals (ISIs) comparable to those of normal peer controls (150 msec or less). This was found to hold for complex nonspeech tones as well as for speech sounds (phonemes). The investigators also found that dysphasic children had an equal amount of difficulty when the task called merely for same-different discrimination. They concluded that "the apparent sequencing difficulty . . . could be regarded as entirely secondary to the defect of discrimination" (Tallal and Piercy, 1973).

2. Discrimination problems are associated with short duration of stimulus and rapidly changing features of the stimulus event. Tallal, Stark, and Curtiss (1976) found that dysphasic children were impaired in their ability to process rapidly changing nonverbal auditory events. In this study they also reported investigations in which dysphasic children demonstrated adequate response ability for processing synthesized steady-state vowels but performed poorly in processing synthesized stop consonants in CV syllables that required auditory processing of rapidly changing formant structures. However, the dysphasic children performed adequately by making correct discriminations when the duration of the CV syllables was extended artificially. Specifically, the dysphasic children performed adequately when the duration of the initial portion of the spectrum that incorporated the acoustic information was elongated. To achieve such elongation, the investigators employed a speech synthesizer under computer control.

Tallal, Stark, and Curtiss (1976) speculate that the primary disorder in dysphasic children may be a disruption in the processing of rapidly changing acoustic signals. "Because the ability to process such signals is essential for the perception of certain speech sounds, its disruption could seriously retard the acquisition of language." (p. 306) It is assumed here that developmental failure to establish this processing ability rather than disruption might be more indicative of the underlying problem in congenital dysphasia.

3. Tallal, Stark, and Curtiss (1976) also report that production errors in speech in an imitative task were related to errors in perception, especially when sounds were presented in clusters. Some of the dysphasic subjects (5 of 12) were able to discriminate between single stop-consonants and vowels. These children performed as well as normal control subjects in their imitative production of single vowels and stop-consonants. All 12 dysphasic children showed significant production errors when the stop-consonants were presented in clusters. The perceptually impaired dysphasic children were significantly worse than the perceptually unimpaired in their imitative speech production. Tallal and Piercy (1978) summarize the implications of this study:

> These findings suggest that the speech production deficits of these dys-phasic children mirror their defects of speech perception. Those speech sounds incorporating rapid spectral changes critical for their perception are most difficult for dysphasic children to perceive and are also most often inaccurately produced. These results add further support to the hypothesis that developmental dysphasia can be accounted for, at least in part, by a failure to develop an auditory perceptual process necessary for the percep-tion of speech. (p. 75)

In a later study, Tallal and Newcombe (1978) report that adult males with chronic focal brain wounds showed impairments in perception and language comprehension similar to those found in developmental dysphasic children. The adults had difficulty in auditory tasks requiring rapid temporal order processing, regardless of whether the stimuli were verbal or nonverbal events.

As an important observation, Tallal and Newcombe (1978) refer to their findings as a counterargument to the criticism that there is little hard evidence to establish developmental aphasia as a diagnostic entity. They say: "It is all the more striking . . . that the pattern of impairment in nonverbal as well as verbal acoustic processing is so similar in both the childhood and adult groups that we have studied" (p.22).

In reviewing the studies by Tallal and her co-investigators, it is important to recognize their use of the term *dysphasia* as indicating a lesser degree of impairment than that of many of the children in the Stanford University studies. Furthermore, developmental aphasia is considered "a deficit in the acquisition of normal language function in children of normal or above-normal intelligence with adequate hearing to permit the perception of verbal sounds. . . ." (Wyke, 1978). It is all the more impressive that the dysphasic children studied in England by Tallal and associates who were not as severely impaired nevertheless showed many of the perceptual dysfunctions of the Stanford population. This is not surprising because some of the Stanford subjects who had completed the program and were recalled as subjects for the study were no longer aphasic (severely linguistically impaired) but were dysphasic. Nevertheless, in novel experimental situations their performances in perceptual tasks were inferior to those of normal controls. A possible explanation is that their knowledge of language, resulting at least initially from direct teaching, permitted fair-to-adequate functioning in verbal teaching situations. However, strategies were poor for novel (experimental) situations where linguistic knowledge was not of great help, so that their basic improficiencies again dominated their performance. One of these improficiencies is probably for recall, especially for speech events.

RELATED PROBLEMS: DEFECTIVE STORAGE (MEMORY)

Fortunately, developmentally aphasic children can be trained to discriminate between isolated speech sounds (McReynolds, 1966) and to make correct discriminative responses when given an immediate opportunity to do so. However, their storage systems for such signals may be defective. It is often found that, when even short periods of delay are introduced, many aphasic children seem unable to retain what they hear. In contrast to tasks for speech-sound discrimination, there is usually better performance for discrimination of other environmental sounds. The implication of these observations is that speech events call for different storage and control than do other auditory events. This, as indicated earlier, is supported by the observations of the Haskins Laboratories investigators.

Another explanation for the actual difference in performance of aphasic children for nonauditory events is that in the real (nonlaboratory-experimental) world, events that can be seen or touched do not pass immediately into the past as they are being produced and presented for response. One may almost always take another look or another touch, or continue to look or to touch as long as needed by the responding individual. In the visual world, sights, pictures, and print do not fade bit by bit. Their features and the information provided ordinarily remain as long as needed without change. Because nonauditory events remain longer, they can be stored and compared with what has previously been stored more easily and more confidently than can auditory events. It is possible to be a slow reader and still comprehend the written word, but it is not comparably possible to be a slow listener.

In experimental situations, Stark, Poppen, and May (1967) studied a population of eight aphasic children (mean age 8 years, 3 months) and eight normal controls approximately 3 years younger (mean age 5 years, 3 months). The experimental task required that the subjects press three keys with pictures on them in the same order as the items were presented auditorally by the experimenter. Five of the eight experimental (aphasic) subjects did less well than the controls. When the experimental task was modified to stress the first item of the series, the aphasic children improved their performance. Stark, Poppen, and May (1967) concluded that the poor performance of five of the aphasic children demonstrated impaired memory for sequences. It is possible to interpret the findings as an indication of impaired memory function when three events have to be processed and reproduced from memory. In such an experimental situation, the first item tends to be forgotten by both normal and aphasic children, but about twice as often (40.6 percent compared with 76.0 percent) for the five aphasic children. However, three aphasic children scored slightly better (37.7 percent error compared with 40.6 percent) than the normal subjects.

EXPRESSIVE DISTURBANCES

It is evident from a review of the studies just reported that the underlying dysfunction of congenitally aphasic children is for intake of rapidly changing stimuli, especially for auditory events, that constitute speech signals. Expressive (encoding) disturbances are the reverse side of the linguistic coin; they too are manifestations of faulty intake or impaired auditory-perceptual processing for oral language. Nevertheless, there are dysphasic children who continue to have residuals or word-finding and syntactic errors in their productive language ability.

As developmentally aphasic children begin to acquire speech, their productions tend to lag behind their comprehension. In a significant sense, they are like normal children who understand many words and multiple word utterances before they produce their first real words to label or identify the objects and events important in their lives. Aphasic and even postaphasic children may continue to find some words that they have learned are still elusive and the children may appear to be suffering from *dysnomia*. This difficulty in word finding closely parallels that found in older children and adults with acquired aphasia as well as in most of us who on occasion suffer from a tip-of-the-tongue frustration. The word we are trying to articulate is not readily recalled, though we can find synonyms or synonymous phrases as substitutes. The child without an extensive inventory of words has no available substitute verbal token and so is functionally more impaired than is a normal speaker.

As aphasic children build up their inventory of words (lexicons), they must also learn how to put the words together according to the conventions (syntax) of the language or the languages of their culture. During this process, which most normal speaking children have under fair, but by no means complete, control by age 4 or 5, aphasic children may still seem to be hunting for words. In reality, they may be trying to organize a construction of words to make an acceptable sentence. Early constructions are likely to resemble the agrammatical utterances of young children who are just beginning to put two words together. Grammatical markers and function words are usually omitted.

Studies by Morehead and Ingram (1973) on populations of aphasic and normal children indicate that differences relative to proficiency in syntax between the two groups tend to increase with age. Aphasic children, even with training, tend to use shorter utterances and grammatically less complex ones than normal children at all ages up to almost 10. At this age, aphasic (dysphasic?) children are about where most normal children half their age usually are in syntactic proficiency. The word *about* must be used generously in regard to the congenitally aphasic population. Compared with normal children, they use fewer sentence types and may still have difficulty with negative-interrogative structures and with embedded phrases and clauses. However, the instructed congenitally aphasic children do show the results of their teaching, so that in time their language constructions resemble the well-formed sentences of normal, but considerably younger, children.

We do not wish to suggest that all congenitally aphasic children share equally all the problems in language acquisition that may be inferred from group results of experimental investigations. Some children, especially those with above-average intelligence, make rapid progress once they get underway. Other children, perhaps a strong majority, continue to have some of the described difficulties well into adolescence. Some have reading problems that begin to become undeniably evident in the third or fourth grade of school and that may underlie many of their learning disorders. Menyuk (1978) seems to sum up the situation:

> Research has indicated that different children labelled as cases of developmental dysphasia have different problems, as suggested by their performance in different experimental situations. On the surface at least, the nature of their problem affects which aspects of the language they have difficulty with (structural and/or segmental), and whether their problem is one of analysis as well as output, or simply one of output. The nature of the problem appears to affect also the rate at which language develops and the direction it takes (i.e., which aspects show comparatively greater or lesser development). Although a number of suggestions have been made concerning *the* way to solve the language problems of children with developmental dysphasia, it is clear that since their language processing difficulties vary, there is no consensus of the ways in which their defect can be remedied. In every instance the particular difficulties of a child should be examined and therapy adopted with more insight into his particular needs. (p. 156)

Oral (Articulatory) Dyspraxia and Apraxia

Some children who have continued difficulties in speech production may in fact be suffering from oral (articulatory) dyspraxia rather than from aphasia. This impairment may also be congenital and may be associated with the aphasic involvement. Less frequently, oral dyspraxia or even more severe oral apraxia may exist as a discrete impairment.

Congenital oral dyspraxias are impairments in the ability to establish voluntary movements involving muscles of the larynx, pharynx, tongue, lips, palate, and cheeks for an intended speech act (a sequence of movements). Oral apraxia implies severe impairment. If comprehension of oral language is not impaired, then the child is left with potentially good intake (capacity for decoding) but difficulty in output (the expressions of encoding). It is not surprising, however, to find that some children will reduce or totally cut off their involvement with linguistic communication because normal interchange is not possible for them. With such awareness, it is still important to appreciate the distinction between the congenitally aphasic involvements that are primarily decoding (comprehension) impairments for spoken language and the motor (productive) impairments that may exist in association with them or as a separate problem. The problem, however, is not without dynamics that may have negative influence on the attitudes and efforts for linguistic communication. In a later chapter, we will consider therapeutic approaches for children with oral apraxia and dyspraxia. At this point, we will consider the implications for therapy from the findings of the reviewed studies on congenitally aphasic children. Later chapters will take up details of therapeutic intervention.

IMPLICATIONS FOR THERAPY

Congenitally aphasic children are those regarded as being perceptually inefficient and lacking in appropriate strategies for dealing with auditory linguistic events at the rate and quantity at which such events are normally produced. What are the therapeutic implications of this position? The following pertain for this special population:

1. They need to be remotivated—invited, induced, seduced—to listen to speakers from whom they may have turned away.
2. The situations for listening should be real and practical and related to the child's ongoing and developing needs.
3. Language exposure should be in reduced quantity and at a slower-than-normal rate of utterance, but not at the cost of distorted speech melody (prosody) or labored, unnatural articulation.
4. A model for teaching the comprehension for linguistic content and form (what is to be decoded and in what constructional forms or syntax) must be established as the basis for oral production.

Chapters 7–9 will present approaches for children with varying degrees of aphasic involvement. Where to begin language therapy will depend, of course, on where the individual child is found to be after informal and formal assessment. For the most severely impaired children, therapy may have to begin with nonverbal procedures. For children who have some language, therapy may begin with approaches and content that are described in Chapters 8 and 9. We reiterate that comprehension (decoding) of language, whatever the content and form, must be established before production (encoding) is expected. However, any linguistic production, if used appropriately, whether spontaneously uttered or evoked after teaching, should be accepted as evidence of comprehension.

REFERENCES AND SUGGESTED READINGS

Albert, M. L., Goodglass, H., Helm, N. A., Rubens, A. B., and Alexander, M. P. *Clinical Aspects of Dysphasia.* New York: Springer-Verlag, 1981.
Benton, A., "The Cognitive Functioning of Children with Developmental Dysphasia," in Wyke, M. A. (ed.), *Developmental Dysphasia.* New York: Academic Press, 1978.

Bloom, L., and Lahey, M. *Language Development and Language Disorders*. New York: Wiley, 1978.

Brown, S. F. "Retarded Speech Development," in Johnson, W. (ed.), *Speech Handicapped School Children*. 3rd ed. New York: Harper and Row, 1967.

Critchley, M. "Aphasiological Nomenclature and Definitions," *Cortex,* 3(1), 1967, 3–25.

Eisenberg, R. B. *Auditory Competence in Early Life*. Baltimore: University Park Press, 1976.

Eisenson, J. "Perceptual Disturbances in Children with Central Nervous System Disfunctions and Implications for Language Development," *British Journal of Disorders of Communication,* 1(1), 1966, 21–32.

Eisenson, J., and Ogilvie, M. *Communicative Disorders in Children*. 5th ed. New York: Macmillan, 1983. Chap. 16.

Ferry, P. C. "Neurological Considerations in Children with Learning Disabilities," in R. W. Keith (ed.), *Central Auditory and Language Disorders in Children*. Houston: College-Hill Press, 1981.

Forrest, T., Eisenson, J., and Stark, J. "EEG Findings in 113 Nonverbal Children" (abstract), *Electroencephalographic Clinical Neurophysiology,* 22, 1967, 291.

Geschwind, N. "Specializations of the Human Brain," *Scientific American,* 421(3), 1979, 180–189.

Goldstein, R., Landau, W. M., and Kleffner, F. R. "Neurological Assessment of Deaf and Aphasic Children," *Transactions of the American Otologic Society,* 46, 1958, 122–136.

Hardy, J. C. "Neurologically Based Disorders," in J. F. Curtis (ed.), *Processes and Disorders of Human Communication*. New York: Harper and Row, 1978.

Hardy, W. G. "On Language Disorders of Young Children: A Reorganization of Thinking," *Journal of Speech and Hearing Research,* 8, 1965, 3–16.

Keith, R. W. "Audiological and Auditory Language Tests of Central Auditory Function," in R. W. Keith (ed.), *Central Auditory and Language Disorders in Children*. Houston: College-Hill Press, 1981.

Kenny, T. J., and Clemmens, R. L. *Behavioral Pediatrics and Child Development*. Baltimore: Williams and Wilkins, 1975.

Liberman, A. M. "On Finding that Speech Is Special," *American Psychologist,* 37(2), 1982, 148–167.

Liberman, A. M., Cooper, F. S., Shankweiler, D. P., and Studdert-Kennedy, M. "Perception of the Speech Code," *Psychological Review,* 74, 1967, 431–461.

Lowe, A. D., and Campbell, R. A. "Temporal Discrimination in Aphasoid and Normal Children," *Journal of Speech and Hearing Research,* 8(3), 1965, 313–314.

Luria, A. R. *The Higher Cortical Functions of Man*. New York: Basic Books, 1966.

McReynolds, L. V. "Operant Conditioning for Investigating Speech Sound Discrimination in Aphasic Children," *Journal of Speech and Hearing Research,* 9, 1966, 519–528.

Menyuk, P. "Linguistic Problems in Children with Developmental Dysphasia," in M. A. Wyke (ed.), *Developmental Aphasia*. New York: Academic Press, 1978.

Morehead, D., and Ingram, D. "The Development of Base Syntax in Normal and Linguistically Deviant Children," *Journal of Speech and Hearing Research,* 16, 1973, 330–352.

Morley, N. E. "Developmental and Receptive Expressive Aphasia," *Speech Pathology and Therapy,* 3(64), 1960.

Rapin, I., and Wilson, B. C. "Children with Developmental Language Disability: Neurological Aspects and Assessment," in M. A. Wyke (ed.), *Developmental Aphasia*. New York: Academic Press, 1978.

Rees, N. S. "Saying More Than We Know," in R. W. Keith (ed.), *Central Auditory and Language Disorders in Children*. Houston: College-Hill Press, 1981.

Rosenthal, W. S., and Wohlert, K. L. "Masking Level Differences (MLD) Effects in Aphasic Children." Paper presented at the American Speech and Hearing Association Convention, 1974.

Rosenthal, W. S., and Eisenson, J. "Auditory Temporal Order in Aphasic Children as a Function of Selected Stimulus Features." Paper presented at the American Speech and Hearing Association Convention, November 1970.

Satz, P., and Bullard-Bates, C. "Acquired Aphasia in Children," in M. T. Sarno (ed.), *Acquired Aphasia*. New York: Academic Press, 1981.

Springer, S. P., and Eisenson, J. "Hemispheric Specialization for Speech in Language Disordered Children," *Neuropsychologia*, 15, 1977, 287–293.

Stark, J., Poppen, R., and May, M. Z. "Effects of Alteration of Prosodic Features on the Sequencing Performance of Aphasic Children," *Journal of Speech and Hearing Research*, 10(4), 1967, 849–855.

Tallal, P., and Newcombe, F. "Impairment of Auditory Perception and Language Comprehension in Dysphasia," *Brain and Language*, 5, 1978, 13–24.

Tallal, P., and Piercy, M. "Developmental Aphasia, Impaired Rate of Non-verbal Processing as a Function of Sensory Modality," *Neuropsychologia*, 2, 1973, 389–398.

Tallal, P., and Piercy, M., "Defects of Auditory Perception in Children with Developmental Dysphasia," in M. A. Wyke, (ed.), *Developmental Dysphasia*. New York, Academic Press, 1978.

Tallal, P., Stark, R., and Curtiss, B. "The Relation between Speech Perception Impairment and Production Impairment in Children with Developmental Dysphasia," *Brain and Language*, 1, 1976, 305–317.

Wyke, M. A. (ed.). *Developmental Dysphasia*. New York: Academic Press, 1978.

Zangwill, O. L. "The Concept of Developmental Aphasia," in M. A. Wyke (ed.), *Developmental Aphasia*. New York, Academic Press, 1978.

chapter *6*

Assessment of Severely Linguistically Impaired Children

The primary purpose in the assessment of children who are severely delayed in their linguistic development is to determine the factors related to the delay and the implications of these factors, if they can be determined, for treatment. The information obtained from these evaluations has immediate and possibly future value. The immediate value is to help us make decisions about whether, when, and how to initiate a training and educational program for the child who is to be assessed. The future value is related to the accumulation of a body of information and insights about children who are severely delayed or impaired in their language acquisition. Such information, when shared, may permit improved classification and, if we and the children are fortunate, more individually designed and productive educational programs than are presently possible.

Assessment of severely linguistically impaired children is multifaceted. The assessors may include a pediatrician or a pediatric neurologist, a child psychiatrist, a psychologist, a speech/language clinician (speech/language pathologist), and an audiologist. If the child is of school age and is attending or has attended school, the judgments of a teacher as to behavior and learning abilities make a significant contribution to the overall evaluation.

All evaluations should be sufficiently recent so that the information obtained will be currently relevant rather than historical; however, comparisons with older evaluations are important because they provide evidence of possible changes over time. Improvements have an obvious positive implication; evidence of decrements in function may imply a process of ongoing pathology.

In all assessment procedures, it is essential that the clinician-examiner observe and note how the results of the evaluation were obtained as well as what was obtained. All results should be considered tentative, implying that evaluations must be repeated periodically and that impressions should not be fixed after an initial trial of an evaluation, however productive it may seem to be. Moreover, all language and educational assessments should include a period of training to permit the clinical team to learn whether and how, at a given time and under a given set of conditions, the child shows what she or he is capable of learning.

PEDIATRIC-NEUROLOGICAL ASSESSMENT

In broad terms, the pediatric-neurological assessment should provide information about how the child is functioning as a physical being and information for making decisions and recommendations as to what other medical examinations may be required to complete the work-up.

The specialized contribution of the pediatric neurologist is, of course, the determination of the integrity or impairments of the child's neurosensory system. Jones (1975) provides guidelines and details on the evaluation of the infant and young child who are suspected of or show definite delay in oral communication. The guidelines include information regarding the family heredity and mother's pregnancy history, defects (anomalies) of the newborn's ear, nose, mouth, and throat, and birth weight. Also important are any unusual features related to pre-, peri-, and postnatal birth events. Especially important would be respiratory distress at birth, difficulty in delivery, evidence of jaundice, need for placing child in a respirator, or any other pertinent factor, such as drugs taken by the mother during pregnancy or immediately before or during delivery. Information of this sort has implications for high risk and possible associated brain damage for the newborn. Jones emphasizes the need to observe early responses of the newborn to light, sights, and sounds.

The following is an outline of background and ongoing information considered important in the evaluation of children referred because they are believed to be severely delayed or impaired in language acquisition or production (aphasic or apraxic). (See Appendix for the detailed Case History Form.)

1. Medical (health) history:
   a. Pre-, peri-, and postnatal information: details of all childhood illnesses and age of child at time of illness; severity of symptoms and after-effects of illness.
   b. Developmental history: sitting up unaided, standing, walking, hand and spoon feeding, including feeding problems; expression of hand preference; prelingual sound making and early verbal acquisitions; adaptive and personal sound development; comparison, if possible, with siblings, parents, or other close relatives.
   c. Family history, including detailed information pertaining to the family

constellation, cultural background, specific interpersonal (familial) dynamics, emotional stresses, and any unusual family or environmental features.

2. Physical examination:

a. General: the purposes are to evaluate the overall physical condition of the child and to note whether there is any evidence of a systemic disease. In particular, the evaluation should include an examination of the oral mechanism for nonspeech and of speech movements; hearing, including speech reception threshold and localization of sound; vision, including acuity, ocular motor control, and visual tracking; balance; and eye-hand coordination

It should be evident that the general physical evaluation is essentially a team approach that calls upon the expertise of a physician and other professionals concerned with children who are severely linguistically retarded. Some aspects of the general physical traditionally are the province of the physician; others obviously call for the expert judgments of an audiologist; still others of a speech pathologist. There need be no rigid lines as to who performs what aspect of the evaluation, provided that the individual assessor has both the training and professional responsibility for what is done.

b. Neurological: beyond the implications of the findings of the general physical examination, the neurological examination is intended to evaluate the child's neurological functioning and to determine whether there is any evidence of a specific disorder of the nervous system. Because the examinee is a young child, the developmental aspects of neurological integration are of fundamental importance, especially in regard to integrated motor acts rather than simple reflex responses.

Routine aspects of the neurological evaluation should include observations of the child's motor status (walking, standing, hopping), the child's awareness of body sense, and his or her relationship of self in space, balance with eyes open and closed, and expression of preferred laterality (hand, foot, eye, and, if possible, ear preference).

It is obvious that such a medical examination cannot be completed in the usual short period of a routine office visit; however, many aspects of the examination can be performed by a nurse or paramedical assistant.

Special additional examinations for a child suspected of being slow or deviant include an electroencephalographic evaluation, ophthalmalogical, otological, and psychiatric assessments, and whatever other evaluations the pediatrician considers necessary from the information and impression obtained during the primary examination. A psychological assessment would also be routinely included.

Part of the responsibility of the pediatrician is the interpretation of the results of the examination to the parents, insofar as such information will help in the understanding and treatment of the child. Similarly, the medical data are reported to the other participants in the assessment process and, of course, are included in the written summaries in each child's case history.

PSYCHOLOGICAL ASSESSMENT

Much of the assessment of the clinical psychologist is, in effect, an extension of the work of the pediatrician and so may be considered part of an extended neurological or, perhaps better, a neuropsychological evaluation. The following is the core of a psychological evaluation:

1. A comprehensive, individual assessment of the child's intellectual (cognitive) functioning under usual and optimal conditions.
2. Evaluations of the child's sensory-motor-perceptual functioning, including differences between single and multiple modality intake.
3. Behavioral observations in a variety of settings, including, if possible, the child at home.
4. Additional indications of learning and social behaviors, including conditions associated with positive and negative expressions.

In regard to the first guideline, it is probably better to consider the assessment of intellectual functioning as one for estimating potential or capacity to learn. Presumably, a linguistically impaired child's potential is greater than the immediately manifest ability. Emphasis, we believe, should be on tests and procedures that do not require verbal mediation. Fortunately, there are many standardized tests that may be administered without oral language, and others that may be adapted for use with nonverbal and severely language-delayed children. In the presentations that follow, selected tests and procedures will be reviewed that we consider representative, but not all-inclusive, of what is available. For more detailed discussions of available assessment instruments and procedures, the reader may consult Darley and Spriestersbach, *Diagnostic Methods in Speech Pathology* (1978), and Darley, *Evaluation of Appraisal Techniques in Speech and Language Pathology* (1979). The latter includes critical reviews of 87 published tests that are widely used by professional clinicians in the field of speech and language pathology. Peterson and Marquardt (1981) describe currently used tests and procedures for the evaluation of children for language and speech proficiency and for developmental skills.

DEVELOPMENTAL INVENTORIES

Inventories that assess the developmental status of a child may include direct sampling and observation of performance ability with peer norms or reports of a parent or caretaker and comparisons with peer expectations.

The Gesell Developmental Schedules

The Gesell (1949) Developmental Schedules, now of historical importance, estimate the intellectual potential of a child based on observations of motor and perceptual functioning. The estimates or projections assume that there is a reliable correlation between motor and perceptual ability and intelligence. The

Gesell Schedules constitute a procedure rather than a formal test. Anastasi (1982) considers that procedures such as the Gesell "may be regarded as a refinement and elaboration of the qualitative observations routinely made by pediatricians and other specialists concerned with infant development" (p. 267). The age range for the Gesell Schedules is 4 weeks to 5 years.

The Bayley Scales of Infant Development

The Bayley (1969) Scales of Infant Development represent a considerable advance over such schedules as the Gesell. The Bayley Scales are intended for the assessment of early mental and psychomotor development of babies and young children up to 30 months of age. These scales provide for differences based on age, sex, color, and urban-rural upbringings. The age period covered in the Bayley Scales includes most of the months that are critical for normal language acquisition. The Bayley Scales yield results that provide a mental developmental and psychomotor developmental index.

The Denver Developmental Screening Test (DDST),*
Revised Edition

The DDST (Frankenburg, Dodds, Fandal, Kazuk, and Cohrs, 1975) is designed as an evaluation instrument to aid in the detection of possible delayed development in children in the age range of 16 to 72 months.[1] Direct observation as well as parent (caretaker) reports of sample behaviors provide the bases for assessment. Four types of behaviors are evaluated: personal-social, motor-adaptive, gross motor, and language.

The DDST is a standardized test. Its norms are based on a population of 1036 normal children in the Denver, Colorado, area. Hubbell (1979) notes that the reliability and validity of the test vary somewhat with the age of the child, "but are comparable with those of other developmental screening instruments" (p. 258). Furthermore, Hubbell suggests that "speech-language pathologists will probably find the test most useful in initial evaluation of children between three and six years, particularly children suspected of possible delay in articulation or language development."

Developmental schedules and scales such as those just presented are important if two related assumptions are accepted. The first is that the potential for language comprehension and production is human-species–specific.[2] The second is that, at least in the early stages, responses to human sights and sounds that are or may become symbolic are expressions of maturational development. These assumptions are essential to an understanding of contemporary cognitive theory, and particularly to an appreciation of the

---

[1]Critical reviews of this test and other tests and inventories discussed herein and indicated by an asterisk(*) may be found in Darley (1979).

[2]Although the success some investigators have had in teaching chimpanzees and primates to sign and to "read" visual symbols is impressive, these accomplishments do not yet pose a threat to human beings, even to an average 2-year-old.

cognitive psychology. Jean Piaget emphasized that differences between younger and older children are qualitative (Piaget and Inhelder, 1969). Such differences in terms of language and thinking should not be quantified. Developmental differences need to be studied and evaluated not only by what the child understands and uses of language, but also by how the child manipulates materials when presented with an opportunity to solve a problem.

It may be difficult to resist the temptation to oversimplify, overgeneralize, and overextrapolate some of the implications of Piaget's psychophilosophy as incorporated in his developmental-cognitive stages. Nevertheless, just as the language correlates of Piaget's early developmental states were presented in Chapter 1, the table of correlates will be extended here to another stage to encompass normal expectations of children from approximate ages 4 to 7. For the sake of convenience, the first two stages will be included in Table 6.1.

Table 6.1   COGNITIVE STAGES (PIAGET): BIRTH TO 4 YEARS

Piaget developmental stage	Linguistic stage
Sensorimotor period (from birth to approximately 18 months): Movements related to sensory intake (perceptions); toward end of period, children arrive at notion of object permanence (out of sight is *not* out of mind)	a. Prelinguistic sound production, crying, vocal play, babbling, lalling, echolalia, and first words; gesturing, mostly pointing and pulling, but also evidence of anticipatory movements in response to caretaker language b. Toward end of stage, single-word productions for labeling and commanding; for some children, two-word utterances
Early preconceptual period (18 to 48 months): Beginnings of symbolic representations; in the early months, most mental activity is about the ongoing present—the here and now; in the later months, the child is able to appreciate (comprehend and deal with) the past and the future; considerable evidence of symbolic play	a. In the early months (18 to 24), two-word utterances, usually without grammatical features b. Gradual increase to three- and four-word and longer utterances that incorporate grammatical features of word order and syntax; verbal productions approximate those of older speakers and are likely to be well-constructed, simple sentences
Early intuitional period (approximately 4 to 7 years): Tasks are solved by immediate perceptual responses; toward end of stage, the child begins to appreciate the concept of reversibility;[a] social play begins to replace egocentric play	Begins to use complex sentences, including relative clauses; the phonetic system of the child's language, including difficult sounds and sound blends, becomes increasingly under control and is likely to be completely or almost completely controlled by age 7

[a]Reversibility implies the capacity to apprehend the essence of a problem so that the problem can be followed through mentally. If required, the direction of the problem can be reversed to its starting point (e.g., $2 + 4 = 6$; $6 - 4 = 2$). Reversibility is markedly accelerated from ages 7 to 12.

Piaget's developmental stages have provided a conceptual framework for a considerable amount of research on the cognitive development of children; however, there are no test inventories, schedules, or scales that can presently be recommended as valid and reliable instruments consistent with Piagetian psychology. Some issues that will have to be satisfied first include determining whether cognition precedes, accompanies, or follows language proficiencies. Does one necessarily need to have appropriate words for a concept to have the concept? In assessment, "correct" answers may be given for "incorrect" reasons. Some children may give idiosyncratic answers (produce unexpected language) that may be quite correct and in keeping with, perhaps, an unexpectedly high level of cognition, but the answers may be considered unacceptable (and so scored as incorrect) because there is no model against which to match the response. Competence for language—a child's knowledge of language—usually precedes performance, but not always.

These issues are not confined to designing an instrument for language assessment peculiar to Piaget's model. The issues do, however, add to the difficulties in devising a valid and reliable Piaget evaluation instrument for language assessment, especially for linguistically and cognitively involved children. For a brief review of the problems and issues, we recommend Schiefelbusch (1972) and Byrne and Shervanian (1977); however, we may do well to go to Piaget himself for his views about formal testing in general and particularly about standardized approaches to language testing of children. Ginsburg and Opper (1979) summarize Piaget's position:

> The testing method has the disadvantage of inflexibility. If a child gives an interesting response, the examiner cannot pursue it. If a child misunderstands the question, the examiner cannot clarify it. If the child's answer suggests an additional topic for investigation, the examiner must leave the matter unexplored. In addition, the test procedure may be suggestive. If the child is asked, "Where did the sun come from?" the question implies that the sun did have an origin, and this idea may not have occurred to the child before. Consequently, his answer may not reveal the spontaneous contents of his thought, but may be merely a hastily considered response to a question encountered for the first time. And finally, the test method does not usually allow the examiner to establish the stability of the child's response. If a child is asked what the sum of 2 and 2 is, and says "4," his answer may be tentative or firm. If he is unsure, further questioning may induce him to change his mind. If his belief is firm, nothing will sway him. In the testing procedure the child gives an answer and that is the end of it: a tentative "4" is as good as a sure one. For these reasons, then, Piaget rejects the testing approach. (p. 92)

If we accept Piaget's position, we would have no choice but to abandon the use of standardized tests and procedures for language assessment or, for that matter, for estimating intelligence. Piaget recommended and employed a clinical approach that permitted an in-depth investigation of why as well as what a child says or does in a given testing situation. Thus, there are no incorrect responses; rather, there are *different* responses according to the situation in which the child is involved. Piaget did find that many of the responses were qualitatively different from some that are characteristic of the ages of the children. This key observation resulted in a rejection of a quantitative definition (concept) of intelligence, one that is based essentially on the number of correct (expected) responses to a test item obtained from a representative population.

On the surface, this qualitative developmental approach in assessing any behavior seems to be incompatible with the widely used approach, following Dr. Binet, of assigning quantities (numbers) for elicited responses in carefully controlled testing situations. However, a proficient and confident clinical psychologist or language clinician does not set aside personal judgment merely for the sake of numbers. The psychologist or the language clinician may use both approaches, separately for some assessments and together for others. An unusual answer will not be deemed incorrect because it was not expected or because a given percentage of children of a given age, sex, cultural background, and so forth, did not provide a statistical basis for determining the acceptability of a response. The subjective observations of clinicians are at least as important as those that translate into numbers.

There are other reasons or positions for shying away from standardized assessments. In her book *Teaching Linguistically Handicapped Children*, Mildred Berry (1980) completely rejects the use of formal language assessment. Berry argues:

> Tests do not ferret out the problems the child has in comprehending or expressing his intentions and his dynamic interaction in oral communication with children in his environment. Instead, commercial tests evaluate isolated segments of language: the literal meaning of words and sentences, the comprehension of lexical items, the understanding of grammatical "rules." (p. 7–8)

Furthermore Berry (1980) emphasizes: "The essential aspects of oral language, however, are not appraised: The child's intention in oral communication, his sensorimotor actions surrounding the utterance, and his use of language in interacting with children (not adults) in a natural communicative environment" (p. 8).

Berry recommends the use of videotaping or audiotaping samples of children's language in a free and familiar environment while the children are engaged in a language task or activity. "Such a procedure allows the teaching team to study the use of oral language of children and their linguistic progress in the context of the communicative experience" (Berry, 1980, p. 8).

There are, of course, some limitations to this approach. Some children do little or no talking, and often these are the ones we are asked to assess. Other children turn off when they have any indication of being recorded. Moreover, no situation can pretend to be natural unless the recorder (the person) and the recording equipment are not visible and the usual routine is not changed.

However, there are nonstandardized approaches that permit us to make value judgments that deserve respect and application in our assessment inventories. Some of these are considered by Leonard, Prutting, Perozzi, and Berkley (1978).

MOTOR ASSESSMENT

In the assessment of the child with serious language delay, it is essential that we learn how the child is functioning motorically at the time of the evaluation. Specifically, it is necessary to know whether the child has the motor capabilities for speech production. Such asessment may be done, in part, by direct observation of the child's peripheral speech mechanism—the size and shape of the oral cavity and the articulatory organs, the arrangement of the jaws and teeth, and the ability of the child to elevate the tongue, move the tongue to positions within the mouth, and protrude the tip of the tongue outside of the mouth. Furthermore, the child should be tested for the ability to produce isolated and sequential articulatory movements at a rate approximating what is needed for speech. Observations of this sort may be made by a pediatrician, an otolaryngologist, or a speech and language clinician. Such observations may, in effect, reveal whether a child has oral apraxia and is therefore impaired for oral speech production.

Blakely (1980) assesses oral articulatory functioning in his *Screening Test for Developmental Apraxia of Speech*. Blakely's procedure is a rather rough instrument and may screen only the most severely impaired orally apraxic children.

Important additional information is provided by observations of the child's gross and fine body movements. The child's manner of walking, hopping, skipping, jumping, and so forth, the ability to balance on one foot, and the ability to throw and catch a ball or bean bag, or even to bounce a ball, provide information about eye-hand coordination as well as spatial orientation. Laterality development, which should include eye, foot, and ear preference as well as hand preference, is now an item of increased importance for language clinicians because of the correlations between the establishment of laterality preference, cerebral dominance, and language development. Information on current laterality preference may be obtained as part of the medical examination or as additional assessments by one of the other members of the evaluation team. Guided observations may be made through the use of specially devised tests, such as the Oseretsky Test of Motor Proficiency (Doll, 1947) and the Harris Tests of Lateral Dominance (Harris, 1955).

The Harris Tests of Lateral Dominance

The Harris (1955) Tests are in fact an inventory of procedures for assessing expressions of lateral preferences and so, by inference, of cerebral dominance. The inventory includes several items requiring that the examinee produce simultaneous and coordinated movements of both hands. The principle on which the Harris Tests are based is that when both hands attempt to perform the same movement simultaneously, the nonpreferred hand (Harris calls it "the non-dominant hand") tends to execute a mirrorwise or reverse action of the preferred hand. Hand preference, and so presumably cerebral dominance, is measured by the number of reversals or partial reversals made by either hand. Preference (dominance) is assessed on the basis of the number of reversals for the various acts involved. Young children, those below age 4 or 5, are not expected to be able to perform on all items of the Harris Tests. The intended age range is 7 to adult.

The Harris inventory does not yield a standard score, although trends in percentages are provided for ages 7 and above. The scoring system does provide a systematic basis for a clinician to arrive at a judgment about an examinee's laterality and so, presumably, about cerebral dominance for particular motor functions. Insofar as dominance for some functions may be correlated with cerebral dominance for language, the Harris Tests may be informative to a sophisticated speech and language clinician or psychologist.

The Oseretsky Test of Motor Proficiency

The Oseretsky Test (Doll, 1947) is a scale of six separate tests with separate items according to the subject's age. The scale measures general static coordination, dynamic coordination of the hands, general dynamic coordination, motor speech, simultaneous voluntary movements, and asynkinesia (ability to perform without overflow or superfluous movements).

SOCIAL DEVELOPMENT

The child's social development is another aspect of the psychological assessment. For most children, language acquisition and social maturity are intimately related. For children with severe language impairment, this relationship does not hold. Parents are the primary assessors of the child's social and emotional development. The Vineland Scale and the Preschool Attainment Record are basically questionnaire inventories that provide the interviewer with information to form judgments about the child's social development.

The Vineland Social Maturity Scale

This scale was designed to assess successive stages of social competence from infancy to adult life (Doll, 1965). In essence, it is a series of items arranged in age periods (levels). The informant provides the interviewer with information relative to aspects of motor and perceptual development in the early years and to social competence during adolescence and adult life. When applied to children, it affords a basis for developmental assessment. Items such as the child's ability to laugh, to imitate sounds (first level), and to name familiar objects (second level), as well as toilet habits (second and third levels), help the examiner arrive at clinical judgments about the child. The nature of the scale, which requires parental recall of the child's performances, lends itself to error. Parental reports may be compared with actual performances of the present status of the child to provide some insight into parental judgments. Although the scale is intended to yield a social quotient, the clinical implications about the specifics of what the child is or is not doing according to age expectancy are probably of greater importance.

The Preschool Attainment Record (PAR)

The PAR is intended as a supplement and extension of the Vineland Social Maturity Scale (Doll, 1966). Although the PAR has not been normatively standardized, the scale does permit comparisons of siblings within a family, or comparisons of the child with himself over periods of time. The PAR covers a range of half-year intervals from birth to 7 years for eight aspects of physical, social, and intellectual development—ambulation, manipulation, rapport, communication, responsibility, information, ideation, and creativity. The appraisal is conducted by interview with a parent or other informant who has dependable knowledge about the child's developmental history. The information thus obtained may be supplemented by direct observation of the child if he or she is available and accessible. A record form is provided for a summary and profile.

VISUAL-PERCEPTUAL AND PERCEPTUAL-MOTOR TESTS AND SCALES

Visual-perceptual and perceptual-motor tests have a long history. Their development and employment are related to the need to find tasks that can be administered to individuals who have a limited understanding of language or an impairment for the reception or production of oral language. Practically, visual tasks (the perception of visual events) can also be administered because, unlike auditory events, they are stable rather than ephemeral. The nature of the task performance required can be demonstrated, and the administration—the directions—can be given in pantomime. Several visual-perceptual tests are included in such scaled tests of intelligence as the Wechsler batteries, the Stanford-Binet (Terman and Merrill, 1960), and the Merrill-Palmer (Stutsman, 1949). This discussion will be confined to tests in frequent use.

The Bender Visual-Motor Gestalt Test

The Bender (1938) Visual-Motor Gestalt Test requires drawings by the subject to assess visual perception. The stimulus items are nine line-drawing figures presented one at a time to the subject for copying. Bender found that brain-damaged subjects perform in characteristically different ways (produce different kinds of figures and make different kinds of errors) from normal and emotionally disturbed subjects. It is essential, of course, that the clinician take into account any motor disability a child may have in the execution of the drawings. Some children who are unable to copy (reproduce) a satisfactory drawing may nevertheless show their perceptual competence in a match-to-sample (multiple-choice) situation, so that it is possible in clinical assessment to separate the visual-perceptual aspect of the task from the motor aspect and therefore to avoid an assumption that a distorted or different product necessarily represents the child's perception of the stimulus event. Only a clinical judgment can be derived from this procedure, however, because it departs from the one employed by Bender.

The Bender Test assumes that normal persons will perceive figures according to gestalt laws of perception and organization. Deviations, with due allowance for possible visual impairments and motor disabilities, are interpreted as indicators of abnormality. As indicated earlier, some deviations are interpreted as indicators of brain damage (organicity) and others of emotional disturbance.

Bender intended her test to be appropriate for an age range of from 4 years to adult. Norms for the assessment of young children have been developed by Koppitz (1964). Hutt (1969) published his adaptation of the Bender Gestalt Test. Hutt and Gibby (1970) provide a detailed scoring system and specific examples of scoring records for the adaptation.

The Developmental Test of Visual-Motor Integration (VMI)

The VMI consists of 24 geometric figures arranged in increasing degree of difficulty (complexity), each to be copied with pencil directly beneath the form (Beery, 1967). The test was designed primarily for children in the preschool and early primary grades. However, the author states that the VMI can be administered in the age range of 2 to 15 years. Scoring is done by comparing a child's production of the copied form with illustrations or by evaluating on the basis of stated criteria.

The VMI was devised "as a measure of the degree to which visual perception and motor behavior are integrated in young children." Beery believes that the geometric forms, unlike letter forms, "are equally familiar to children of varying backgrounds."

Beery (1967) found the VMI to have a higher correlation with mental age than with chronological age. However, on the basis of his gathered data for the VMI, he obtained a correlation of .89 for the 2- to 15-year age range. The correlations are higher for the first-grade children than for the older children. Age equivalents based on raw scores are provided in the administration and scoring manual.

Form Board Tests

There are several adaptations and variations of form board tests, based for the most part on the original Seguin form boards. The Arthur (1947) Point Scale includes adaptations of Seguin form boards as part of a scale of performance tests. These may be easily employed with children with severe language impairment. The Gesell Form Board, 1949, (Gesell and Amatruda 1957) is a revision of an earlier model developed at the Vineland Training School. The Gesell Form Board, 1952, (Gesell and Amatruda, 1957) is especially appropriate for younger children or for those suspected of being mentally retarded. It requires the insertion of three forms—a circle, a triangle, and a square—each approximately 3 inches in diameter, into an opening in a board.

As has been noted in regard to some other tests that were reasonably free of cultural influence when initially produced, many form boards have become puzzle games for young children. Experience, therefore, may influence results, especially if time for solution is a factor in scoring.

Block-Design Tests

Wechsler, among others, includes block-design tasks as part of his performance scales. The original Kohs (1923) block designs included figures (designs) made up with the colors red, yellow, blue, and white. Modifications such as Wechsler's reduce the colors used to red and white and use relatively simple designs.

Block-design tasks require that the subject be able to perceive a pattern or design of different colors as a gestalt or whole configuration, to analyze the pattern into component parts, and to reproduce the pattern, presented on a card, with an arrangement of colored blocks.

The standard method for administering the block-design tests is to present a card with the design—the stimulus item—and several colored blocks. The examinee is expected to arrange the blocks so that the result (the top colors on the blocks) reproduces the design. The procedure should be illustrated once or more for the subject. If the subject fails, it is recommended that a block arrangement rather than a card be used for reproduction—that is, copying. If this is done successfully, the card design should be tried again, with a second demonstration.

In testing young children, it is recommended that only simple designs be used and that the colors be limited to two, as in the Wechsler (1974) Intelligence Scale for Children and the Wechsler (1967) Preschool and Primary Scale of Intelligence.

Other tests of visual perception that are included in many general inventories of intelligence include the ability to draw a cross, a square, or a diamond.

Knox Cube Imitation Test (Grace Arthur Modification)

The Knox cube test calls for the imitation of a sequence of block-tapping movements on four blocks (Arthur, 1947). The test begins with a sequence of two taps (1-4) and progresses finally to a sequence of seven taps (4-1-3-4-2-1-4). The test can be administered with verbal directions—"Now you do what I did"—or by imitation without verbal direction. It constitutes a basis for assessing visual sequencing through a simple motor response. This test is included in the Arthur (1947) Point Scale of Performance Tests, Revised Form II.

Frostig Developmental Test of Visual Perception

The Frostig Test is designed to assess five operationally defined visual-perceptual functions: visual-motor coordination, figure-ground perception, perceptual constancy (the perception of invariant properties such as shape, size, and position despite the variability of sensory impressions), position in space, and spatial relationships (Frostig, Lefever, and Whittlesley, 1964).

By this inventory, according to the authors, a clinician can chart a child's strengths and weaknesses in visual perception and thereby constitute the basis for a remedial program.

As a diagnostic instrument, the Frostig Test is intended to be helpful in directing attention to possible visual-perceptual impairments or delays in children of primary school age. However, the clinician must be certain that the child understands the task necessary for an appropriate performance.

General Comment on Visual-Motor Perceptual Tests

Is visual perceptual functioning directly or even indirectly related to an individual's ability for perception of the kinds of auditory events that constitute spoken language? Visual perception and visual sequencing, functions that are assumed to be assessed by the instruments just considered, are obviously incompatible with blindness. Nevertheless, the blind, as a total population, have no conspicuous difficulties in learning to speak. It may be that visual-perceptual functioning is correlated with general intelligence, and this with the capacity for language acquisition. If this is so, then tests of visual perception are measures of whatever contributes to general intelligence, rather than assessments of functions that are specific to language.

AUDIOLOGICAL ASSESSMENT

Routine audiometric evaluation is only a small part of what we need to learn from the audiologist in regard to the hearing and listening capacities of the linguistically delayed or impaired child, and particularly the aphasic child. Many such children are known to have some degree of hearing loss, as determined by routine audiometry. Unless such hearing loss is moderately severe or severe (above 60 dB in the crucial pitch range), a report that is restricted to results of pure-tone signal assessment is of limited value. What we need to know is the child's reception for speech and the ability to perceive and to discriminate speech signals, vowels, consonants, and syllable combinations of vowels and consonants in a variety of environmental conditions. We also need to know whether the child responds to a signal when it is initially presented and then adapts and ceases to respond on the second or third presentation of the same signal. Furthermore, we need to know whether there is any evidence of perceptual deafness to some types of signals but not to others. If, for example, the audiologist obtains a reliable threshold of response for a pure-tone signal but an inconsistent response to speech signals, we are provided with information about the child's capacity for listening as well as for hearing.

Additional assessment is needed of the child's ability to sequence a series of speech signals—for example, to determine not only the child's auditory memory span for consonant-vowel (CV) combinations but also the ability to keep the order of the phonemic presentations in mind so that he or she can discriminate between a CV combination versus a second combination of consonant-vowel or vowel-consonant. The number of phonemes a child can process correctly, through either a matching or, if the child is capable of it, an oral reproduction, helps shed light on what the auditory perceptual abilities of the child may be and provides a basis for deciding where training should begin.

The audiologist cannot expect to assess a child suspected of being aphasic or more generally severely linguistically impaired as quickly as is usually possible with most other children. The audiologist must anticipate the need for some conditioning training as well as for teaching the child how to respond to the presented auditory stimuli. The audiologist must be patient, resourceful, seductive, and yet firm in getting the child-patient involved in the task of assessment. As for all other members of the evaluation team, the audiologist needs to report not only the results obtained but also the conditions under which they were obtained. Clinical observations and judgments are as important as objective findings.

The audiological evaluation for a child with severe language delay should provide the clinician with information about the subject's presumed ability to receive a variety of auditory signals, especially those for speech. Reception and perception (phonemic discrimination and sequencing for the kinds of auditory events that constitute speech) are more informative and thus more important than responses to pure tone signals. Environmental conditions that may be controlled by the audiologist, such as competing noises (ambient sounds, airplane or truck noises, signal-to-noise ratios), provide information about the circumstances that impair listening and therefore have implications for speech comprehension. Essentially, what clinicians need to learn in order to plan their intervention strategies is whether a child has auditory difficulties that include or go beyond simple acuity in responding to an auditory signal.

Auditory Discrimination and Perception

Normal language acquisition requires the ability to process signals that are received by our distance receptors—our eyes and ears. The unique character of speech signals and the knowledge we now have about the processing of such signals by the central nervous system are still so meager and limited that we cannot yet expect to have reliable tools and measurements for the assessment of perceptual functions that may underlie speech perception. Tests such as digit span, which is included in most inventories or scales for the assessment of intelligence, are obviously not relevant in the evaluation of a truly nonverbal child. Children with some language ability may be assessed with such items as digit span, nonsense syllable span, and the widely used Wepman test. Each is, in effect, a procedure that measures immediate recall for an auditory event or series of events. Auditory perception will again be considered in our review of assessment procedures for articulation.

Several procedures intended to address this area of auditory processing will be considered. As a preliminary general observation, many of the instruments and procedures would benefit from continued field testing and validation. Some procedures may be regarded as first-order attempts to respond to a recognized assessment need; these tests have found publishers before they themselves were sufficiently tested to meet recognized criteria of validity and reliability.

The Goldman-Fristoe-Woodcock Auditory
Selective Attention Test*

This test is intended to measure the ability of an individual to attend to a listening task (situation) in the presence of a competing noise (Goldman, Fristoe, and Woodcock, 1976). The competing (distracting) sound (noise) is systematically controlled so as to vary in intensity level and type (human voice, ambient cafeteria noise, moving fan). The initial items are presented without a competitive noise.

The test task requires that the examinee point to appropriate pictures (one of four) according to recorded instructions. The test compares a subject's correct responses with basic data from an experimental population, age range 3 to 80 years. Most of the data were generated from a population of children from 3 to 12 years of age. Presumably, therefore, the test has relevant implications for the assessment of children who are identified as linguistically delayed as well as for most children in the same age range.

Leach (1979), in his evaluation of this procedure for auditory inattention, states: "The authors present some preliminary validity data that suggest that the instrument is sensitive to some types of communication problems. However, the validity of the instrument is still in question until sufficient numbers of clinicians and sufficient research data establish it as a sensitive index for auditory selective problems. These data are yet to be collected" (pp. 148–149).

The Goldman-Fristoe-Woodcock Test
of Auditory Discrimination (G-F-W TAD)*

The G-F-W TAD is a rather widely used instrument designed to assess speech-sound discrimination under favorable (quiet) conditions and controlled noise (Goldman, Fristoe, and Woodcock, 1970). It is intended for use with subjects aged 3 years 8 months to older adults.

The test task, to which each examinee is first trained, calls for pointing to appropriate pictures (one of four) for associated words presented by tape recording. Each associated word is one syllable in length, either consonant-vowel-consonant or consonant-vowel. Each picture plate has two items for which associations are to be made by pointing. In essence, the G-F-W TAD assesses 'auditory discrimination by a pointing response that reflects recognition memory. Vetter (1979), commenting on the test, says: "The Quiet Subtest and Noise Subtest permit auditory discrimination under ideal listening conditions as well as under more real-life listening conditions. In general the test appears to have content or face validity" (p. 160). Test results yield scores that may be transformed into percentile or standard scores by comparison with normative tables supplied in the test manual.

Vetter (1979) suggests that clinical data other than those provided by the authors of the G-F-W TAD need to be collected and made available for critical examination so that the test can be better evaluated. He states: "If it is used as a test of an individual subject's auditory discrimination ability, interpretation should be made with caution" (p. 160).

In his review of widely used tests for auditory (speech-sound) discrimination, Locke (1980) makes a general observation of procedures that employ pictures to assess phonemic perception: "The major problem with picture tests, one which makes them practically useless for most clinical purposes, is that most production-relevant contrasts cannot easily be represented with pictures." Research by Snow (1963) cited by Locke shows that "only three of the 36 most commonly confused contrasts are tested, even though the test uses four pictures per trial instead of two."

To generalize from Locke's observation, most tests that purport to evaluate phonemic discrimination fail to assess the kinds of phonemic errors that children tend to produce and so possibly to perceive as they mature in their control of the sounds of their language. Whatever the instruments do test may be of much less import and significance than what they fail to measure.

The Wepman Auditory Discrimination Test*

The Wepman (1973) Auditory Discrimination Test (ADT) is included in the author's battery for assessing perceptual behavior. The ADT consists of 40 single-syllable word pairs, 10 of which are identical (e.g., *ball-ball*) and 30 of which differ by a single phoneme (e.g., *bum-bun*). The subject is asked to indicate whether the pairs are the same or different. The score is based on the number of correct responses to the syllable (word) pairs. Each word pair is equated for length to avoid the possibility of a discrimination response on the basis of span (length) rather than audition.

The ADT has two equated forms to permit retesting after a short period following an initial evaluation or for a second testing if the examiner believes that the responses to the first may have been inappropriate.

The ADT is not an exception among the several auditory tests that fail to consider and sample the sound feature contrasts of the speech sounds of our language. Thus, the question of validity is raised. Wepman, aware of such reservation in regard to the ADT, presents evidence in the manual of improvement in test results correlated with age in the 5- to 8-year range.

The ADT is used as a screening instrument for children who have or may have problems in language acquisition, articulation, and reading. It is unclear whether the nature of the test or some coincidental but not identified feature gives it the value Wepman and others attribute to it. Locke (1979) concludes his evaluation of the ADT with the statement: "Individual clinicians may decide for themselves, as they always have, whether they wish to use the test in the service of their clients."

The Auditory Sequential Memory Test (ASMT)

The premise of the ASMT (Wepman and Morency, 1975), as stated in the manual, is that "the ability to recall the exact order of an auditory stimulus is a unique aspect of perceptual auditory memory." The authors employ digit span—the number of digits a child can repeat in order of presentation immediately after hearing them. The position taken by Wepman and Morency is that sequential-order recall of digits is perceptual in nature "because it simply requires repetition without meaning attached." This test is as strong or as weak as its premise and its related assumption that sequential reproduction of digits is a perceptual and presumably noncognitive function. Furthermore, this process is presumed to be important in speech accuracy, syntactic proficiency, phonic reading, written language, and mathematics.

Digits are presented at the rate of one per half-second for test spans of from two to eight digits. Each span has two series of numbers. A span response is correct if a child succeeds on either series. A response is incorrect if there is an error of omission, addition, or production in an order not presented by the examiner.

In their manual, Wepman and Morency (1975) state: "Children who show auditory imperception, whether in sequencing, discrimination or memory should be given special consideration." Furthermore, they recommend: "Whenever this specific auditory imperception—sequential memory—is discovered, the other auditory perceptual functions should be studied and the auditory modality as a whole given special attention."

Perhaps future research will determine whether the claims for the findings and implications of the ASMT are justified. As of now, it would seem best to accept the test for what it is—a simple test of auditory sequential memory for a span of digits. Such a subtest is part of the most widely used batteries for assessing intelligence. Along this line, Wepman and Morency (1975) observe: "Where judgment about a child's intelligence or his achievement is based on auditory instruction, there may be a need to re-interpret the results obtained by such testing. School psychologists and classroom teachers should recognize the effect of auditory imperception of any kind on the reliability of assessments where instructions are given orally."

TESTS AND SCALES FOR COGNITIVE AND INTELLECTUAL ASSESSMENT

With due awareness of the limitations of formal testing, as indicated in the preceding discussion, we will present some published tests, test inventories, and scales that are in fairly wide use for young school-age children. Emphasis will be on instruments that may help a teacher or clinician of linguistically retarded children arrive at judgments of surface deficiencies and, more important, of possible underlying problems. The published instruments are by no means intended to be all-inclusive of what is presently available. They are instruments with which we have had some experience in the related responsibilities of a speech and language clinician, a clinical psychologist, and an administrator of speech and language clinics. Noninclusion of any assessment procedure should not be interpreted as having a negative implication; neither should the inclusion of a given test or scale constitute a positive recommendation for its use.

The Boehm Test of Basic Concepts (BTBC)*

The Boehm (1971) Test employs pictures that are designed primarily to assess young children's (ages 5–7) mastery of concepts that the author believes to be essential for understanding oral communication in kindergarten and first grade. Boehm considers her test to be appropriate as well for second-grade children who may be socially disadvantaged.

The BTBC is a screening device for cognitive functioning that enables a teacher and clinician to determine where a child is cognitively and what a given child may need to be taught to function on age-grade level. The BTBC, available in two alternative forms for the same concepts, is a standardized instrument and is adequately reliable. Norms are provided in percentages and percentiles for grades and socioeconomic levels. Directions for test administration are also available in Spanish.

The BTBC is not an appropriate instrument for children with severe language delay. It is appropriate for children who may have difficulty in learning in classroom situations, presumably because of underlying cognitive deficits and associated lack of language proficiency. To the degree that this presumption may have merit, and with due regard for the possibility that discovered deficits may not in fact be expressions of cultural differences, the BTBC is a useful instrument.

Wechsler Scales

David Wechsler was the author of several test scales for the assessment of the intelligence of children and adults. Only those scales standardized on populations of children will be reviewed here. All of the Wechsler scales have a common feature, in that each is, in effect, two separate tests—one to measure verbal intelligence (verbal directions as well as verbal responses required) and one to measure performance intelligence (instructions may be verbal or by gesture, but responses call for a performance) without associated oral language. Full scale intelligence quotients are a product of combining the results of the two parts of the scale.

In the test standardizations, Dr. Wechsler was aware of the possible effects of cultural differences and cultural bias. Although no assessment instrument can ever completely avoid some degree of injustice to some segment of a population, the Wechsler tests probably do as well as any published assessment instrument. All of the Wechsler tests are based on scaled scores for each age level, rather than on a hypothetical mental age, as in the Terman-Merrill revisions of the Stanford-Binet Test.

The Wechsler (1967) Preschool and Primary Scale of Intelligence (WPPSI) is intended for children in the age range of 4 to 6½ years. This scale includes five verbal subtests plus one alternate and five performance test items. The verbal test items are obviously inappropriate for children who are severely linguistically impaired. The performance items, especially those that can employ gestures or imitation for administration, are more appropriate for the population with which this book is concerned.

Some of the subtests are also found in Wechsler's (1974) WISC and in other test batteries. These test items have been adapted, however, for use with children aged 4 to 6½ years.

The WPPSI and the other Wechsler test scales have enjoyed wide use among psychologists who accept the usefulness of intelligence tests as a valid indicator of functioning levels of intelligence. Whether the WPPSI or any other test can in fact predict or prognosticate whether a given child has or will have the capacity "to understand and cope with the world"—and how well—may still need some time for resolution.

The Wechsler (1974) Intelligence Scale for Children, Revised (WISC-R), is intended for children and adolescents in the age range 6 years to 16 years 11 months. The standardization sample was based on the proportion of white and nonwhite children in the 1970 census. The standardization results obviously may vary somewhat according to changes in the proportions of population since 1970.

The WISC-R yields verbal and performance IQs based on scaled scores for each of ten tests and two alternate tests if needed. Our comments for the WPPSI hold also for the WISC-R. The performance items of the WISC-R have been standardized for deaf children (Anderson and Sisco, 1977).

The Merrill-Palmer Scale (MPS)

The MPS (Stutsman, 1949) is one of the older test scales for preschool children (ages 2 to 5 years). Most of the test items can be administered by pantomime or by example. The MPS uses simple form boards, puzzles, and pictures as well as tasks calling for manual dexterity (e.g., cutting with scissors). Some language items, such as questions, call for simple comprehension of everyday events (e.g., "What does a kitty say?") Others call for imitation (repetition) of words or phrases.

At the time of initial standardization (1931), most of the test items were considered culture-free. Contemporary children who are not culturally under-privileged are likely to have considerable experience with the test items as games. This experience assumes special significance because many of the items have time limits for successful scoring. The scale is not appropriate for children with manual-motor problems.

If scored in keeping with instructions for administration, the MPS yields mental ages and percentile ranks. If administered to help a clinician arrive at a clinical judgment of a child's approximate intellectual potential, the MPS is a useful instrument.

NONVERBAL TESTS FOR ASSESSMENTS OF INTELLECTUAL FUNCTIONING

The Porteus Maze (PM) Test

The Porteus (1965) Maze Test is, in effect, a series of tests (initial tests and extensions for retesting) designed to assess mental ability through a nonverbal approach. The basic inventory employs 12 mazes of increasing degree of difficulty for solution. The test task (problem) requires that the subject find the way out of a maze diagram, using a pencil to show the path taken for the solution. The PM may be used for children in the age range 3 to 12 years. A manual published in 1965 includes directions for administration and scoring.

Use of the PM assumes that the child can see the test item (no visual problem) and can hold and control a pencil or other marker to indicate the solution. Because the mazes are abstract and not eye-catching, they may not interest young children. Motivation may therefore be a problem that examiners should anticipate.

The Raven Coloured Progressive Matrices (CPM)

There are several Raven nonverbal inventories intended for retarded and non-English–speaking persons in ages ranging from 5 years upward to older adults. One of these inventories, the CPM (Raven, 1962), was initially published in 1947 for a population from 5 to 11 years old. The CPM assesses mental ability through the use of colored pictures and designs. The test items call for a solution of a visual-perceptual problem by arranging pieces to create pictures or designs. The tests become increasingly abstract and difficult in the upper levels.

Raven's norms and percentile scores are based on a British population. It is suggested that the examiner be mindful of the possibility, if not the likelihood, that some of the test items are much like those that have become puzzle games for many children and so are not free of cultural influences.

The Hiskey-Nebraska Test (HNT) of Learning Aptitude

The Hiskey-Nebraska Test (Hiskey, 1966) was designed to assess children with severe oral-language problems, including the deaf. The HNT has an age range of 3 to 16 years. All test items are nonverbal and thus do not require either verbal comprehension or production. The test yields a learning age rather than an IQ.

The Leiter International Performance Scale (LIPS)

The LIPS (Leiter, 1948) has a rather broad age range (2 to 18 years). The scale items in the tests to be administered first call only for perceptual matching. Later test items require higher mental processes, including analogy and application of a principle, to complete a sequence of forms. The testing directions may be given through pantomime or in simple language. No language is required for response to the directions.

The LIPS is a useful instrument for assessing the cognitive potential of nonverbal children. Our experience suggests that IQs derived from this scale are considerably more reliable for children above age 5 or 6 than for younger ones.

The Columbia Mental Maturity Scale (CMMS)

The CMMS is intended for children in the age range of 3 years 6 months to 10 years (Burgemeister, Blum, and Lorge, 1972). The test items are three or more geometric forms or pictures on rectangular cardboards, each 6 by 19 inches. The scale has 92 items arranged in eight overlapping levels. The initial level is determined by the child's chronological age. (We would recommend one level below the age level, except, of course, for younger children.). Directions for the CMMS may be given through pantomime. The only response required is for the child to point to the correct time. Correctness involves a decision as to which geometric form or picture does not belong with the other two or more representations on the cardboards.

Because neither administration nor response calls for language, the CMMS is particularly suitable for nonverbal children or for children who speak a language other than the examiner's. The scale is also suitable for deaf and motorically handicapped children.

The CMMS provides age deviation, percentile, and stanine scores. Norms for this scale were obtained by testing a national sample according to sex, parental occupation, and geographic area. Its ease of administration and applicability for the nonverbal, as well as its reliability, make the CMMS one of the better instruments for assessing the intellectual potential of preschool children.

MODALITY TESTS FOR FUNCTIONS RELATED TO LANGUAGE

The Illinois Test of Psycholinguistic Abilities (ITPA)*

Since its publication, the ITPA has been one of the most widely used inventories for assessing children with developmental disabilities, including the mentally retarded and those who are linguistically delayed (Kirk, McCarthy, and Kirk, 1968). Lately, the ITPA has been criticized for the types of subtests used, the rationale for what is included, its failure to measure what it purports to measure, its failure to indicate clearly what is meant by psycholinguistic abilities, and the failure of the various subtests to assess subprocesses of whatever the psycholinguistic abilities are supposed to be. (See Prutting, 1979, for a critical review of the ITPA and Kirk and Kirk, 1978, for a response to recent criticisms.)

The ITPA was intended by the authors as an evaluation instrument for young children. Norms are provided for the age range of 2½ to 10 years. The authors hold, however, that the greatest usefulness of the ITPA is for children in the 4- to 8-year age range because "the norms at both extremes were obtained to increase the ceiling for eight year olds or to show a deficit for three and four year olds" (Kirk and Kirk, 1978, p. 60).

Kirk et al. (1968) emphasize that their test is intended to be a clinical indicator to help in determining differential abilities and disabilities among cognitive, perceptual, and memory functions in young children, preferably those in the 4- to 8-year age range. They caution: "One of its greatest abuses is to consider it a solution to all problems and to use scores as a final diagnosis instead of another possible aid to clinical judgment" (Kirk and Kirk, 1978, pp. 60–61).

They postulate three dimensions of cognitive ability as a model for their approach:

1. *Channels of communication:* These are the routes or sensory modalities "through which the content of communication flows." The ITPA deals specifically with the auditory and visual input modalities; the tests of the ITPA assess for expression of input through the auditory-vocal, auditory-motor, visual-motor, and visual-vocal approaches.

2. *Psycholinguistic processes:* Three main processes are considered in analyzing the child's language acquisition: (a) the receptive process, or the ability of the child to recognize and understand what has been presented orally; (b) the expressive process, or the skills requisite to the expression of ideas by either vocal (oral) or visible (gesture) performance; and (c) the "organizing process which involves the internal manipulation of percepts, concepts, and linguistic symbols. It is a central mediating process elicited by the receptive process and preceding the expressive process.

3. *Levels of organization:* These are determined by the degree "to which habits of communication are organized within the individual. . . ." The ITPA model postulates two levels: (a) the representational, which calls upon the established complex mediating process of utilizing symbols (verbal mediation) that "carry the meaning of an object," and (b) the automatic level, which calls upon less voluntary but highly automatic functions. Automatic functions or expressions of a "chain of responses" are involved in activities such as visual and auditory closure, speed of perception, ability to reproduce a sequence presented visually or orally, rote learning, the synthesizing of isolated sounds into words, and utilizing (applying) the redundancies of experience. In essence, whether the test item is visual or auditory, the child is required on the

basis of presumed exposure and experience to identify an event—for example, an object partially concealed—or to complete a verbal expression. Auditory-sequential memory is tested by digit span, with digits presented at half-second intervals. Visual sequencing is tested by requiring the child to reproduce an arrangement of nonmeaningful figures (chips) after a 5-second exposure.

In response to current criticism that the ITPA is not, in fact, a psycholinguistic instrument, Kirk and Kirk (1978) explain:

> The ITPA was designed as a diagnostic test to delineate intraindividual variations in functioning in those areas involved in language and other forms of communication. We called it a psycholinguistic test because it was concerned with psychological functions of information processing, perception, and memory as well as the use of linguistic codes. The term may not now be an adequate designation of the test, but it was suitable in 1961 before linguists developed their own use of the term. (p. 60)

In regard to the population and intended function of the ITPA, Kirk and Kirk (1978) emphasize:

> The functions it tests are designed to denote deficits that require remediation. If the child has difficulty in communication because he cannot translate the code used in spoken language, that is, if he does not understand auditory language (receptive aphasia), then a remedial program should be organized to teach him to understand language. If he is delayed in talking (expressive aphasia), he should be taught techniques for expressing himself verbally. If he has a deficiency on a number of auditory vocal tests and is average or above on visual motor tests, remediation should be organized to improve the whole range of auditory vocal abilities. Furthermore, if the child has superior abilities in some functions, they should be used to develop parallel abilities in the deficient areas. (p. 60)

When the revised ITPA was published, its authors believed:

> The psycholinguistic model on which the ITPA is based attempts to relate those functions whereby the intentions of an individual are transmitted (verbally or nonverbally) to another individual and reciprocally, functions whereby the environment or the intentions of another individual are received and interpreted. (ITPA Examiner's Manual, p. 7)

More space has been given here to the ITPA than to the other assessment approaches because, despite its serious limitations, it continues to be one of the most frequently used tests available to speech and language clinicians. If used appropriately, with all the proscriptions and prescriptions of the Kirk and Kirk (1978) article "The Uses and Abuses of the ITPA," the test will have continued but more restricted use. This use may be more in keeping with the initially intended use of the instrument—to identify functional areas of strengths and weaknesses of children who are regarded as mentally retarded. The ITPA may be useful in assessing children with a moderate amount of linguistic delay, but not children who are seriously delayed in comprehension or production of language. For whomever it is used, we agree with Prutting (1979), who states: "This test should be used only as a supplement to accurate observation of any given child in a variety of communicative settings in which the need to communicate is maintained" (p. 165). This same observation is relevant, of course, to the use of any test or assessment procedure.

RECEPTIVE LANGUAGE TESTS AS MEASURES OF INTELLECTUAL FUNCTIONING

The Full-Range Picture Vocabulary Test (FRPVT)

The FRPVT assesses receptive (comprehension) vocabulary through the use of line drawings (pictures) on cards (Ammons and Ammons, 1958). The task calls for the child to point to one of four drawings appropriate to the key word presented by the examiner. The FRPVT has two forms to permit reassessment or continued evaluation in the event that the examiner believes the first testing session was not indicative of the subject's ability. The age range is 2 years through adult level.

The authors view their test as an instrument to determine intelligence based on verbal (vocabulary) comprehension. It is best, however, to think of the FRPVT as a measure of approximating receptive vocabulary. Unfortunately, because the test has not been revised since its publication, the pictures and some of the key words are not as representative as they might be for a contemporary population of children or young adults.

The Peabody Picture Vocabulary Test (PPVT-R)

The PPVT-R is a revision of the widely used Peabody Picture Vocabulary Test, intended for an age range of 2½ years through adult (Dunn and Dunn, 1981). Like its predecessors, the PPVT-R has two forms, L and M. Administration calls for the examiner to point to one of four pictures on a page that is appropriate to the verbal instruction. The authors state: "The PPVT-R is designed primarily to measure a subject's receptive (hearing) vocabulary for Standard American English."

A second function is "to provide a quick estimate of one major aspect of verbal ability for subjects who have grown up in a standard English-speaking environment. In this sense, it is a scholastic aptitude test." The authors acknowledge that the PPVT-R is not a comprehensive test of general intelligence, but it does measure vocabulary, an important facet of general intelligence. The Dunns caution that performance on a vocabulary test should not be equated with innate or fixed ability.

The PPVT-R manual provides raw scores and standard score equivalents, by age as well as percentile, and stanine scores that correspond to standard score equivalents.

It is apparent that the authors of the PPVT-R are aware of the limitations of their test for assessing subjects who do not speak or who have not been exposed primarily to standard American English.

Dunn and Dunn (1981) provide some words of caution in the use, interpretation, and implications of assessment with the PPVT-R:

> Ironically, the same characteristics that make the PPVT-R appealing—its convenience, its shortness, and its simplicity—can also be serious limitations if they result in casual administration and scoring. More importantly, examiners run the danger of overgeneralizing from a screening device that measures only hearing vocabulary, which is just one aspect of the complex linguistic and cognitive domains. Instead, this test should be seen only as suggesting the level of present functioning of a person, leading to a comprehensive study of the individual, or as part of a test battery. (p. 4)

From our point of view, the greatest value of the PPVT-R is that the instrument requires either pointing or a simple gesture of "yes" or "no" (if the examiner does the pointing) to arrive at a level of word comprehension (receptive vocabulary). Thus, the PPVT-R can be used as an approximation of the extent of linguistic retardation in children who may be seriously delayed in language or, because of a motoric problem, impaired in their ability to indicate what they may know, at least minimally, of language. Obviously, the PPVT-R is a guide to where more extensive assessment should begin.

The Preschool Language Scale (PLS)

The PLS appears to be modeled after the Stanford-Binet scales in that a basal age is determined at a level at which a child passes all test items, and testing continues until a level at which all items are failed (Zimmerman, Steiner, and Evatt, 1969). A value in months (the value varying with the age level) is given for each correct response. Again, in the manner of determining IQs on the Stanford-Binet, a language quotient is determined by dividing the total earned age scored by the child's chronological age.

The PLS is, in effect, two tests—one for assessing auditory comprehension (CA) and the second for productive verbal ability (VA). The two can be combined into a single "language age" by determining the average of the CA + VA.

Auditory comprehension tasks call for the child to follow an instruction that does not require expressive verbalization (pointing to a picture or part of a picture). Verbal comprehension tasks require that the child identify something or respond to an instruction verbally (e.g., providing names for six animals).

The age range covered in the PLS is from 1.5 to 7 years; thus, children who are delayed in language development can be assessed. We consider it especially important for such children, and preschool children, to have their auditory comprehension evaluated separately from their verbal production.

AUDITORY COMPREHENSION OF LANGUAGE STRUCTURE

The Assessment of Children's Language Comprehension (ACLC), Revised Edition*

The ACLC (Foster, Giddan, and Stark, 1973) is intended to assess the comprehension of syntactic units of children in the age range of 3 through 7 years. The test is based on three related assumptions derived from the authors' experience with linguistically retarded children:

1. Language learning progresses from the simple to the complex.
2. Linguistically retarded children are likely to have short auditory memory spans.
3. As a result of the restraints imposed by short auditory memory spans, most linguistically retarded children are not proficient processors of what they hear.

The ACLC employs a vocabulary of 50 common words, including nouns, verb forms, prepositions, and modifiers. Each critical word is illustrated on a card that contains five different pictures. The initial task (Part A of the test) calls for the child to point to the appropriate picture according to the verbal direction of the examiner—for example, "Show me the _____."

Parts B, C, and D of the ACLC call for the child to point to the appropriate picture according to verbal directions that incorporate a number of critical elements that increase from two to four. A critical element is a grammatical unit.

The first level tests single words that may be used as nouns, progressive verb forms, prepositions, and modifiers. The second level introduces two critical items. A correct response is intended to reveal the child's understanding of the relationship of the items—for instance, "cat walking" in a display that includes a cat walking, a cat sitting, a man sitting, and a horse walking. The third level includes three critical items, with the addition of a preposition, such as "ball under the table." At the four-critical-element level, the sentence types represent expanded noun phrases and agent-action relationships, such as "happy little girl jumping" and "cat standing under the bed." Through the critical element approach, the authors intend to assess (1) the child's receptive vocabulary for common words, (2) the number of critical elements (information words) the child can process, and (3) the pattern in the breakdown (failures) of critical sequences.

The 1973 edition of the ACLC provides norms based on the responses of 365 children in the 3- to 6.5-year age range. The ACLC has been found to be a useful clinical instrument in differentiating linguistically retarded children from normal children. Nevertheless, the test has been criticized for rather weak standardization and a lack of supporting statistical data for its norms or strong evidence of validity (Longhurst, 1979). Our own experience with it has been positive. The ACLC is a useful, relatively quick test (about 15 minutes) to administer. Nevertheless, it is not at all certain whether, for many children, it is verbal memory rather than syntactical proficiency that is being assessed.

The Northwestern Syntax Screening Test (NSST)

The NSST is intended, as the name implies, as a quick screening instrument to identify children "who are sufficiently delayed in syntactic development to warrant further study" (Lee, 1969, 1970). The NSST assesses both receptive and productive (expressive) use of syntactic forms, using identical linguistic structures in both parts of the test.

Receptive items are tested by having the child point to pictures that correspond to a presented statement (e.g., "Show me *the cat is under the chair*," "Now show me *the cat is behind the chair*").

Expressive items are tested by adding the task of expression to the initial task of reception. The instructions call for the examiner to present the pictures by saying something along this line: "I will tell you about these pictures. When I am done, you copy me. Say just what I say. Don't talk until I tell you. Ready?" The examiner then shows the first page of pictures and says, "*The baby is sleeping. The baby is not sleeping.* Now, what's this picture?" The examiner points to the key picture, *the baby is sleeping,* and waits for the child to reply; then the examiner points to the other picture and waits for a reply.

The task for the expressive items is essentially that of *elicited imitation,* with pictures used as a visual reinforcement. The scores are based on correct verbatim imitation of sentences or on responses that, though not verbatim reproductions, "accomplish the grammatical test item but which alter the sentence insignificantly and preserve grammatical correctness." The examiner should note all errors of omission or modification of the presented sentence.

Percentile ratings for receptive and expressive items are provided based on a population of 242 children ranging in age between 3 years and 7 to 11 years. The children came from middle- and upper-class communities and from homes where a standard American dialect was spoken. According to the manual for the NSST, "Any child whose score is below the 10th percentile would warrant further study and a consideration for a remedial language training program, unless his performance in other language areas were satisfactory." The test author emphasizes that "it is important that the examiner consider this test a screening instrument only and not a detailed analysis of a child's syntactic skill."

In reply to criticism, Lee (1977) admitted that the norms for the NSST are of doubtful value for children beyond age 6 years, 11 months. The test should be limited to children whose dominant language exposure is to standard American-English.

It appears that the NSST is an early experimental approach to a new kind of language-assessment procedure. It is limited to assessment of syntax. With a larger and broader population sampling, which should result in revised norms and percentile scores, the value of the NSST should increase. At present, it does have merit in providing a clinician with material for arriving at a guided judgment about a child's comprehension and performance relative to a number of syntactic formulations that differ in level and complexity.

The NSST is not intended for children of preschool age who are severely retarded in language acquisition. It is intended as a screening instrument for children who will require further assessment to complete their evaluation.

The Test for Auditory Comprehension of Language (TACL)*

The TACL (Carrow, 1973) is another widely used instrument intended to assess a child's auditory comprehension of language (vocabulary and linguistic constructions). The test consists of a set of cards, each of which contains three black-and-white line drawings. The drawings are designed to "represent referential categories and contrasts that can be signaled by form classes and function words, morphological constructions, grammatical categories, and syntactic structure." The child indicates his or her response by pointing to one of three line drawings on the stimulus card. There are 101 card plates. A briefer version of the TACL, recommended only as a screening test, consists of 25 items. Both tests are available in English and Spanish versions for populations of children in the 3 through 6 age range.

The test items for the TACL are arranged by grammatical category, so that all items in each category must be presented before proceeding to the next. Carrow reports that, when so administered, the TACL requires about 20 to 30 minutes.

The manual for the TACL provides norms for children aged 3 through 6 from a middle-class socioeconomic background, so that comparisons based on these norms and percentile ratings can be determined. The types (classes) of errors a child makes afford information that makes it possible to plan a language therapy program.

The TACL manual does not provide separate norms for girls and boys. This is a limited reservation in the light of the once commonly held assumption that girls in the age range of this intended test population are ahead of boys in overall language proficiency. A second reservation is based on the population—economic middle class—on which the TACL was standardized. Overall, this test seems to deserve its wide acceptance and use as an assessment instrument for determining the auditory comprehension of linguistically retarded children.

The Carrow Elicited Language Inventory (CELI)*

Testing the use of elicited imitation—the repetition or attempted imitation of a linguistic structure presented by an adult—is based on the assumption that such production will reveal a child's proficiency in language (Carrow, 1974). This assumption is derived from findings, such as those of Brown and Fraser (1963), that in the range of 25 to 35 months, children's repetitions (imitations) of presented adult sentences have the same mean number of words and the same syntactic character as their spontaneous utterances. Somewhat older children (those between 37 and 43 months), however, were found by Fraser, Bellugi and Brown (1963) to be able to imitate sentences that they could not comprehend. In using elicited imitation for the assessment of syntax in children under 3 years of age, and for children with severe language delay, we need not be concerned with the matter of production without comprehension. Our assumption is that such children do, in fact, reveal their proficiency for syntax in their elicited imitative productions.

The key problem in the use of elicited imitation is producing a series of model sentences that incorporate syntactical features according to a developmental schedule based on the syntactic development of normal children.

Elicited imitation is used as the procedure for the CELI to assess children's grammatical productions. The test consists of 52 constructions, one phrase and 51 sentences, each presented to the child to elicit an imitative production. The CELI does not attempt to sample all sentences children may use spontaneously, even children in the 3- through 8-year-old age range. Sentence constructions and types that are sampled include active voice (all but four), passive voice (four), negatives, interrogatives, and imperatives. Grammatical categories are more representative and include all the forms children in the 3- through 8-year-old range may be expected to use.

When the CELI is administered, the child's responses are recorded on tape and later transcribed and classified according to grammatical categories. The child's score is determined by the number of errors made. The manual for the CELI provides percentile scores and stanines that permit comparisons of the examined child with other children in the same age range.

The CELI has a limitation that is inherent in all tests that assess language—they cannot sample everything without exhausting both examinee and examiner. As it is, it takes from 20 to 30 minutes to administer the CELI and about twice as long to score it. However, the information derived is worth the effort.

Prutting and Connolly (1976) reviewed the use of elicited imitation in studies in which the procedure was employed as an assessment instrument. They conclude:

A critical review of the studies indicates that the role of spontaneous imitative behavior and elicited imitation performance in language acquisition is unclear. . . . Elicited imitation alone may underestimate, overestimate, or accurately describe the child's language performance. It therefore seems necessary that elicited imitative assessment procedures be used in conjunction with a spontaneous language sample. In this manner elicited imitation tasks may be compared to a representative sample of the child's language performance.

LANGUAGE SAMPLING

A promising and relatively new approach to language assessment is the procedure of language sampling. Ideally, the kind of language children use spontaneously can be obtained only by recording their utterances in a variety of natural conditions and settings. This is not always practical, however, unless the instruments for recording are concealed and the parents or other caretakers are not themselves influenced by the awareness that there is ongoing recording. Awareness, even on a minimal level, is likely to modify what an adult says to a child and what the child, in turn, will say. In reality, most language sampling procedures elicit responses from the child through conversation, pictures, toys, or play activities. All of these circumstances are controlled to an important degree by the person obtaining the language sample. Ideally, there should be no such control.

A language sample is supposed to provide the clinician with information about what a child uses and presumably knows of language as well as what the child may not use and possibly or probably does not know. To make certain that the failure to use certain language forms and structures is not a product of circumstances—that the child had no need or wish to produce certain forms— an elicited imitation procedure such as the CELI (Carrow, 1974) may be used as a supplement. A general assumption relative to language sampling is that comprehension of a linguistic structure may be assumed if the child uses it on his or her own initiative. This assumption would rule out possible echoic responses.

There is no consensus on how large a sample should be considered adequate and representative of a child's language production. For practical reasons, especially if the sample is obtained in a clinical setting, from 50 to 100 utterances are usually recorded. On occasion we may have to do with less if we are dealing with a reluctant child or with one who is obviously at a single-word stage. Time constraints, especially if the sample is taken in a clinic, may well determine the size of the sample. If the parent or other observer feels that a child's language production is not representative, however, a second or even third recording session is in order. A time-saving alternative may be the use of elicited imitation to supplement the sample.

Recording and Analysis

It is essential that the child's language sample be recorded so that analysis may be done at leisure and so that opportunities for comparing impressions with another clinician are possible. There are several procedures for approximating a child's linguistic, essentially grammatical, proficiency based on the elicited language sample. The procedures share a common assumption—that certain linguistic (grammatical) categories are acquired by most normal speaking children in a fairly orderly, though not rigid, developmental sequence. Thus, Lee (1974) has a detailed procedure for comparing a given child's utterances with sentences that are types or representations of normal children's language. According to Lee (1974):

> Developmental Sentence Analysis is a method for making a detailed, readily quantified and scored evaluation of a child's use of standard English grammatical rules from a tape-recorded sample of his spontaneous speech

in conversation with an adult, in this case with his clinician. It provides another way of measuring a child's growth and progress throughout the period of clinical teaching. Because it is constructed upon developmental stages of language acquisition, it allows a clinician to select appropriate teaching goals based upon an individual child's performance. (p. xix)

Lee cautions that her procedure for analysis and teaching is appropriate only for children who are exposed to and learning standard American English grammar. Children from bilingual homes or children "from communities where dialects differ significantly from standard English should not be evaluated by this technique." This is an important caution to observe, so that the teacher or clinician will not confuse dialect difference with lack of grammatical proficiency.

Lee provides representative "sentences," from two-word asyntactic utterances to elaborated constructions that include conjunctions, pronouns, negative forms, interrogatives, and interrogative reversals. Lee's *Developmental Sentence Analysis* (1974) explains the rationale and method for her analysis and scoring system.

Tyack and Gottsleben, in their *Language Sampling, Analysis and Training* (1977), recommend obtaining 100 utterances to be analyzed and compared with information based on recent research on grammatical acquisitions in normal children. They compute a mean length of utterance and a word-morpheme index from the sample, according to which they place a child at a developmental linguistic level (LL). The particular level is based on a study by Morehead and Ingram (1973), "The Development of Base Syntax in Normal and Linguistically Deviant Children." Five developmental linguistic levels are postulated by Morehead and Ingram.

Tyack and Gottsleben (1977) recommend that when analyzing a language sample, the clinician should make note of the morphological inflections and the basic construction (sentence) types the child produces and should enter these on a score sheet at the expected linguistic level. Forms and constructions not produced are also noted. The forms and constructions that did not occur in the child's sample but are expected to be at or below the child's assigned LL become the immediate goals for intervention.

It is recommended that the clinician employ an elicited imitation approach, such as the CELI, to determine whether the absence of expected forms or constructions is peculiar to the particular sample or is actually an indication of delay in acquisition.

Bloom and Lahey (1978) describe a procedure for analyzing a language sample that considers form (language construction) as related to content and use. They emphasize: "If goals of intervention are to include content/form/use/interactions, then analyses that lead to goals must include all three" (p. 456).

The Bloom and Lahey approach is more demanding than either Lee's or Tyack and Gottsleben's. However, it does provide more information about what a child knows or does not know of language, or at least produces, and the circumstances (control and situation) that govern the language the child does use.

Language sampling is almost always more time-consuming than other forms of assessment that employ standardized tests. Learning how to take and analyze a language sample also requires a greater investment in time than learning how to administer most tests. We believe that the difference in the information obtained through language sampling justifies the investment in time; however, if only a short and limited period is available to the clinician or teacher, standardized testing that includes elicited imitation still produces valuable information for clinical intervention.

PHONOLOGICAL AND ARTICULATORY ASSESSMENT

There is probably no area of child language in which any knowledge, however limited, is so far ahead of assessment procedures as in phonological assessment. This might be a result of a sudden growth of knowledge regarding how children acquire their phonological systems, what the deviancies in sound production mean beyond their surface indications, or how the deviancies relate to lexical and syntactic proficiencies. We suspect that all three factors are involved and that other factors will emerge when we learn more about child language. Still more will emerge when we learn what we need to know about deviancies in language that tend to persist beyond the time when infantilisms, in the form of sound substitutions and varieties of lisps, either do or do not improve, whether spontaneously or with directed intervention.

The high incidence of phonological deviancies in the oral productions of linguistically retarded children is impressive. Studies such as those by Ingram (1976) constitute an important first step in understanding the phonological productions and systems of linguistically retarded children. At present, we can identify articulatory differences, and it would appear that the differences or deviancies are lawful rather than random. It is possible to appraise linguistically retarded children clinically but we still cannot assess them with any great feeling of assurance that what we hear and observe is not so individualized that generalizations must be made with extreme caution.

Locke (1980a, 1980b) presents a rationale and tentative criteria for an approach to assessing the auditory perception of children who present phonological disorder problems. Essentially, Locke's position is that speech perception deserves clinical interest to the extent that production difficulties are linked to problems of perceptual processing, and that the elicitation of perceptual responses is one of the few good ways of inferring what a child knows about the phonological structure of language (Locke, 1980, p. 445). In his essay, Locke presents his criteria for an assessment procedure for speech perceptual functioning when performed for the projected purpose of treating an articulatory disorder.

The kind of assessment that Locke proposes is likely to be time-consuming or, perhaps better, to be a justifiable investment in a considerable amount of time. We look forward to the development of such procedures for auditory assessment. Until they become available, there is little choice other than to do the best possible with what is available, with awareness that it is necessary to do better.

These reservations should be kept in mind when reviewing the several published tests and procedures for the assessment of articulation and children's phonological systems.

The Templin-Darley Tests of Articulation, Second Edition*

The Templin-Darley (1969) Tests represent a well-accepted, traditional approach to assessing articulation. The tests have 141 items that use colored pictures as stimuli. The screening part of the tests includes sounds and sound clusters "associated with significant progress in development of articulation." There is a special test for assessing and predicting palatopharyngeal competence.

One of the stated purposes of the Templin-Darley Tests is to enable the clinician to obtain a detailed description of a child's articulation to permit analysis and prescription for speech therapy when intervention is indicated. The test manual provides norms based on Templin's 1957 investigation of language development in children.

The Templin-Darley Tests will not meet the expectations of clinicians who look for phonemic feature distinctions or aberrant rules in their analysis of a child's phonological errors. As has already been observed, no presently published test meets such criteria. So, perhaps, Craven's (1979) closing sentence in her evaluation of the tests may be accepted: "For the speech-language pathologist whose purposes match those of the authors and whose population is similar to the normative group, these tests will continue to be useful" (p. 119).

The tests may be less useful in assessing numerous and deviant articulation errors in children who are severely linguistically retarded and whose phonological systems are aspects of overall deficient linguistic proficiency.

A Deep Test of Articulation

McDonald's (1964) test is based on the principle that a syllable rather than a discrete sound is the basic unit in articulatory coding. Pictures are used in pairs to connect syllables so that combinations such as *tubvase, tubsheep,* and *teethsheep* may be elicited. Each sound is tested in combinations that McDonald considers to be fundamental phonetic contexts. A score sheet and instructions are provided to determine the child's percentage of correct articulation.

McDonald's test employs a picture form as stimulus items for children whose reading level is below the third grade and a sentence form for children with higher than third-grade reading ability. A screening deep test is intended to assess an examinee's ability to articulate the nine most commonly misarticulated sounds.

McDonald's approach, because it does deep test, is useful as a diagnostic instrument for articulatory proficiency in brief contextual utterance. The nature of the procedure requires more training of the subject than does the Templin-Darley or most other published tests.

The Fisher-Logemann Test of Articulation Competence (TAC)

The TAC (Fisher and Logemann, 1971) represents an instrument and procedure that move in the direction of feature analysis of articulatory production. Consonant features are (1) place of articulation (oral articulators involved in the production of the sound), (2) manner of articulation, and (3) voicing (voiced or voiceless). Vowel features are (1) place of articulation, (2) height of tongue, (3) degree of tension (tense or lax), and (4) degree of lip rounding.

The TAC approach for speech-sound analysis is probably well known to clinicians whose experience goes back to the 1950s and 1960s. It is far from the presently developing distinctive feature theory systems. Nevertheless, the TAC approach does provide information useful to the clinician, especially regarding whether common features underlie several articulatory errors.

The TAC employs a picture form and a sentence form for eliciting single words that incorporate the selected sound (consonant, sound blend, vowel, or diphthong). Errors of omission, substitution, and distortion are recorded on test forms.

An interesting aspect of the TAC is that the assessment procedure provides for the effect of a speaker's dialect. The authors made the point that misarticulations are deviations not from an idealized standard dialect but from the speaker's native dialect, whatever it may be. In keeping with this position, the manual for the TAC includes characteristic regional (United States) dialect patterns and black English (Negro dialect).

The TAC picture form can be used to assess young school-age children, including those who have moderate language delay. Although it may not assess enough to help clinicians with severely linguistically retarded children, the TAC does measure and provide useful information for what it intends to achieve.

Phonological Analysis

Recent approaches for the systematic analysis of children's phonological systems include three key publications: Shriberg and Kwiatkwoski's (1980) *Natural Process Analysis* (NPA); Ingram's (1981), *Procedures for the Phonological Analysis of Children's Language;* and Weiner's (1979) *Phonological Process Analysis.* All three describe procedures that are intended to provide a complete and detailed description of a child's developing phonological system—normal, delayed, or deviant—as expressed in articulatory production.

Phonological analysis of children's speech determines the rules that a given child uses for his or her sound system. Shriberg and Kwiatkowski (1980) state: "Phonological rules simply describe observed regularity in behavior. Rules provide the phonologist a means for organizing, analyzing, and discussing phonological data" (p. 3). A child's phonology, whether it is developmentally normal or deviant, expresses the rules that are being used when that child is trying to communicate something—to signify meaning.

Phonological process analysis is a long and detailed procedure that requires considerably more training than does the administration of the usual articulation test. Because the procedure generates considerably more information about what the child is doing in the process or articulation, however, phonological analysis is usually worth the time and the effort it entails.

McReynolds and Elbert (1981) urge investigators and clinicians to define and establish criteria and standards for determining when detailed phonological analysis is justified: "Otherwise, much time and effort will be expended on material and procedures that offer no more useful information than our present evaluation procedures."

TRIAL TEACHING

Perhaps the best assessment procedure, as well as the best test of assessment, is trial teaching. Optimally, if not practically, every child who is of the proper age and who does not have clear indications of sensory and motor disabilities that might explain failure for speech onset should be given several weeks of trial teaching. Routine testing, even if it is testing in depth and over a period of a week or more, assesses the results of the child's exposure, experiences, and influences up to the time of the formal assessment. In some instances, we may be assessing the effects of the child's environment as much as we are assessing the child. Trial teaching adds a dimension of new experiences in a new setting with a different person. Under this new set of conditions, children may be helped to express their potentials rather than initial limitations. Thus, a greater sampling of behavior may be assessed, and insights may be gained that may be of therapeutic significance in that they go beyond the findings of formal assessment. In the final analysis, the purposes of assessment for a child with severe language delay is to determine not only what has been acquired or has not been acquired in language but also whether, what, and how more can be acquired with the intervention of direct instruction. This is the purpose of trial teaching, including intervention to improve speech intelligibility through articulation training.

REFERENCES AND SUGGESTED READINGS

Ammons, R. B., and Ammons, H. S. *The Full Range Picture Vocabulary Test.* Missoula, Mont.: Psychological Test Specialists, 1958.

Anastasi, A. *Psychological Testing,* 5th ed. New York: Macmillan, 1982.

Anderson, R. J., and Sisco, F. H. *A Standardization of WISC-R Performance Scale for Deaf Children.* Washington, D.C.: Office of Demographic Studies, Gallaudet College, 1977.

Arthur, G. *A Point Scale of Performance Tests, Revised Form II.* New York: Psychological Corporation, 1947.

Bayley, N. *The Bayley Scales of Infant Development.* New York: Psychological Corporation, 1969.

Beery, K. E. *Developmental Test of Visual-Motor Integration,* Chicago: Follett, 1967.

Bender, L. *A Visual-Motor Gestalt Test and Its Clinical Use.* New York: American Orthopsychiatry Research Monograph no. 3, 1938.

Berry, M. F. *Teaching Linguistically Handicapped Children.* Englewood Cliffs, N.J.: Prentice-Hall, 1980.

Blakeley, R. W. *Screening Test for Developmental Apraxia of Speech.* Tigard, Ore.: C. C. Publications, 1980.

Bloom, L., and Lahey, M. *Language Development and Language Disorders.* New York: Wiley, 1978.

Boehm, A. E. *Boehm Test of Basic Concepts.* New York: Psychological Corporation, 1971.

Brown, R., and Fraser, C. "The Acquisition of Syntax," in C. N. Cojer and B. S. Musgrave (eds.), *Verbal Behavior and Learning Problems and Processes.* New York: McGraw-Hill, 1963.

Burgemeister, B., Blum, L., and Lorge, I. *Columbia Mental Maturity Scale.* New York: Harcourt, Brace, Jovanovich, 1972.

Byrne, M. C., and Shervanian, C. C. *Introduction to Communicative Disorders.* New York: Harper and Row, 1977.

Carrow, E. *Test for Auditory Comprehension of Language.* Boston: Teaching Resources Corporation, 1973.

Carrow, E. *Carrow Elicited Language Inventory.* Boston: Teaching Resources Corporation, 1974.

Craven, D. "The Templin-Darley Tests of Articulation," in F. L. Darley (ed.), *Evaluation of Appraisal Techniques in Speech and Language Pathology.* Reading, Mass.: Addison-Wesley, 1979.

Darley, F. L. (ed.). *Evaluation of Appraisal Techniques in Speech and Language Pathology,* Reading, Mass.: Addison-Wesley, 1979.

Darley, F. L., and Spriestersbach, D. C. *Diagnostic Methods in Speech Pathology,* 2d ed. New York: Harper and Row, 1978.

Doll, E. A. (ed.). *The Oseretsky Test of Motor Proficiency.* Minneapolis: Educational Publishers, 1947.

Doll, E. A. *Vineland Social Maturity Scale.* Circle Pines, Minn.: American Guidance Service, 1965.

Doll, E. A., *Preschool Attainment Record.* Circle Pines, Minn.: American Guidance Service, 1966.

Dunn, L. M., and Dunn, L. M. *Peabody Picture Vocabulary Test (PPVT),* Rev. ed. Circle Pines, Minn.: American Guidance Service, 1981.

Fisher, H A , and Logemann, J. A. *The Fisher Logemann Test of Articulation Competence.* Boston: Houghton-Mifflin, 1971.

Foster, C. R., Giddan, J. J., and Stark, J. *Assessment of Children's Language Comprehension.* Palo Alto, Calif.: Consulting Psychologists Press, 1973.

Frankenburg, W. K., Dodds, J. B., Fandal, A. A., Kazuk, E., and Cohrs, M. *Denver Developmental Screening Test (DDST),* Rev. ed. Denver: Ladoca Project and Publishing Foundation, 1975.

Fraser, D., Bellugi, U., and Brown, R. "Control of Grammar in Imitation, Comprehension, and Production," *Journal of Verbal Learning and Verbal Behavior,* 2, 1963, 121–135.

Frostig, M., Lefever, D. W., and Whittlesley, R. R. B. *Marianne Frostig Developmental Test of Visual Perception.* Palo Alto, Calif.: Consulting Psychologists Press, 1964.

Gesell, A., *Gesell Developmental Schedules.* New York: Psychological Corporation, 1949.

Gesell, A. and Amatruda, H. *Developmental Diagnosis.*, 2d ed. New York: Paul Hoeber, 1957.

Ginsburg, H., and Opper, S. *Piaget's Theory of Intellectual Development,* 2d ed. Englewood Cliffs, N.J.: Prentice-Hall, 1979.

Goldman, R., Fristoe, M., and Woodcock, R. W. *Goldman-Fristoe-Woodcock Auditory Selective Attention Test.* Circle Pines, Minn.: American Guidance Service, 1976.

Harris, A. J. *Harris Tests of Lateral Dominance.* New York: Psychological Corporation, 1955.

Hiskey, M. S. *Hiskey-Nebraska Test of Learning Aptitude.* Lincoln, Neb.: Union College Press, 1966.

Hubbell, R. D. "Denver Developmental Screening Tests," in Darley, F. L. (ed.), *Evaluation of Appraisal Techiques in Speech and Language Pathology.* Reading, Mass.: Addison-Wesley, 1979.

Hutt, M. L. *The Hutt Adaptation of the Bender-Gestalt Test,* 2d ed. New York: Grune and Stratton, 1969.

Hutt, M. L., and Gibby, R. G. *An Atlas for the Hutt Adaptation of the Bender-Gestalt Test.* New York: Grune and Stratton, 1970.

Ingram, D. *Phonological Disability in Children.* New York: Elsevier; and London: Edward Arnold, 1976.

Ingram, D. *Procedures for the Phonological Analysis of Children's Language.* Baltimore: University Park Press, 1981.

Jones, M. H. "Habilitative Management of Communicative Disorders in Young Children," in E. L. Eagles (ed.), *Human Communication and Its Disorders.* New York: Raven Press, 1975.

Kirk, S. A., and Kirk, W. D. "Uses and Abuses of the ITPA," *Journal of Speech and Hearing Disorders,* 43(1), 1978, 58–75.

Kirk, S., McCarthy, J. J., and Kirk, W. D. *Illinois Test of Psycholinguistic Abilities,* Rev. ed. Urbana: University of Illinois, 1968.

Kohs, S. C. *Intelligence Measurement.* New York: Macmillan, 1923.

Koppitz, E. M. *The Bender-Gestalt Test for Young Children.* New York: Grune and Stratton, 1964.

Leach, E. A. "Goldman-Fristoe-Woodcock Auditory Selective Attention Test," in Darley, F. L. (ed.), *Evaluation of Appraisal Techniques in Speech and Language Pathology.* Reading, Mass.: Addison-Wesley, 1979.

Lee, L. L. *Northwestern Syntax Screening Test.* Evanston, Ill.: Northwestern University, 1969.

Lee, L. L. "A Screening Test for Syntax Development," *Journal of Speech and Hearing Disorders,* 25, 1970, 103–112.

Lee, L. L. *Developmental Sentence Analysis.* Evanston, Ill.: Northwestern University, 1974.

Lee, L. L. "Reply to Arndt and Byrne," *Journal of Speech and Hearing Disorders,* 42, 1977, 323–327.

Leiter, R. G. *Leiter International Performance Scale.* Washington, D.C.: Psychological Service Center, 1948.

Leonard, L. B., Prutting, C. A., Perozzi, J. A., and Berkley, R. K. "Nonstandardized Approaches to the Assessment of Language Behaviors," *ASHA,* 20(5), 1978, 371–379.

Locke, J. L. "The Inference of Speech Perception in the Phonologically Disordered Child. Part I: A Rationale, Some Criteria, the Conventional Tests," *Journal of Speech and Hearing Disorders,* 45(4), 1980a, 431–444.

Locke, J. L. "The Inference of Speech Perception in the Phonologically Disordered Child. Part II: Some Clinically Novel Procedures, Their Uses. Some Findings," *Journal of Speech and Hearing Disorders,* 45(4), 1980b, 445–468.

Longhurst, T. M. "Assessment of Children's Language Comprehension." in F. L. Darley (ed.), *Evaluation of Appraisal Techniques in Speech and Language Pathology.* Reading, Mass.: Addison-Wesley, 1979.

McDonald, E. *A Deep Test of Articulation.* Pittsburgh: Stanwix House, 1965.

McReynolds, L. V., and Elbert, M. "Criteria for Phonological Process Analysis," *Journal of Speech and Hearing Disorders,* 2(46), 1981, 197–203.

Morehead, D. M., and Ingram, D. "The Development of Base Syntax in Normal and Linguistically Deviant Children," *Journal of Speech and Hearing Research,* 1973, 16, 330–352.

Peterson, H. A., and Marquardt, T. R. *Appraisal and Diagnosis of Speech and Language Disorders.* Englewood Cliffs, N.J.: Prentice-Hall, 1981.

Piaget, J. and Inhelder, B. *The Psychology of the Child.* New York: Basic Books, 1969.

Porteus, S. D., *Porteus Maze Tests, Vineland Revision.* New York: Psychological Corporation, 1965.

Prutting, C. A. "The Illinois Test of Psycholinguistic Abilities, Revised Edition." in F. L. Darley, (ed.), *Evaluation of Appraisal Techniques in Speech and Language Pathology.* Reading, Mass.: Addison-Wesley, 1979.

Prutting, C. A., and Connolly, J. E. "Imitation: A Closer Look," *Journal of Speech and Hearing Disorders,* 3(4), 1976, 412–422.

Raven, J. C. *Guide to Using Progressive Matrices (1949),* Rev. ed. London: Lewis, 1962.

Schiefelbusch, R. "Language Disabilities of Cognitively Involved Children," in J. V. Irwin and M. Marge (eds.), *Principles of Childhood Language Disabilities.* New York: Appleton-Century-Crofts, 1972.

Shriberg, L. D. and Kwiatowski, J. *Natural Process Analysis* (NPA), New York: Wiley, 1980.

Snow, K. "A Detailed Analysis of Articulation Responses of 'Normal' First Grade Children," *Journal of Speech and Hearing Research,* 6, 1963, 277–290.

Stephenson, W. T. "The Boston University Speech and Sound Discrimination Test," in F. L. Darley, (ed.), *Evaluation of Appraisal Techniques in Speech and Language Pathology.* Reading, Mass.: Addison-Wesley, 1979.

Stutsman, R. *The Merrill-Palmer Scale.* New York: Harcourt Brace Jovanovich, 1949.

Templin, M. C. *Certain Language Skills in Children.* Minneapolis: University of Minnesota Press, 1957.

Templin, M. C., and Darley, F. L. *The Templin-Darley Tests of Articulation,* 2d ed. Iowa City: University of Iowa, Bureau of Education and Service, 1969.

Terman, L. M., and Merrill, M. A. *Stanford-Binet Intelligence Scale, Form L. M.* Boston: Houghton-Mifflin, 1960.

Tyack, D., and Gottsleben, R. *Language Sampling, Analysis and Training,* Palo Alto, Calif.: Consulting Psychologists Press, 1977.

Vetter, D. K. "Goldman-Fristoe-Woodcock Test of Auditory Discrimination." in F. L.

Darley, (ed.), *Evaluation of Appraisal Techniques in Speech and Language Pathology*. Reading, Mass.: Addison-Wesley, 1979.

Wechsler, D. *Wechsler Preschool and Primary Scale of Intelligence*. New York: Psychological Corporation, 1967.

Wechsler, D., *Wechsler Intelligence Scale for Children (WISC-R)*. New York: Psychological Corporation, 1974.

Weiner, F. *Phonological Process Analysis*. Baltimore: University Park Press, 1979.

Wepman, J. M. *Auditory Discrimination Test*. Palm Springs, Calif: Language Research Associates, 1973.

Wepman, J. M., and Morency, A. *The Auditory Sequential Memory Test*. Palm Springs, Calif.: Language Research Associates, 1975.

Zimmerman, I. L., Steiner, V. G., and Evatt, R. L. *Preschool Language Scale*. Columbus, Ohio: Charles E. Merrill, 1969.

chapter 7

Phonological Deficiencies in Aphasic and Dysphasic Children

The chapter on the assessment of linguistically retarded children notes the need to investigate the presence of possible dialect and syntactic differences when a child's surface (apparent) presenting problem appears to be in the area of articulation. The use of a sound or the simplification of a sound cluster (blend) that does not meet standard expectations but is consistent with age, specific environmental influence, or broader dialect difference may sometimes need consideration and possible remediation. Such differences, however, are only occasionally related to deviant phonology. We will consider a child to be deviant in phonology when there is evidence of failure or limitations in the knowledge expressed in the practices (rules) that govern the sound system of the language the child is exposed to and trying to produce.

This observation is not to be interpreted as inconsistent with recent positions summarized by Ingram (1976): "Evidence . . . suggests that deviant phonology may be not just a phonemic disorder, but a more global linguistic one" (p. 122). The awareness that a child has a deviant sound system should put the clinician on the alert for associated deviancies in the use of syntax and in the semantic component of language (Shriner, Holloway, and Daniloff, 1969; Panagos, 1974; Menyuk and Looney, 1972). In brief, it is necessary to distinguish between a child who has difficulty with articulating a sound or sounds, either in isolation or in relatively consistent contextual situations, and one whose rules in regard to the sounds of the language are deviant. The child who lisps is not the same kind of child as the one who can sometimes produce sibilants appropriately but substitutes another sound or omits the sibilant in contexts where most peer-age children, including those who lisp, do not. Furthermore, the child with a truly simple articulatory defect, such as a lingual protrusion lisp or a *w* for an *l* or *r* substitution, is very different from the one with severe articulation disorders. The latter child reveals limitations—serious delays, sound substitutions, and sound combination simplifications—that are not in keeping with the developmental patterns of normal young children.

This chapter will be concerned primarily with the phonological deviancies of aphasic and dysphasic children. These deviancies are sometimes quantitative—maintenance of infantile tendencies—and sometimes qualitative, in that they appear to be individual expressions of tendencies that do not follow developmental patterns of normal children (Ingram, 1976). Fortunately, however deviant the aphasic and dysphasic children may be in their phonologies, each tends to be fairly lawful unto himself or herself; that is, each child usually follows rules that are individually consistent. Fortunately, also, there are some common trends that permit discerning clinicians to break the code and arrive at the child's rule system. Because this can be done, therapeutic intervention becomes possible. Ingram (1976) notes: "Virtually every study that has undertaken the linguistic analysis of a child with a phonological disability has revealed system in the child's speech" (p. 99). Later, we will consider a number of types of phonological processes that Ingram found to be most common in investigations of deviant children.

NORMAL PHONOLOGICAL DEVELOPMENT

Before considering the deviant phonology of aphasic and dysphasic children, we shall review normal phonological development. At the opening of the chapter, we presented a negative definition of what characterizes a child with deviant phonology. Such a child shows evidence of failure or limitation in the knowledge of or use of the rules that govern the sound system of the language or languages of his or her environment. In normal phonological development, a child has such knowledge and intuitively applies (uses) the rules that pertain to the sound system or systems he or she speaks. Normally, children learn the sound system—the rules, structure, and function of speech sounds—along with other linguistic information and practices relating to the morphemic, syntactic, and semantic systems of their language or languages. Normally, also, children are not aware of how or what they learn as they become speakers of a language and are happily innocent of how rule-abiding they are as they acquire the language or languages of their culture.

As suggested earlier, aphasic children are either delayed in acquiring such knowledge of the rules of their spoken language system or, in some instances, use different rules and so have idiosyncratic phonologies. With such awareness on the part of the clinician, it becomes possible to decode what the child is trying to say and to modify the child's utterances so that they become intelligible.

THE SOUNDS (PHONEMES) OF AMERICAN ENGLISH

Most children reach the normal adult level of articulation proficiency between ages 8 and 9; however, intelligible speech—the utterance as a whole being understood even though some sounds are not proficient—is usually achieved by age 3. Vowel production is usually well controlled by age 4. Delay or failure in vowel production may imply hearing loss and in some instances may be associated with overall delay in language acquisition.

Consonant sounds are produced with essentially normal proficiency at different ages, according to the place and possibly the relative difficulty (precision of and action of the articulators) required for their production. Shriberg (1980) shares an observation made by many linguists and phoneticians: "Interestingly, sounds that are not frequently used as phonemes in languages of the world are also those that children learn later or tend to misarticulate" (pp. 274–275). Although no child has an obligation as an individual to observe this tendency, the information provided in the tables in this chapter suggests that this is so. In essence, sounds that are difficult to discriminate are also difficult to produce, are controlled later than sounds that are more readily discriminated (they may be seen as well as heard), and are among the first to be correctly articulated.

Table 7.1 presents the common phonemes of American English, with key words and International Phonetic Alphabet (IPA) symbols. Tables 7.2 and 7.3 present the order of consonant sound proficiency for children, including a comparison in Table 7.2 between Templin (1957) and Prather, Hedrick, and Kern, (1975). Table 7.3 gives a developmental listing for consonants controlled between ages 2 and 6, with more lenient criteria than are usually expected as indications of proficiency.

An examination of the tables indicates that there are differences as well as similarities among the studies in the order of articulatory proficiency. The more recent studies generally find an earlier age of proficiency than do the older studies. Differences may be accounted for by several factors, including (1) youngest age of subjects, since Templin (1957) did not include children below age three, hence gave no age of proficiency for younger children, as in the Prather, Hedrick, and Kern (1975) and Sander (1972) studies; (2) Templin tested for sounds in initial, medial, and final position, whereas Prather et al. tested for sounds in the initial and final position; (3) judgments regarding what constitutes articulatory proficiency; and (4) differences in the socioeconomic and educational backgrounds of the subjects and of the members of their home environments.

Despite differences, there is a general orderly pattern of sound development in the studies. There is also a fair amount of correspondence with the pattern of phonemic development (Table 7.4), based on Jakobson's (1968) distinctive feature theory. Jakobson states unequivocally: "Whether it is a question of French or Scandinavian children, of English or Slavic, of Indian or German, or of Estonian, Dutch or Japanese children, every description based on careful observation repeatedly confirms the striking fact that the relative

Table 7.1 THE COMMON PHONEMES OF AMERICAN ENGLISH

Key word	IPA symbol	Key word	IPA symbol
	Consonants		
*p*it	p	*c*at	æ
*b*ean	b	*ho*t	ɒ or ɑ
*t*in	t		depending upon regional or individual variations
*d*en	d		
*c*ook	k		
*g*et	g	*s*aw	ɔ
*f*ast	f	*o*bey, s*ew*	o or ou
*v*an	v	b*oo*k	ʊ
*th*in	θ	b*oo*n	u
*th*is	ð	c*u*t	ʌ
*s*ea	s	*a*bout	ə
*z*oo	z	supp*er*	ɚ
*sh*e	ʃ		by most Americans and ə by many others
mea*s*ure	ʒ		
*ch*ick	tʃ		
*j*ack	ʤ	h*ear*d	ɝ
*m*e	m		by most Americans and ɜ by many others
*n*o	n		
si*ng*	ŋ		
*l*et	l		
*r*un	r		*Diphthongs*
*y*et	j	s*igh*	aɪ
*h*at	h	n*oi*se	ɔɪ
*w*on	w	c*ow*	aʊ or ɑʊ
*wh*at[a]	ʍ or hw		depending upon individual variations
	Vowels	*may*	eɪ
s*ee*	i	t*oe*	ou
s*i*t	ɪ	r*efu*se	ɪu or ju
c*a*ke	e		depending upon individual variations
m*e*t	ɛ		
b*al*m	ɑ	*u*se	ju
m*a*sk	æ or a depending upon regional or individual variations		

[a]If distinction is made in pronunciation of words such as *what* and *watt, when* and *wen.*

142

Table 7.2 COMPARISON OF ORDER OF SOUNDS (ARTICULATION DEVELOPMENT) IN CHILDREN AGED 2 TO 4 YEARS

| Sound | Age | | Sound | Age | |
	Prather, Hedrick, and Kern (1975)	Templin (1957)		Prather, Hedrick, and Kern (1975)	Templin (1957)
m	2	3–0	s	3	4–6
n	2	3–0	r	3–4	4–0
h	2	3–6	l	3–4	6–0
p	2	3–0	ʃ (sh)	3–8	4–6
ŋ (ng)	2	3–0	tʃ (ch)	3–8	4–6
f	2–4	3–0	ð (voiced th)	4	7–0
j (y)	2–4	3–6			
k	2–4	4–0	ʒ (measure)	4	7–0
d	2–4	4–0	ʤ (jump)	4+	7–0
w	2–8	3–0	θ (voiceless th)	4+	6–0
b	2–8	4–0			
t	2–8	6–0	v	4+	6–0
g	3	4–0	z	4+	7–0

Source: Adapted from Prather, E. M., Hedrick, D. L., and Kern, C. A. "Articulation Development in Children Aged Two to Four Years," *Journal of Speech and Hearing Disorders,* 40, 1975, 179–191.

Table 7.3 ORDER OF CONSONANT SOUND PROFICIENCY BASED ON SANDER'S (1972) CRITERIA

Age	Sounds[a]
2	h, m, n, w, b, p, t, k, g, ng, /ŋ/, d
3	f, y /j/, s, r, l
4	ch /tʃ/, sh /ʃ/, j /ʤ/, z, v
5	voiceless th /θ/, voiced th /ð/
6	zh /ʒ/

[a]Correct articulation for a sound in two of three word positions and 50% rather than 75% correct performance.

Table 7.4   PATTERN OF PHONEMIC DEVELOPMENT (DISTINCTIONS)

1. The presence or absence of consonants in syllables: [bɑk] and [ɑk], [vek] and [ek].
2. Stop and fricative sounds with sonorants (nasals, vowellike consonants): *b–m, d–r, g–n, v–y* /j/.
3. Nasal and liquid sounds: *m–l, m–r, n–l, n–r, n–y, m–y.*
4. Intranasal distinctions: *m–n.*
5. Intraliquid distinctions: *l–r.*
6. Fricative and nonfricative: *z–m, v–n.*
7. Labial and nonlabial: *b–d, v–z.*
8. Stop and fricative: *b–v, d–z, k–f.*
9. Lingual and velar: *d–g, t–k.*
10. Voiceless and voiced cognates: *p–b, t–d, k–g, f–v, s–z.*
11. Blade and groove sibilants: s–sh /ʃ/, z–zh /ʒ/.
12. Liquid and glide: *r–y, l–y.*

Source: Based on a study by Shvachkin of the development of phonemic proficiency in early childhood (see Slobin, 1967).

chronological order of phonological acquisitions remains everywhere and at all times the same" (p. 46). This orderliness does not hold for aphasic children with deviant phonologies.

DISTINCTIVE FEATURES

Jakobson (1968) and Chomsky and Halle (1968) view a phoneme—a basic speech sound of a language—as a bundle of features that enable a listener to distinguish one sound from another. The features are products of the place (articulatory organs and place of involvement in the production of the sound), manner of production, and acoustic impression. Although Jakobson and Halle's distinctive sound features are by no means unanimously accepted by phoneticians and speech pathologists, they do provide a basis for understanding how speech sounds are learned and produced. There is increasing acceptance of the notion that when children learn to produce speech sounds, what in fact occurs is that they learn to perceive and produce sets of distinctive features (McReynolds and Engmann, 1975; Singh, 1976; Winitz, 1975).

A distinctive speech sound feature is either present (+) or absent (–) and in this sense is considered binary in the bundle of features that constitute a given phoneme. Table 7.5 provides the terms most frequently used in distinctive feature analysis; Table 7.6 presents the distinctive features for American English consonants; and Table 7.7 presents examples of the distinctive features for the bilabial consonants /p/, /b/, and /m/.

A sound feature analysis of phonemes that emphasizes place and manner of production is presented in Table 7.8. This basis of analysis is sufficiently close to the Jakobson-Halle approach and provides an adequate number of features to be practical for the purposes of perceptual training and articulatory

Table 7.5 TERMS USED IN DISTINCTIVE FEATURE ANALYSIS

Term	Characterized by
Consonantal	Interference of breath stream and abrupt movements of formants.
Vocalic	No interference of breath stream and steady or slow moving formants.
High	Front or back of tongue being raised from neutral position.
Low	Front or back of tongue being lowered from neutral position.
Back	Back of tongue being retracted from neutral position.
Anterior	Production in the front position of mouth, tongue, or lips.
Coronal	Involvement of the tip or blade, which is raised from neutral position.
Continuant	Partial obstruction of air stream, which continues to flow.
Voicing	Accompanying vocal fold vibration.
Nasal	Lowering of the velum with the air stream passing through the nose.
Strident	High degree of turbulence or noisy sound where articulated.
Sonorant	Absence of any interference with flow of glottal sound.

Source: Reprinted with the permission of Macmillan Publishing Company from *Communicative Disorders in Children*, 5th ed., by Jon Eisenson and Mardel Ogilvie. Copyright © 1983 by Macmillan Publishing Company.

Table 7.6 DISTINCTIVE FEATURES OF VARIOUS PHONEMES (CONSONANTS)

Phoneme

Feature	p	b	t	d	k	g	tʃ	ʤ	f	v	θ	ð	s	z	ʃ	ʒ	m	n	ŋ	r	l	j	h	w	ʍ
Consonantal	+	+	+	+	+	+	+	+	+	+	+	+	+	+	+	+	+	+	+	+	+	−	+	−	+
Vocalic	−	−	−	−	−	−	−	−	−	−	−	−	−	−	−	−	−	−	−	+	+	−	−	−	−
High	−	−	−	−	+	+	+	+	−	−	−	−	−	−	+	+	−	−	+	−	−	+	−	+	+
Low	−	−	−	−	−	−	−	−	−	−	−	−	−	−	−	−	−	−	−	−	−	−	+	−	−
Back	−	−	−	−	+	+	−	−	−	−	−	−	−	−	+	+	−	−	+	−	−	−	−	+	−
Anterior	+	+	+	+	−	−	−	−	+	+	+	+	+	+	−	−	+	+	−	−	+	−	−	+	+
Coronal	−	−	+	+	−	−	+	+	−	−	+	+	+	+	+	+	−	+	−	+	+	−	−	−	−
Continuant	−	−	−	−	−	−	−	−	+	+	+	+	+	+	+	+	−	−	−	+	+	+	+	+	+
Voicing	−	+	−	+	−	+	−	+	−	+	−	+	−	+	−	+	+	+	+	+	+	+	−	+	−
Nasal	−	−	−	−	−	−	−	−	−	−	−	−	−	−	−	−	+	+	+	−	−	−	−	−	−
Strident	−	−	−	−	−	−	+	+	+	+	−	−	+	+	+	+	−	−	−	−	−	−	−	−	−
Sonorant	−	−	−	−	−	−	−	−	−	−	−	−	−	−	−	−	+	+	+	+	+	+	−	+	−

Source: Reprinted with the permission of Macmillan Publishing Company from *Communicative Disorders in Children*, 5th ed., by Jon Eisenson and Mardel Ogilvie. Copyright © 1983 by Macmillan Publishing Company.

Note: Some authors use [č] for [tʃ] [ǰ] for [ʤ] [š] for [ʃ] [ž] for [ʒ] [y] for [j]. Based on Jakobson and Chomsky and Halle (1968).

Table 7.7   DISTINCTIVE FEATURES OF /p/, /b/, AND /m/

	Voice	Nasal	Continuant	Labial
p	−	−	−	+
b	+	−	−	+
m	+	+	+	+

production of aphasic children. A large number of studies have been generated by the Jakobson (1968) distinctive feature approach—for example, McReynolds and Engmann (1975), Williams and McReynolds (1975), Singh (1976), Ruder and Bunce (1981), Weiner (1981), and others that are reviewed in Bernthal and Bankson (1981) and Eisenson and Ogilvie (1983). Most of the reported studies had as subjects children who, despite their articulatory defects, were not considered to be conspicuously deficient in language acquisition. Experience indicates that, for practical purposes, the phonemic features included in Table 7.8 are sufficient for establishing speech-sound discrimination and intelligible production for aphasic children.

Walsh (1974) has reservations about acoustic distinctive feature approach, holding that this system has practical shortcomings that "constitute a considerable obstacle to diagnosing and treating speech disorders." Walsh asserts that the distinctive features include "contrived acoustic properties and are motivated by a concern for optimal notational economy." Walsh presents a tentative set of speech-sound features that are based on articulatory activity rather than on acoustic impressions.

Earlier, we indicated that one of the major concerns in this book would be with children who are severely linguistically retarded and designated as aphasic. The most severely linguistically retarded may be essentially nonverbal. Although such children present no phonological problems, they are more likely than most others to have deviant phonologies as they begin to acquire language. Among these aphasic children may be found some who have been turned off and turned away from oral language and who need to be encouraged and, if necessary, seduced to listen so that they may learn to speak. Other aphasic children, as well as those who are less impaired and may be designated as dysphasic, are also likely to have deviant phonologies.

The approaches that will be described later are intended for the population of aphasic children that is likely to have deficient phonologies as they begin to acquire or increase their linguistic acquisitions. Children with congenital oral (articulatory) apraxia—those who may understand spoken language but cannot themselves produce intelligible speech because their organs of articulation literally do not do their bidding—will be considered separately in chapter 10.

Most linguistically retarded children who have phonological disorders may have a variety of difficulties in both the perception and the production of speech. Some children with a history of linguistic retardation appear to have acquired deviant phonological systems that require special decoding abilities on the part of the listener in order to make sense of their oral utterances.

Table 7.8 FEATURES OF PRODUCTION OF CONSONANTS IN AMERICAN ENGLISH SPEECH

Manner of articulation	Articulators used				
	Lips (bilabial)	Lip–teeth (labiodental)	Tongue–teeth (linguadental)	Tongue point–gum (lingualveolar)	Tongue–hard or soft palate (palatal)
Voiceless stops	p			t	k
Voiced stops	b			d	g
Voiceless fricatives	hw (ʍ)	f	θ (th)	s, /ʃ/ (sh)	
Voiced fricatives		v	ð (th)	z, /ʒ/ (zh)	
Nasals (all voiced)	m			n	/ŋ/ (ng)
Vowellike consonants	w			r, l	j (y), rᵃ

Note: The features of sound production included in this table are voicing, nasality, affrication, duration, and place of articulation.
ᵃIn combinations such as *k* or *g* followed by *r*, the *r* sound may be produced in this position.

Ingram (1976) raises two related questions about the child who is identified as having phonological problems. First, does the child so identified show evidence of functioning with essentially the same phonological system as that of a younger child—one whose phonology is just developing as part of normal language acquisition? If this is so, then this is a matter of developmental delay. The second question suggested by Ingram is whether children with phonological problems "acquire a phonological system in a unique way, showing patterns of acquisition that never appear in young normal children." If the answer to the second question is in the affirmative, there should be observable characteristics in an individual child's phonological system that are different from those of the younger normal child but are nevertheless "lawful." The implication of *lawful* is that, for a given child, the characteristics occur with determinable regularity relative to contextual phonetic situations.

It is possible that some linguistically retarded children who are deviant in phonology show both tendencies—delay in some respects and differences in others. However, each child must necessarily be studied for what each child shows. Therapy needs to be individualized in the light of clinical findings. It should be noted that Ingram does not question that phonologically deviant children have a system for their production. Ingram's questions are related to the nature of the child's system. Once this is determined, there are available procedures for therapeutic intervention. The following cases illustrate this approach.

Delayed Phonology in a Child Aged 3 Years, 11 Months   Keith, age 3 years 11 months, is described by his parents as "jabbering jargon." Unless he points to what he wants, or occasionally gestures, the parents profess not to understand him. Keith's almost 6-year-old sister does much better and often acts as his interpreter. According to his parents, Keith did not begin to talk until he was almost 38 months of age. It is interesting that they had less difficulty in understanding him then than they do now.

Evaluation procedures, employing standardized and informal testing, revealed that Keith did have a phonological system, one that was little changed in the year since the onset of his first words. The child was essentially using only seven identifiable sounds, that including /t/ for all voiceless stops, /b/ for voiced stops, /m/ for nasals, /f/ for fricatives, an occasional /g/, and the vowels /ʌ/ and /u/. These are sounds that more normal children produce in the first few months of their speaking careers, usually as part of what Ingram (1976) refers to as "the phonology of the first fifty words."

Rick, Aged 4 Years, 4 Months   Rick, a few months older than Keith, also had a history of delayed onset of speech (age 3 years 1 month) but had speech that was decodable. Rick was also beginning to put words together in two- and occasionally three-word utterances. His success in communicating was more dependent on acceptable vowel production and in overall intonation pattern than in proficiency with consonants. Rick tended to omit final consonants, substituted /w/ for /r/ and /l/, and generally reduced sound clusters to single sounds so that *spoon* became /pu/ and *stove* became /to/.

Rick, too, was assessed as having a delayed phonological system, more advanced than Keith's but still essentially infantile (developmentally delayed) as well as deviant in some aspects of phonology.

In working out remedial clinical programs for Keith and Rick, and children like them, we follow the procedures advocated by Shriberg (1980). This program recognizes and applies some of what we know about normal phonological development, including processes (rules) observed by Ingram (1980) in his study of deviant phonology.

Shriberg (1980, p. 279) summarizes some of the natural processes[1] that are represented in normal early child language as belonging to one of three types, each of which serves to simplify a child's speech production. These types are as follows:

1. Reduction of the complexity of syllables within a word through deletion. This may be accomplished by (a) deleting an unstressed syllable (e.g., *nana* for *banana, way* for *away*); (b) deleting a sound in a consonant sound cluster, which is usually a more difficult or later-controlled sound than the one that remains (e.g., *pot* for *spot, dink* for *drink*); or (c) deleting a final consonant (e.g., *da* for *doll*).
2. Assimilation, showing the influence of one sound within a word on another sound. The likely result is a substitution, usually of the sound the child has under control or had under earlier control, rather than the assimilated sound. The production of *bubby* for *bunny* represents *progressive (forward) assimilation* (the first consonant influencing the second); *nunny* for *bunny* represents *regressive (backward) assimilation* (the later consonant influencing and so substituted for the earlier one).
3. Phonemic substitutions other than those resulting from assimilation. Frequent among such substitution processes are (a) stopping, whereby stop sounds, acquired early, replace other sounds that are usually acquired later—for example, *tay* for *say* and *dis* for *this* have alveolar stops substituted for fricatives, and *dady* for *lady* is a stop substitution for a liquid sound; and (b) fronting, in which palatal and velar sounds are replaced by alveolar sounds, as in *do* for *go* and *bite* for *bike*.

The information that follows should serve as a guide to the types of errors a linguistically delayed child may be making in articulatory efforts. These are by no means all-inclusive, but they are consistent with recognized universal simplification strategies that are common to normal children. Insofar as a particular child's articulations seem to be instances of the use of these strategies, that child may be considered delayed in speech. What is the task of the

---

[1]*Natural processes* are the tendencies that children express in the errors of articulation as they acquire a language system.

speech and language clinician in regard to such information and applied assumption? We agree with Shriberg (1980) that the task of the speech pathologist (speech and language clinician) is "to analyze delayed speech with the goal of producing a set of descriptive statements (rules) that summarize a child's phonological system (p. 280). Such statements become the basis for the prescription—the remedial procedures—for a given child's phonological errors. Such an analysis and description (Shriberg refers to it as a natural process analysis) will be directed to answering three related questions:

1. In the light of a child's age, which natural processes are normal? It might be added as an additional consideration that "normality" may also be related to the age of onset of first identifiable words and onset of speech in other members of a child's family.
2. Are there any processes that would be normal (typical) of a younger child?
3. Do the child's articulatory productions reveal phonological rules (idiosyncratic processes) that are not characteristic and thus normal for most younger children? We should note the assumption that, however idiosyncratic, there is evidence that the child is observing some rule, and so the errors or deviancies are neither random nor isolated. Because of this assumption, it follows that the rule the child is using is discoverable, and so the productions in turn become decodable. The discovery process becomes the basis for therapeutic intervention, whether it is on the basis of question 1 or 2 above or of idiosyncratic processes.

THERAPEUTIC INTERVENTION FOR CHILDREN WITH PHONOLOGICAL DEFICIENCIES

In working out an individual program to improve the phonemic proficiency of children who are severely delayed in language development, several basic assumptions are made. These assumptions need to be tested for each child, of course, so that no clinical time will be invested in teaching a child to do what she or he is already reasonably able to do. The first of these assumptions is that most of the children with whom we are concerned are likely to have difficulty in making phonemic discriminations and probably greater difficulty in sequencing (processing the correct order) of speech signals at the rate at which such signals normally occur in conversational speech (Rosenthal, 1970; McReynolds, 1966; Tallal and Piercy, 1978; Stark and Tallal, 1981). The second corollary assumption is that motor performance of the organs of articulation is also likely to be less proficient than for nonlanguage delayed children. Shriberg (1980) summarizes his view, which is based on published research of perceptual-motor functioning of children with severely delayed speech, with the observation: "The average performance of a group of children with *severely* delayed speech is likely to be lower than the average performance of normal children on conventional tests of auditory discrimination, tongue and lip mobility, and oral sensation" (p. 283).[2]

A third assumption is that the perceptual-motor dysfunctions, both for making discriminative distinctions and for sequencing, are subject to improvement by training. These basic and rather broad assumptions may be translated into guidelines for a training program for phonemic processing when assessment procedures have determined the needs of an individual child.

GUIDELINES FOR PHONEMIC TRAINING

1. With rare exception, hearing (the physical reception of sound) is not a significant problem. Although some linguistically retarded children may show mild-to-moderate hearing loss, they can hear normal conversational speech.
2. Discrimination of isolated vowels presents no problem that cannot be dealt with in early training.
3. Consonant sound discrimination difficulty is greatest for glides, fricatives, and affricates, next greatest for stops, and least for nasals.
4. Linguistically retarded children have greater difficulty in processing (discriminating between) speech sounds that are different in regard to a single feature or characteristic than they do in processing sounds that differ by two or three features.
5. In general, severely linguistically retarded children—particularly those who are so retarded and perceptually impaired as to be considered dysphasic or, more severely, aphasic—require a longer time interval between speech signals for correct processing (discrimination and determination of temporal order) than do normal speaking children.

THE CHILD'S LEXICON AND PHONOLOGICAL TRAINING

The ultimate goal in phonological training is to improve the child's ability to communicate in spontaneous, normal situations. Simulating normal social situations is therefore a necessary part of the program. However, before this can be accomplished for and with a child who is also linguistically retarded, practice must be provided that progresses from words to phrases to sentences, to be incorporated as soon as possible in conversational situations.

If the child has a working vocabulary, it is the answer to where to begin in word selection. If the lexicon is small, then it may be expanded in keeping with Lahey and Bloom's (1977) suggestion, "Planning a First Lexicon: Which Word to Teach First," as well as with the suggestions of Holland (1975) in her article "Language Therapy for Children: Some Thoughts on Context and Content."

---

[2]The perceptual problems are most severe for children who are dysphasic or aphasic; the motoric problem is comparably most severe for children who have oral (articulatory) apraxia. A small percentage of children have both aphasic and apraxic involvements.

Also recommended is the article "Environmental Language Intervention," by MacDonald and Blott (1974), for a philosophy of a selection of words that have semantic relevance. In essence, the choice of words with due regard for the phonemic context should also make it possible for the child to be an improved communicator. Words that are taught only as labels must soon be supplemented by words (they may be the same as when they were initially used as labels) and used to bring about something of interest or concern to the child. Useful words will be practiced words that can be extended from a clinic situation to the other environments in which a child functions. Thus, words such as *cup, doll, mama, dada, papa, water, doggy, cookie, kitty,* and *ball* may be good for starters or expanders of a child's own lexicon. These words may be used as labels or as words to make something happen (to control someone's behavior) according to the child's wishes. Add to these such words as *now, more, no, up,* and *down,* and *down,* and we have important imperatives. All of these words, we may note, include consonants that are normally controlled and proficiently produced by most 3-year-olds. The selected words are high in frequency with normal children, because they are useful in serving their needs. Of course, if a child has a working vocabulary that is not readily decodable, then determining what the child's rules are would provide a basis for correction.

However much we would like to recommend an environmental approach to language training, it appears that the rationale and philosophy of the environmental approach would be pushed beyond its applicable limits. An environmental teaching program is intended primarily to establish and encourage language use in natural settings. Remediation to improve the intelligibility of communication by correct articulation, except by example may result in discouraging a child's efforts. The correction may be mistaken for rejection. It is recommended, therefore, that training to establish a lexicon and appropriate syntactic utterance in the interest of semantics be separated in time and, if possible, in place from articulatory training. If at all possible, different clinicians should also be employed.

First, of course, it is necessary to analyze and determine where a child is phonologically, using the discussion in the preceding pages and what immediately follows as guides. Important aspects of analysis include the need to learn whether a child perceives sounds and differences between sounds, whether the child perceives them in some contexts and not in others, and the relationship between what a child perceives and can distinguish and what the child incorporates and expresses in his or her articulatory productions.

SPEECH-SOUND PRODUCTION
AND PERCEPTUAL PROCESSING

Locke (1980) sets down eight criteria for determining how a child's production of speech sounds is linked to possible problems of perceptual processing. Locke emphasizes the need for eliciting perceptual responses as "one of the few good ways of inferring what a child knows about the phonological structure of language." An assessment procedure should meet the following criteria. It should:

1. Examine the child's perception of the replaced sound in relation to the replacing sound, that is, the target phoneme versus its substitution phoneme, or, as in the case of complete omission, silence;
2. Observe the same phonemes in identical phonetic environments in production and perception;
3. Permit a comparison of the child's performance on target and replacing sounds with his discrimination of target and perceptually similar control sounds;
4. Be based on a comparison of an adult's surface form and the child's own internal representation;
5. Present repeated opportunities for the child to reveal his perceptual decisions;
6. Prevent nonperceptual errors from masquerading as perceptual errors;
7. Require a response easily within a young child's conceptual capacities and repertoire of responses; and
8. Allow a determination of the direction of misperception. (p. 445)

Based on evidence from their study of published articulation tests, Shriberg and Kwiatkowski (1980) conclude that "*natural process analysis is best based on a sample of continuous speech.* Procedures that involve responses to a word list evoked spontaneously or by immediate or delayed imitation . . . yield unstable data" (p. 9). We have no quarrel with this observation, provided that a sample of continuous speech is possible. When dealing with a population of aphasic children, or any other young and severely linguistically retarded children, it is possible to find youngsters who are essentially nonverbal or are at a single- or two-word stage, with utterances evoked only by direct stimulation. There may be little or no spontaneous speech, either in the clinical setting or, as the parent may report, in the home. We must therefore be prepared to employ elicitation procedures in order to provoke and evoke verbal responses. Procedures may include the use of puppets, dolls, or toys in play situations. Picture or toy identifications or elicited imitation of an adult or a verbal peer instructed by the adult—with or without visual prompts—may also be used. These procedures permit the clinician to know what the target words are and in what way, if elicitation is attained, the child's productions are deviant. Ingram (1981) also suggests the use of a phonological diary, which he defines as "a diary that is completed over a period of days during which the analyst writes down in phonetic form the child's production of adult words" (p. 12).

In *Procedures for the Phonological Analysis of Children's Language,* Ingram (1981) provides a detailed approach for analyzing the phonologies of children's speech. McReynolds and Engmann (1975) describe procedures for distinctive feature analysis and for analysis of articulation errors. Bernthal and Bankson (1981) describe several approaches for articulatory assessment, including procedures for obtaining language samples.

It should not be assumed that children's articulatory products necessarily represent their discriminative perceptions of what is presented to them. Phonological analysis should therefore include perceptual processing to learn what the child hears and how the sounds produced relate to what is presented. Locke's (1980) guides for assessment procedures should be helpful for this purpose. As a general observation, we should be aware that even for verbal children with articulation deficiencies, speech-sound production is not a reliable guide to perception; nevertheless, there is some relationship. On the basis of a survey of studies on speech-sound production and discrimination, Bernthal and Bankson (1981) conclude: "A relationship appears to exist between speech sound discrimination skill and articulation in subjects with impaired articulation, although the precise nature of the relationship has not been determined" (p. 116). Williams and McReynolds (1975) investigated the functional relationship between discrimination and production in the context of a training study. Their subjects were four children in the age range of 5 years, 1 month, to 6 years, 10 months. They found that "production training was effective in changing both articulation and discrimination; however discrimination training was effective in changing only discrimination."

AUDITORY PROCESSING: A MULTILEVEL PROGRAM FOR SEVERELY LINGUISTICALLY RETARDED (APHASIC) CHILDREN

The remaining pages of this chapter will present training programs for severely linguistically retarded (aphasic) children. Where to begin will be determined by what the clinician finds in the assessment process. The initial findings and the findings of ongoing assessments as the training progresses will inform the clinician of what steps and at what levels procedures need to be taken. In addition, the clinician will learn what the child acquires in the course of training that may not have been directly taught. Some children, who tune in to spoken language and once again learn to listen may establish considerably more articulatory proficiency than can be considered a direct result of the training itself. Again, we note that the programs are not intended for children with oral (articulatory) apraxia. These children will be considered separately in a later chapter.

It is possible that some children (fortunately, a very small percentage of even those who are aphasic) have developed perceptual defenses, usually unconscious ones, against spoken utterance. In effect, these children behave as if they were functionally deaf to speech (hard-of-listening). For these children, and perhaps for others of preschool age, auditory (listening) training may begin with mechanical and animate (nonspeech) sound discrimination. This level of approach provides an opportunity for success in auditory discrimination as well as establishing a procedure that may be followed later for phonemic training. We assume success because the capacity to process nonspeech auditory events is a right cerebral hemisphere function. Unless a child has been turned off from all meaningful environmental sounds and does, in fact, behave as if functionally deaf, the approach should work and should reinvite the child to become a listener, at least to those auditory events that are at the outset nonsymbolic and decodable.

AUDITORY DISCRIMINATION FOR ENVIRONMENTAL (NONSPEECH) EVENTS

Mechanical Noise Discrimination

This program is intended for children who have been turned off and away from spoken language, for nonlisteners or "hard-of-listening" children who may have established perceptual defenses against spoken language because they could not understand what they were physically able to hear. Solely as an introduction and seduction to getting the child to listen, we begin by establishing an association (identification) between mechanical noises and their source. In effect, we are helping the child to be aware of what he or she is able to identify among the many nonspeech sounds in the environment. Thus, a child is shown a bell that is rung or a horn that is blown. After the demonstration, the noise of the object may be recorded and produced from a tape recording or by the clinician while the child's back is turned. The child is then invited to make the same noise with one of two objects from a display. Even if the child points to the correct object, he or she should be encouraged to produce the noise for the pleasure of the deed. Thus, also, sound discrimination becomes associated with sound production, with the child being active in both processes.

Animate Noise Discrimination

The approach described for mechanical noise discrimination may also be used for animate noise discrimination, using toy animals that produce reasonably close approximations of real animal noises. Thus, a child can make a discriminative response between a cat's meowing and a dog's barking, a bird's chirping and a rooster's crowing, a cow's mooing and a lamb's bleating, a lion's roaring and an elephant's trumpeting, and so on. An even better approach would be to select sounds that the clinician knows are present in the child's community—the sounds of pets and birds and bees, and so forth—as a basis for creating awareness of the real sounds.

Sequential (Temporal Order) Training

If the approaches just described are to have any carryover to prepare the child for listening to spoken language, it is important to teach not only discrimination but also the processing of a series or sequence of sounds. At this stage the noise signals may be played back from tapes and the child instructed to point to the appropriate objects or pictures of the objects in the order of the sounds they make. We would begin with a two-noise series, with a half-second interval between the noises, and then progressively reduce the interval to about one-tenth second. When the child is successful with the processing of two noises, we would increase the task to three, and then to four. When four-noise sequences are correctly processed, we consider the child ready to become involved in applying the techniques she or he has learned to speech-sound perception.

SPEECH-SOUND (PHONEMIC) PROCESSING

In our projected program for phonemic processing, we will be guided by some of the published information on the phonologies of normal children while they acquire their first 50 words. This acquisition usually occurs during the age range (approximate) of 12 to 18 months. Ingram (1976) notes: "During this period, the child comes to acquire about 50 words before his vocabulary begins to grow very rapidly" (p. 17). Ingram also notes: "The nature of the child's phonology is very primitive during this time, and can be discussed as a separate period of acquisition."

Although we shall use Jakobson's generalizations regarding the universality of normal phonologies, we cannot ignore the observations of Ferguson and Farwell (1975): "Since children have different inputs and utilize different strategies, the gradual development of phonological organization and phonological awareness may proceed by different routes and at different paces." In essence, we must consider the influence of a given child's lexicon as the items relate to phonemic and phonological acquisitions. In a population of children whose vocabularies are extremely limited and who are being directly taught, input is highly selective, as are language experiences and awarenesses. In effect, the clinician, at least at the outset, is likely to be the one who determines the route and the rules that a child in treatment is apt to follow.

Jakobson's generalizations still serve as a guide, but we hope not so rigidly as to delay the introduction of words and, in due time, syntactic structures that a child needs in order to acquire functional verbal utterance at the earliest possible time. What the child cannot use to advantage away from a clinical setting will not be reinforced by natural practice. What the child can use will make clinical practice meaningful.

Based on Jakobson's generalizations, Ingram (1976) noted a common order of phonemic acquisition in normal children as they learn to produce their first 50 words. The likely, but not invariable, order is as follows:

1. First syllables are consonant-vowels (CV) or reduplicated as CVCV.
2. The first consonants are likely to be labials, usually /p/ or /m/.
3. Stop sounds, usually /t/ or /k/ follow bilabial acquisitions.
4. The first vowel is likely to be /a/, followed by /i/ or /u/.
5. Fricatives are acquired after stops.

Ingram also cited Ferguson and Garnica (1975) to the effect that the sounds /h/ and /w/ are among the first usually produced by children in their early verbal acquisitions.

With these observations and reservations noted, we will present a developmental program for speech sound (phonemic) processing for children who are severely linguistically delayed in language acquisition. Our target population will continue to be aphasic children. We will emphasize the desirability of establishing phonemic discrimination and associating discrimination with production. We accept the principle that perception normally precedes production in early language development and we acknowledge that this principle (assumption) may be applied with positive results in our program for phonemic processing.

FIRST CONTRASTS FOR PHONEMIC PROCESSING

Consonant-Vowel (CV) vs. Vowel

The first phonemic discrimination task calls for the child to establish a discriminative response between a consonant-vowel (CV) unit and an isolated vowel (e.g., [m + i] vs. [i]). Our immediate purpose for this task is to create awareness of two units that are different, though they share a common feature in the vowel. We do not initially require that the child articulate the units. However, if the child spontaneously produces them, we learn not only that she or he perceives the units as different but that she or he is also capable of producing them in keeping with the perception of the difference. It is assumed that in the early stages of the training program, most children who are in need of auditory training will not be able to produce what they are exposed to and might perceive. Consequently, it will be necessary to obtain a nonoral response in order to determine whether they are responding differentially to the auditory event. This can be established either by teaching the child to associate auditory signals with objects or pictures—the child is taught to point out the correct association—or by teaching the child to make a yes or no response by a head gesture or a hand gesture (thumb up or thumb down) for same or different.

Slobin (1967) describes a well-established approach for testing discrimination with small children:

> The general procedure for testing a discrimination with small children is to provide some objects they can discriminate easily, and to give them different names. With small children, the easiest discriminations are between different shapes like triangle and circle, and big differences in size. So make a list of the syllables to be used in the testing, and see to it that every pair tested has a "named object" easily discriminated by a child from the object named by the syllable paired with it. There are three steps in the learning: a) the child learns that there are two different objects; b) the child learns that there will be a reward with only one of the objects at a time, and that he must choose; and c) the actual test, with a choice based on the *name* of the object rather than another one. Example and method: a large triangle is "too"; a small triangle is "tea." Use as rewards trinkets, colored sticky paper, or some other objects which don't readily satiate as do foods. Variation might be a good idea.

In the section on the syndrome of developmental aphasia, we presented evidence that aphasic children require more time for making correct discriminative and temporal order judgments for auditory events than do their nonlinguistically impaired age peers. With experience in the experimental situation, the interstimulus interval (ISI) tends to be reduced. Our program incorporates the implications of this information in training the aphasic children to listen and process auditory speech events.

The syllables—actually, consonant plus vowel words—chosen for the initial level of training, when and if necessary, include sounds that appear early in the phonemic acquisitions of normal children. Our observations indicate that these sounds are also easiest for aphasic children to discriminate. Even for aphasic children, the perception of a nasal or stop consonant followed by a vowel should present no problem and should require little training. We begin there, for the most severely impaired children, to establish a technique or procedure for listening and to provide opportunity for the child to experience success. The materials that immediately follow, presented phonetically and orthographically, are sample units for this probably positive experience.

C + V		V		C + V		V	
[mi]	(me)	[i]	(ēē)	[ti]	(tea)	[i]	(ēē)
[mei]	(may)	[ei]	(ay)	—		—	
[mu]	(moo)	[u]	(ōō)	[tu]	(too)	[u]	(ōō)
[mai]	(my)	[ai]	(ī)	[tai]	(tie)	[ai]	(ī)
[ma]	(ma)	[a]	(ah)(ä)	—		—	

Note that most of the CV syllables selected for this training experience are usable words that are fairly high in frequency among normal children.

If these CV units are presented for a yes or no response, the order should be randomized in a sequence, such as:

[ma]	[ma]		[ma]	[a]
[ma]	[ma]		[ma]	[a]
[ma]	[a]		[ma]	[ma]
[ma]	[ma]		[ma]	[ma]

If the child cannot make distinctions when the units are presented at a normal rate of utterance, the following suggestions for presentation should be followed:[3]

1. Present the units with a just-discernible interval between consonant and vowel and about a half-second interstimulus interval (ISI) before producing the isolated vowel, (e.g., m-a - - - - a.
2. Repeat, reducing the ISI to a quarter-second or less and finally to a just-discernible pause.

[3]See Table 7.1 for phonetic and diacritical representations of the phonemes of American English. Our practice materials, from this point on, will be presented in phonetic symbols.

3. When the contrasts are established, present the first units on a single-breath impulse as a vowel-consonant syllable. Allow a half-second interval before presenting the vowel. Repeat, reducing the ISI to a quarter-second and finally to a just-discernible pause.
4. Repeat as in 2 and 3, replacing /m/ by /t/ or /k/. If the child has difficulty in these contrasts, repeat as in 1. Continue until achieving a minimum of 75 percent (preferably 90 percent) correct response.

Nasal Consonant + Vowel vs. Vowel + Nasal Consonant

At this point we are concerned with having the child become aware of the order or sequence of sounds. Thus, the stimulus items consist of pairs of a vowel and a nasal consonant, or a nasal consonant and a vowel, with only the order of the sounds changed. The surface task is for the child to indicate whether what he or she receives is the same or different. The stimulus items should be presented in a random order so that the child will not be likely to guess, except by chance, whether a given pair is in fact the same or different.

The items should be presented initially as two-phoneme syllables. If it appears that the child has difficulty with such presentations, then a just-discernible interval may be introduced between the phonemes for each pair. If the child succeeds with such presentations, then the pairs should again be presented as syllables, with a slower-than-normal rate of production. Sample sequences follow:

1. [m + vowel], [vowel + m]

[mɑ]	[mɑ]	[ɑm]	[ɑm]
[mɑ]	[ɑm]	[ɑm]	[mɑ]
[mɑ]	[ɑm]	[mɑ]	[mɑ]
[ɑm]	[mɑ]	[ɑm]	[ɑm]
[mu]	[mu]	[mu]	[um]
[mu]	[um]	[um]	[um]
[um]	[um]	[mu]	[mu]
[um]	[mu]	[mu]	[mu]
[mu]	[mu]	[um]	[mu]

The same can be done for combinations of [m + vowel] or [vowel + m] with the vowels /l/, /ɔ/, /o/, /i/, /e/, /ɛ/, and /ʌ/.

2. [n + vowel] and [vowel + n] Make combinations as in 1 above for these pairs. The /ŋ/ will not be used for sequence of sound training at this stage, because the sound does not occur as the initial sound of a syllable in English. We are omitting the /ŋ/ to avoid any possibility that the child may carry over any expectation that this sound may be the initial consonant of an English word.

Stop Consonants (/k/, /t/, /p/, /g/, /d/, /b/) in Contrast with Nasals

The strategy at this stage is to present sound combinations that are distinctively different by at least two features in syllables that comprise a consonant plus a vowel (CV combination). As indicated earlier, stop consonants are acquired and we assume, therefore, also perceived earlier than fricatives, so that the first contrasts will be between stops plus vowels and nasals plus vowels. The minimum contrast units will be for two-phoneme syllables.

1. [m + vowel] vs. [k + vowel]   If we begin with [mɑ] vs. [kɑ], we have two syllables in which the feature differences for the consonants include place of articulation, voicing, nasality, and duration. Theoretically, and we hope practically, the child should have little difficulty in perceiving the differences (discriminating) between these syllables, or any others that are combinations of the voiceless stop (k + vowel] and the voiced bilabial [m + vowel]. Following are some samples of syllable contrasts that the clinician will present with a discernible ISI to elicit same or different responses from the child:

| [mɑ] | [kɑ] | [mi] | [ki] | [mo] | [ko] |
| [kɑ] | [mɑ] | [mu] | [ku] | [mɑɪ] | [kɑɪ] |

The same can be done with substitution of other vowels, as in sample materials for [m + vowel], [vowel + m].

For the purpose of economy of space repeated pairs of syllables will no longer be presented. The clinician should be reminded of the need to randomize presentations so that child will not select same or different on the basis of the order of presentation rather than as a result of active perceptual processing.

2. [m + vowel] vs. [t + vowel]   Following the establishment of the foregoing contrasts, we suggest the substitution of /t/ for /k/ so that the basic units for discrimination constitute [m + vowel] vs. [t + vowel]. In combination, then, we would arrive at units that would include the following:

[mɑ]	[tɑ]	[ti]	[mi]
[mu]	[tu]	[tai]	[mai]
[mo]	[to]	[te]	[me]
[mɔ]	[tɔ]	[tʌ]	[mʌ]

3. [m + vowel] vs. [p + vowel]   The consonants /m/ and /p/ are both bilabials. Thus, this contrast reduces the feature difference by one, since both are articulated in the same place. However, the remaining features are numerous enough that the child should have no difficulty in discriminating the syllable combinations. There is a possibility that children who have been trained to become careful visual observers may assume that they see what they do not hear, and so may confuse the /m/ and /p/ because both are produced with bilabial activity. If this turns out to be so, we recommend that the child's hand be placed in front of the clinician's mouth to feel the plosive quality for the /p/ and at the sides of the nose for the humming quality of the /m/. This procedure should help establish the differences between these two bilabial phonemes.

Sample pairs for the contrasts include the following:

[mɑ]	[pɑ]	[pɛ]	[mɛ]
[mo]	[po]	[pʌ]	[mʌ]
[me]	[pe]	[pu]	[mu]
[mi]	[pi]	[pɔ]	[mɔ]

The foregoing syllable contrast and those that follow include nonsense syllables. In extended practice, however, syllables that are also functional words may be emphasized. As soon as possible, the syllables that are words should be incorporated into two-word utterances in practical situations; for example, *pay me* should result in a payment that is meaningful to the child, and *my pie* might produce a taste of a piece of pie. This procedure may help enhance the related processes of perceptual discrimination, decoding, and production.

4. [m + vowel] vs. [g + vowel] The /g/ is the sound as in the word *go*. All the contrast pairs presented include the feature difference of voicing between the consonants; that is, /m/ is voiced, and /k/, /t/, and /p/ are voiceless. The consonant /g/, like /m/, is voiced. Thus, there is a reduction in one of the distinctive features between the consonants.

Syllable contrast pairs to be presented in keeping with the suggestions for [m + vowel], [vowel + m], and [p + vowel] include the following:

[mɑ]	[gɑ]	[geɪ]	[meɪ]	[ʌg]	[ʌm]
[mɔ]	[gɔ]	[gɛ]	[mɛ]	[æg]	[æm]
[mo]	[go]	[gʌ]	[mʌ]	[um]	[ug]
[mu]	[gu]	[gæ]	[mæ]	[ɑm]	[ɑg]

In the foregoing samples and those that follow, contrasts for the vowels /ɪ/, /a/, /ɒ/ and the central vowels /ə/ and /ɜ/ and their variants. The vowels omitted present special perceptual problems related to similarity of production, and so also of perception, as for /ə/ and /ɪ/, or because of variation in different regions of the United States. The latter pertain especially for the vowels /a/, /ɜ/ and /ɒ/. However, a clinician who is working with a child and has knowledge of the child's regional dialect may compose appropriate syllables that take into consideration the pronunciations the child is most likely to hear.

5. [m + vowel] vs. [d + vowel] Syllable contrasts are as immediately preceding samples.

6. [m + vowel] vs. [b + vowel]   We now have a further reduction in articulatory features. Both the /m/ and the /b/ are bilabial, and both are voiced. Syllable contrast samples are as follows:

[mɑ]	[bɑ]	[bi]	[mi]
[mu]	]bu]	[bæ]	[mæ]
[mo]	[bo]	[be]	[me]
[mɔ]	[bɔ]	[bʌ]	[mʌ]

7. [n + Vowel] vs. [Stop Consonant (/k/, /g/, /p/, /b/, /t/, /d/) + Vowel]   These syllable combinations can be constructed along the lines suggested for the [m + vowel] vs. [stop + vowel] samples. We could reserve the /t/ and /d/ for the last because of the shared common place of production (tip of tongue and upper gum ridge) for the /n/, /t/, and /d/.

At this stage, many if not most children who were successful in the previous sound discrimination exercises may find the tasks relatively easy and no longer challenging. We would therefore suggest what amounts to a screening test for the [n + vowel] vs. [stop + vowel] to determine whether there is any need for training in discrimination for these combinations. A quick screening test might include the following syllable contrasts:

[nɑ]	[kɑ]	[nʌ]	[gʌ]	[næ]	[tæ]
[ni]	[ki]	[ne]	[ge]	[no]	[to]
[næ]	[pæ]	[nɔ]	[bɔ]	[ne]	[de]
[nɔ]	[pɔ]	[ni]	[bi]	[nu]	[du]

Based on the results of this screening, the clinician can develop practice units specific to the needs of the child. Incidentally, if a child spontaneously produces the sound pairs before indicating the same or different responses, he or she should be given a special reward in recognition of this accomplishment.

8. [Nasal + Vowel] vs. [Fricative + Vowel]   The fricative consonants include /f/, /θ/ (th), /s/, /ʃ/ (sh), and their voiced cognates /v/, /ð/, /z/, and /ʒ/ (zh).

As indicated in the foregoing discussion, we would begin with a screening test to determine whether and where specific training is needed for contrasts with fricative consonants:

[mɑ]	[fɑ]	[mɑ]	[sɑ]	[me]	[ʃe]
[mi]	[fi]	[mi]	[si]	[ma]	[ʃa]
[mu]	[θu]	[mu]	[su]	[mɔ]	[ʃɔ]
[me]	[θe]	[mo]	[so]	[me]	[ʃe]
[mɔ]	[θɔ]	[mo]	[θo]	[mʌ]	[ʃʌ]
[ma]	[va]	[mi]	[ði]	[ma]	[zɑ]
[mi]	[vi]	[mæ]	[ðæ]	[mi]	[zi]
[mu]	[vu]	[mo]	[ðo]	[mu]	[zu]
[mo]	[vo]	[me]	[ðe]	[me]	[ze]

Syllables such as these may be constructed with /n/ substituted for /m/ (e.g., [na] [fa], [nu] [vu], [ne] [θe], [no] [zo], etc.). We would predict that the contrasts with /n/ are likely to be more difficult than those with /m/.

We recognize, of course, that even if a child perceives (discriminates correctly) that a combination such as [ma] is different from [sa], it does not mean that his or her perception is based on an appreciation of the attributes of the consonants that make for the difference. Only when the child begins to produce the sounds, even though the production may be defective, can we assume that the discriminations are based on the individual perceptions of the sounds. It follows that if a child is producing the sounds, there is no longer any need for discrimination training.

The phoneme /ʒ/ (zh) is not included in this screening list because the sound does not occur initially in English words and only rarely in final position. It occurs most frequently in medial position. We do not consider training for contrasts with /ʒ/ necessary at this stage. The clinician may make up syllable contrasts, however, if he or she so desires.

9. [Nasal + Vowel] vs. [Affricate + Vowel]   The affricate (stop plus fricative) sounds are [tʃ] (ch) and [dʒ] (dzh). Again, we recommend determining whether a child needs training in any way for the syllable contrasts that include a nasal and a vowel vs. an affricate and a vowel. Following are some combinations that may be used in a screening procedure. The clinician should randomize the order of the presentations:

[ma]	[tʃa]	[ma]	[dʒa]	[no]	[tʃo]	[na]	[dʒa]
[mi]	[tʃi]	[mi]	[dʒi]	[ni]	[tʃi]	[ni]	[dʒi]
[mu]	[tʃu]	[mæ]	[dʒæ]	[na]	[tʃa]	[nɔ]	[dʒɔ]
[me]	[tʃe]	[me]	[dʒe]	[nʌ]	[tʃʌ]	[nʌ]	[dʒʌ]

Other Consonant-Vowel Contrasts

Up to this point, our CV contrasts have included a nasal plus a vowel and either a stop or a fricative plus a vowel. Nasality has been a constant feature in the sound-discrimination training. Now the contrasts will be with consonants other than nasals, beginning with consonants that are relatively far apart (two or more features) and moving toward those that are different by only one feature. For features in the production of consonants in American-English speech and for the rationale for the choice of these features, see Table 7.3.

10. [Stop + Vowel] and [Fricative + Vowel] (e.g., [pɑ] and [sɑ]   Consonant-vowel (CV) combinations such as [pi], [pe], [pɛ], [pæ], [pu], [po], [pɔ], and [pɑ] may be contrasted with CV syllables with an initial fricative. The contrast syllable pairs should have the same vowel, and the element of voicing should be held constant (e.g., [pɑ] [sɑ] [tu] [su], [ki] [ʃi], [bo] [zo], [dɔ] [vɔ], and [gɑ] [ðɑ]).

We suggest that the order for contrasts between stop and fricative CV syllables follow the sequence of /s/, /ʃ/, /θ/, /f/ and /p/, /k/, /t/. For combinations with voiced consonants, the suggested order is /b/, /g/, /d/ and /z/, /ʒ/, /ð/, /v/.

Table 7.9 CONTRAST COMBINATIONS FOR STOP, FRICATIVE, AFFRICATE, AND SEMIVOWELS

	Stop	Fricative	Affricate	Semivowels
Voiceless	p k + Vowel t	s ʃ θ + Vowel f	tʃ + Vowel	
Voiced	b g + Vowel d	z ʒ ð + Vowel v	dʒ + Vowel	r,l, w,j, + Vowel

Table 7.9 presents the consonants that may be combined with vowels for making syllable contrast practice material.

11. Stop and Affricates (e.g., [pɑ] and [tʃɑ]) The affricates [tʃ] and [dʒ] present special problems because they are, as their phonetic symbols indicate, combinations of a stop and a fricative. The suggested order for training in stop vs. affricate contrasts is /p/, /k/, and /t/ with [tʃ] and /b/, /g/, and /d/ with [dʒ]. Thus, we would have CV combinations such as [pɑ], [kɑ], and [tɑ] to contrast with [tʃɑ] and [bɑ], [gɑ], and [dɑ] to contrast with [dʒɑ].

12. Stop and Vowellike Consonants (Semivowels) The vowellike consonants or semivowels are /r/, /l/, /w/, and /j/ (y). Because these are all voiced sounds, our contrast training will be with the voiced stops /b/, /d/, and /g/, and we may have syllable pairs such as the following:

[bɑ]	[rɑ]	[go]	[ro]	[du]	[ru]
[bɑ]	[lɑ]	[go]	[lo]	[du]	[lu]
[bɑ]	[wɑ]	[go]	[wo]	[du]	[wu]
[bɑ]	[jɑ]	[go]	[jo]	[du]	[ju]

13. Semivowels and Fricative, Affricate Contrasts The sounds /r/ and /l/ are among the later ones produced proficiently by many children. They are also the sounds that continue to present difficulty for many children beyond 7 or 8 years of age. A frequent substitution is a sound that approximates /w/. The difficulty children have in the production of /r/ and /l/ is not, however, related to perceptual or discriminative problems for these sounds (Menyuk and Anderson, 1969).

Training at this stage may begin with semivowel and fricative contrasts and then proceed to semivowel vs. affricates. Following are some combinations:

[ri]	[zi]	[lɑ]	[zɑ]	[wi]	[zi]
[re]	[ze]	[li]	[zi]	[we]	[ze]
[rɔ]	[zɔ]	[lo]	[vo]	[wu]	[ðu]

[ru]	[zu]	[læ]	[væ]	[wɑ]	[ða]
[ri]	[dʒi]	[læ]	[dʒæ]	[we]	[dʒe]
[re]	[dʒe]	[lo]	[dʒo]	[wɑ]	[dʒɑ]
[rɑ]	[dʒɑ]	[li]	[dʒi]	[wo]	[dʒo]

A RATIONALE FOR OTHER SOUND CONTRASTS
IN PHONEMIC TRAINING

It should be apparent at this point that the possible combinations for speech-sound discrimination are so great in number that neither the effort nor the space to present them could be justified. What we shall do now is provide a rationale for the kinds of phonemic discriminations that English-speaking children need to acquire (understand) their language.

Shvachkin's study on the development of phonemic perception in early childhood, referred to earlier, is a basic investigation of receptive discrimination of speech sounds. Shvachkin studied Russian children in the age range between 11 months and 1 year, 11 months, for their understanding of words differing by only a single phoneme. On the assumption, which we consider tenable, that phonological discrimination as well as phonological acquisition (production) remains the same regardless of the language the child learns, we can apply Shvachkin's observations to children exposed to English (see Table 7.4).

Our order of presentation thus far, in general but not in every instance, has been consistent with the pattern of phonemic development indicated earlier. We have tried to reconcile Shvachkin's sequence with observations on the number of distinctive phonemic features severely linguistically retarded (aphasic) children seem to require to discriminate between speech sounds.

Consonant–Vowel–Consonant (CVC) with the Same
Consonant in the First and Third Positions
(e.g., [mam] and [pip])

Our purpose at this stage is to increase the length of the syllable presented to the child in consonant-vowel-consonant units, using the same consonant in the first and third positions of the syllable. The syllable contrasts may be those previously presented for the [nasal + vowel] vs. [stop + vowel], [fricative + vowel], and [affricate + vowel] exercises, with the addition of a repeated consonant to produce a CVC unit. Thus, we might have syllables such as the following:

[mim]	[dɑd]	[pup]	[faf]
[mem]	[kik]	[sæs]	[vov]
[nan]	[kek]	[sas]	[vev]
[nun]	[gʌg]	[ziz]	[tʃʌtʃ]
[tut]	[gɑg]	[zuz]	[dʒadʒ]
[tat]	[pip]	[fif]	[θɑθ]

Syllables such as these may be presented in contrast with [nasal + vowel + nasal] or in reduplicated presentations for same-or-different responses. The intervals between syllable presentations (interstimulus intervals) should at first be clearly discernible—approximately a quarter of a second— and then reduced until they are just discernible. Finally, they should be presented as if they were equally stressed syllables of a two-syllable utterance (e.g., [mam mam], [mam tat], [tat tat], etc.), with different initial sounds for stop-fricative contrasts, as follows:

[bik]	[sik]	[dʌd]	[vʌd]
[bek]	[sek]	[dɑk]	[vɑk]
[kup]	]fup]	[kɪp]	]vɪp]
[pet]	[set]	[pɑz]	[zɑz]
[pɔt]	[sɔt]	[tut]	[θut]

The following features CVC syllables with different third sounds:

[pik]	[pim]	[sap]	[san]
[pek]	[pez]	[sɔm]	[sɔk]
[bɑf]	[baʃ]	[tʃek]	[tʃef]
[tup]	[tuz]	[zup]	[zun]

When it becomes evident that the child can make the discriminations, or can process same and different sound sequences even when they are presented as if they were two-syllable utterances, she or he is ready for the next step in training.[4]

Bisyllables Differing in Vowels (Strong and Weak Vowels)

Weak vowels in unstressed syllables are a feature of spoken English. Thus, either the vowel schwa /ə/ or /ɪ/ is likely to be present in words of two or more syllables. The need for children exposed to English to tune in on the vowel difference and on the stress patterns and prosody of English utterance should be apparent. Following are some two-syllable nonsense combinations that can be used as model forms for practice in a same-or-different procedure or in any procedure in which the child indicates an awareness of vowel or syllable stress difference:

---

[4]If the clinician feels intuitively that the child can process the two-syllable presentations, then these should be presented first. If the child is successful, there is no need to present the CVC units with discernible interstimulus intervals.

First Syllable Stress	Second Syllable Stress	First Syllable Stress	Second Syllable Stress
[mi pɪm]	[mɪ pim]	[ti [sɪt]	[tɪ sit]
[me kɪm]	[mɪ kem]	[te sɪt]	[tɪ set]
[mu səm]	[mə sum]	[pɑ ʃəp]	[pə ʃap]
[mo ʃəm]	[mə ʃom]	[pɛ rəp]	[pə rɛp]
[nɑ sən]	[nə ran]	[su kət]	[sə kut]
[tɑ sək]	[tə sak]	[sɑ dət]	[sə [kɑt]
[pɑ ʃək]	[pə ʃak]	[ru kət]	[rə mut]
[mu rət]	[mə rut]	[lɔ pət]	[lə pɔt]
[so pət]	[sə pot]	[tʃɑ məp]	[tʃə mɑp]

DISCRIMINATION OF MEDIAL SOUNDS IN BISYLLABIC CONTEXT

Moving in the direction of contexts that approximate real words, we would now introduce bisyllables with a weak-strong vowel construction that differ by only a medial sound (e.g., [hə mɑk] and [hə ʒɑk]).[5]

At this point we would look for any evident difficulties in responses when the medial sounds are close together in regard to distinctive features (e.g., [hə sɑk] and [ha ʃak], or [hə sɑk] and [hə zak]), and we would emphasize training to overcome discriminatory weaknesses. The constructions that follow are in approximate order (greatest number to fewest) relative to distinctive sound features:

[hə] + CVC Constructions		Sound Contrasts for First Sound of Stressed Syllable	
[hə][6] [mɑk]	[hə] [ʒɑk]	[hə] [ʃʌp]	[hə] [dʌp]
[mɑk]	[gɑk]	[dʒɑb]	[θab]
[muk]	[suk]	[dʒeb]	[veb]
[pɑk]	[ʒɑk]	[vɑk]	[ʃɑk]
[bik]	[ʃik]	[fub]	[sub]
[mɑg]	[θag]	[set]	[ʃet]
[nup]	[pup]	[feb]	[veb]
[nep]	[tʃep]	[nup]	[mup]
[nuk]	[vuk]	[tak]	[dɑk]
[bek]	[zek]	[kep]	[gep]
[sɑp]	[bap]	[ʂap]	[zɑp]
[sip]	[pip]	[pun]	[bun]
[zup]	[tup]	[tʌm]	[dʌm]

[5]These are the basic constructions used by McReynolds (1966) in her study. McReynolds found that, with training, severely linguistically retarded (aphasic) children can make discriminatory responses to such syllables, but at a slower rate than normal controls.
[6]The first syllable for each member of each pair is [hə].

POSITION (SOUND) SEQUENCING

One of the underlying difficulties in the auditory processing of aphasic children is sequencing (keeping in mind the order of events), so that a word such as *ten* can be distinguished from *net,* or *pats* from *past.* In early language acquisition, sequencing (temporal order) difficulties are common when children begin to use polysyllabic words. Characteristic transpositions such as *aminal* for *animal* and *pasghetti* for *spaghetti* are often maintained for a considerable time. Our concern at this time is not with production, but with reception and perception. Thus, the material presented will require the child not to reproduce a sequence but to recognize and indicate whether the sequences are the same or different. Of course, if the child spontaneously produces the sequences correctly, we may assume that he or she has received and processed them as they were presented. In the lists that follow, the syllables will be presented orthographically and we will not be concerned that many of the syllables are real rather than nonsense words.

It is suggested that, at the outset, the child be given a few items for screening purposes to determine whether quantity (number of phonemes) rather than order, per se, is a basic problem.

Screening Items

kip	pick	pot	top	pats	past
nub	bun	sub	bus	muts	must
nib	pin	lease	seal	nets	nest
bud	dub	stone	notes	claps	clasp

CVC Sample Items for Sequencing

nap	pan	feel	leaf	lag	gal
gun	nug	can	nack	lane	nail
cup	puck	neat	teen	mode	dome
kit	tick	meat	team	pal	lap
bad	dab	face	safe	tack	cat
moon	noom	side	dice	cut	tuck
ash	ax	rust	ruts	animal	aminal
mast	mats	brisk	bricks	elephant	ephalant
pest	pets	must	muts	spaghetti	pasghetti
clasp	claps	nest	nets	telephone	tephelone

SUMMARY

The materials in this chapter are intended to provide a base for understanding normal phonological development—the better to understand the improficiencies of aphasic and dysphasic children. The exercises in the program for training children with difficulties in perceptual processing of speech events—children who may be considered "hard-of-listening"—are intended to overcome their dysfunction, which seriously impairs their capacity for oral-aural linguistic decoding.

We believe our program is developmental and is consistent with the available information about normal children's abilities in their phonological acquisitions. Accordingly, we first determine where the child is in level of perceptual functioning and then move the child to where he or she needs to be in order to perceive (discriminate and make temporal order judgments about) speech signals. The objective, of course, is for the child to understand and produce spoken language. Several instruments described in the chapter on assessment may be used to establish a baseline for the individual child. In many instances, for the most severely impaired children, the clinician will have to exercise subjective judgment regarding where to begin. Trial training provides one basis, perhaps the most reliable one, for exercising clinical judgment.

As a general observation, aphasic children are both delayed and, individually, often deviant in the rules they use for their phonological acquisitions. In general, also, they need greater perceptual distance to make correct discriminative and temporal order decisions than do their normal age peers. Our practice materials are intended to observe the implications of this information. The final sets of exercises are for children who need training in temporal order processing. We believe that children who can make correct temporal order decisions are ready for the programs in language production.

REFERENCES AND SUGGESTED READINGS

Bernthal, J. E., and Bankson, N. W. *Articulation Disorders.* Englewood Cliffs, N.J.: Prentice-Hall, 1981.

Chomsky, N. and Halle, M. *The Sound Patterns of English.* New York: Harper and Row, 1968.

Eisenson, J., and Ogilvie, M. *Communicative Disorders in Children.* New York: Macmillan, 1983.

Ferguson, C. A., and Farwell, C. B. "Words and Sounds in Early Language Acquisition," *Language,* 51(2), 1975, 419–439.

Ferguson, C. A., and Garnica, O. "Theories of Phonological Development," in E. H. Lenneberg and E. Lenneberg (eds.), *Foundations of Language Development.* New York: Academic Press, 1975.

Holland, A. "Language Therapy for Children: Some Thoughts on Context and Content," *Journal of Speech and Hearing Disorders,* 40(4), 1975, 514–523.

Ingram, D. *Phonological Disability in Children.* New York: Elsevier; and London: Edward Arnold, 1976.

Ingram, D. *Procedures for the Phonological Analysis of Children's Language.* Baltimore: University Park Press, 1981.

Jakobson, R. *Child Language, Aphasia and Phonological Universals.* The Hague: Mouton, 1968.

Lahey, M., and Bloom, L. "Planning a First Lexicon," *Journal of Speech and Hearing Disorders,* 42(3), 1977, 340–350.

Locke, J. "The Inferences of Speech Perception in the Phonologically Disordered Child, I and II," *Journal of Speech and Hearing Disorders,* 45(4), 1980, 431–444; 445–468.

MacDonald, J. D., and Blott, J. P. "Environmental Language Intervention," *Journal of Speech and Hearing Disorders,* 39(3), 1974, 244–256.

McReynolds, L. K. "Operant Conditioning for Investigating Speech Sound Discrimination in Aphasic Children," *Journal of Speech and Hearing Research,* 9(4), 1966, 519–528.

McReynolds, L. K., and Engmann, D. L. *Distinctive Feature Analysis of Misarticulations.* Baltimore: University Park Press, 1975.

Menyuk, P. and Anderson, S. "Children's Identification and Reproduction of /w/, /r/ and /l/," *Journal of Speech and Hearing Research,* 12(1), 1969, 39–52.

Menyuk, P., and Looney, P. L. "Relationships Among Components of the Grammar in Language Disorder," *Journal of Speech and Hearing Research,* 15(2), 1972, 395–406.

Panagos, J. "Persistence of the Open Syllable Reinterpreted as a Symptom of Language Disorder," *Journal of Speech and Hearing Disorders,* 39(1), 1974, 23–31.

Prather, E. M., Hedrick, K. L., and Kern, C. A. "Articulation Development in Children Aged Two to Four Years," *Journal of Speech and Hearing Disorders,* 40(2), 1975, 179–191.

Rosenthal, W. S. "Perception of Auditory Temporal Order as a Function of Selected Stimulus Features in a Group of Aphasic Children." Doctoral dissertation, Stanford University, 1970.

Ruder, K. F., and Bunce, B. H. "Articulation Therapy Using Distinctive Feature Analysis to Structure Training Program: Two Case Studies," *Journal of Speech and Hearing Disorders,* 46(1), 1981, 59–65.

Sander, E. K. "When Are Speech-Sounds Learned?" *Journal of Speech and Hearing Disorders,* 37, 1972, 55–63.

Shriberg, L. D. "Developmental Phonological Disorders," in T. Hixon, L. D. Shriberg, and J. H. Saxman, *Introduction to Communication Disorders.* Englewood Cliffs, N.J.: Prentice-Hall, 1980.

Shriberg, L. D., and Kwiatkowski, J. *Natural Process Analysis (NPA).* New York: Wiley, 1980.

Shriner, T. H., Hollaway, M. S., and Daniloff R. C. "The Relationship between Articulation Defects and Syntax in Speech Defective Children," *Journal of Speech and Hearing Research,* 1969, 12(2), 319–325.

Shvachkin, N., in F. Smith and G. A. Miller, *The Genesis of Language* (abstracted by D. I. Slobin). Cambridge, Mass.: M.I.T. Press, 1966.

Singh, S. *Distinctive Features: Theory and Validation.* Baltimore: University Park Press, 1976.

Slobin, D. (ed.). *A Field Manual for Cross-Cultural Study of the Acquisition of Communicative Competence.* Berkeley: University of California, 1967.

Stark, R. E., and Tallal, P. "Perceptual and Motor Deficits in Language-Impaired Children," in R. W. Keith (ed.), *Central Auditory and Language Disorders in Children*. Houston: College-Hill Press, 1981.

Tallal, P., and Piercy, M. "Defects of Auditory Perception in Children with Developmental Dysphasia," in M. A. Wyke (ed.), *Developmental Dysphasia*. New York: Academic Press, 1978.

Templin, M. C. *Certain Language Skills in Children*. Minneapolis: University of Minnesota Press, 1957.

Walsh, H. "On Certain Practical Inadequacies of Distinctive Feature Systems," *Journal of Speech and Hearing Disorders,* 39(1)1, 1974, 32–43.

Weiner, F. "Treatment of Phonological Disability Using the Method of Meaningful Minimal Contrast: Two Case Studies," *Journal of Speech and Hearing Disorders,* 46 (1), 1981, 97–103.

Williams, G. C., and McReynolds, L. K. "The Relationship between Discrimination and Articulation Training with Misarticulations," *Journal of Speech and Hearing Research,* 18(3), 1975, 401–412.

Winitz, H. *Articulatory Acquisition and Behavior*. New York: Appleton-Century-Crofts, 1969.

Winitz, H. *From Syllable to Conversation*. Baltimore: University Park Press, 1975.

chapter 8

Establishing and Developing Language in Severely Linguistically Handicapped Children

Children who are severely delayed in language acquisition may range from those who are essentially nonverbal, who neither comprehend nor produce meaningful language, to those who are at a one-word stage when their age peers are understanding and using appropriate syntactic constructions. The reference is to children who, based on indices other than language, are presumably of an intellectual age (cognitive stage) for whom a greater degree of language proficiency is expected beyond what is evidenced. It is also assumed, for the purposes of this discussion, that the children are not deaf, are not emotionally disturbed, and do have adequate oral mechanisms for articulate language.

Where and when to begin therapy will depend on where the child is in terms of language proficiency and the usually associated cognitive indices. For some children, the starting point may be to establish a basic comprehension vocabulary to be matched, concurrently or as soon as possible, by a vocabulary for expression. For other children, the first step may be to advance them beyond an essentially infantile level of linguistic proficiency. For still others, the beginning may be on a higher level, yet one that, for reasons that are not always readily apparent, is considerably below what we might expect according to other indices of cognitive development.

PRELINGUISTIC COGNITIVE FUNCTIONS

It might help to review, however briefly, some of the cognitive achievements of children who are at the single-word stage, usually arrived at between 9 and 18 months of age. In terms of Piaget's psychophilosophy, normal children in this age range are in the latter months of the sensorimotor stage, culminating in the use of language. In the first months, in the absence of language or symbolic function, sensorimotor intelligence, which is directed at getting results, is essentially practical. Prelingual intelligence at this period

> ... succeeds in eventually solving numerous problems of action (such as reaching distant or hidden objects) by constructing a complex system of action-schemes and organizing reality in terms of spatiotemporal and causal structures. In the absence of language or symbolic function, however, these constructions are made with the sole support of perceptions and movements and thus by means of a sensorimotor coordination of actions, without the intervention of representation or thought. (Piaget and Inhelder, 1969, p. 4)

Usually by the end of the sensorimotor period, or at about 18 months, most children are in the single-word (holophrastic) language stage. At this time—for some children as early as 9 months and for a few as late as 24 months—children's behaviors reveal the following cognitive achievements:

1. They can engage in deferred imitation.
2. Object permanence is established (out of sight is not out of mind).
3. They can engage in symbolic play and so can pretend that they and other things are not what we usually assume them to be.
4. They have discovered the use of tools and can use an intermediary to achieve an end. The intermediary may be a person, usually older, who is available for manipulation.

With these intellectual achievements established, the children are able to represent to themselves actual objects and events. According to Piaget and Inhelder (1969) this is requisite for the acquisition of knowledge and symbolic experience. At this stage, children begin to use their first words, initially usually to label (name or identify) persons, objects, and events, and later to bring about what they were able to label. In effect, children at this age are learning the instrumental use of language.

ESTABLISHING PRELINGUAL REPRESENTATIONAL BEHAVIOR

This chapter and the next will consider approaches and content for establishing representational understanding and behavior in severely linguistically retarded children. We shall begin with the nonverbal child who is identified as having little or no functional language for communicative purpose. At the extreme end, such children show little evidence of comprehending spoken (oral) language and, correspondingly, have little or no productive verbal behavior. These children, for the most part, are ones who are likely to be congenitally or developmentally aphasic.[1]

Our working assumption is that although these severely linguistically retarded children hear, they are impaired in their auditory discriminative and sequencing abilities—in their perceptual functioning for speech—and so cannot establish an oral linguistic system as a basis for representational-symbolic behavior. Fortunately, as Bruner (1967) notes, "images . . . can be infused with the properties of symbolic functioning, as can tool-using involving action."

The program we will outline is intended to establish representational behavior through an approach that initially bypasses the oral modality and then introduces oral-aural (auditory) visual association for nonspeech events. Through this approach, the child may be induced to listen as well as to hear, and ultimately to process speech as well as nonspeech.[2]

LEVEL I: OBJECT-TO-OBJECT ASSOCIATION

Matching of Identical Objects

On this level, the child is presented with identical objects for matching. These objects should be selected so that they are life size and within the child's environmental experience. The object to be matched should be placed in direct view of the child at a distance of 12 to 18 inches, and the object for matching should be immediately in front of the child. The clinician demonstrates that one object is to be placed next to the other. By pantomime, the child is instructed to imitate the action.[3] If the child fails to do this, then the clinician goes through the action with him or her by placing and holding his or her hand over the object and moving it to the object to be matched.

Objects for matching may include pieces of fruit, such as apples or oranges; cups, saucers, spoons; blocks (wood or plastic); combs, large buttons, keys, and other items that the child may be expected to have had exposure to and experience with at home.

This task is obviously an easy one; its purpose is the establishment of a procedure—a simple action based on visual stimulation that will be used in the next steps.

The next step is to have the child select one of two objects to be matched

---

[1]Criteria for congenitally aphasic children were considered earlier (chapter 5.) Briefly, they include failure to acquire language despite evidence of adequate intelligence, adequate hearing; an absence, at least in the younger children, of autistic manifestations or other evidences of emotional instability; and no anomalies of the oral mechanism.

[2]If it becomes quickly apparent in working with a child that he or she has no difficulty with object matching (association), then he or she should be moved directly to visual representation (picture) tasks. These are described later.

[3]Successful (correct) performances will be reinforced by a candy type of reward or by some form of social approval, such as a gentle pat on the back, a smile, or a nod of approval. We suggest beginning with a quickly edible reward.

with the target object. If this step is established, the assortment of objects available for selection may be increased from two to three.

We have found that some children will not perform the task required if the object to be matched is not placed within an enclosed field or structure. Some children will reject the task of placing one object next to another on an open surface but will perform correctly if the target object is in an enclosure, such as an open wooden or cardboard box large enough to receive a second like object.

We recommend that, at first, the selection material contain the like object and one unlike object—for example, a spoon and a block of wood for matching to a spoon. In a later step, related objects, such as a cup and a spoon, plus an unrelated one, such as a comb, may be used to match with a cup.

Matching of Like but Not Identical Objects

This step is intended to establish the notion of near-likenesses despite differences. It is essentially a first step in the development of categorical behavior. The first unlike feature may be one of size, so that the child's task is to match a small spoon—a teaspoon—with a soup spoon, or a small block with a large block. Then, in keeping with therapeutic principles and approaches, changes in features of the objects to be matched should be introduced, one feature at a time, until the child is able to appreciate that likenesses are determined by essential features and not by incidental attributes. Ultimately, what we hope to have the child appreciate is that a ball is to bounce or to throw or to catch, that a block is for building, and so forth. The next step is intended to move the child further toward categorical behavior.

LEVEL II: CATEGORICAL MATCHING

In our earlier discussion of perception, we indicated that perception is a process of categorization or organization of events into classes or categories. A *category* represents a group of experiences that, despite differences, have common features or a common denominator or function. The ability to categorize, which is unconsciously and spontaneously arrived at by normal children, is retarded or impaired in brain-damaged children. If the normal acquisition of language (speech) is affected, as it is in aphasic children, categorization or concept formation is also impeded. Thus, Johnson and Myklebust (1967) observe: "In terms of remedial education, experience indicates that the teacher must be aware that some children form concepts spontaneously when they acquire the necessary verbal facility. On the other hand, many must be assisted in learning to generalize and categorize" (p. 44). The program that follows is intended to help the nonverbal child establish categorical behavior on an elementary level. Actually, a first step in this direction was taken in the matching of like but not identical objects, described earlier. This kind of matching may be continued by providing the child with opportunities to match life-size objects to reduced-size (toy-game) objects, such as spoons, plates, and so forth, made of the same materials, and then with objects made of different materials, such as metal and plastic tableware. A further step in the direction of the representational might be to match real pieces of fruit to wax fruit.

The target for matching is now a group (two or three objects). The object to make the match should be included with one or two other unlike objects for selection by the child. Demonstration by the clinician is in order if the child does not initiate the selection or appears to be making random selections. The clinician may also demonstrate pretended use of the objects.

Following are some suggested objects that may be used to establish categorical matchings:

Target Grouping	Items for Selection
Knife, fork	Block, spoon
Orange, apple	Banana, button
Cup, plate, bowl	Glass (clear plastic), ball, spool of thread
Paper, pencil	Pen, spoon, button
Orange, apple	Lemon, fork, paper clip
Carrot, potato	Pea pod, pencil, block
Orange, apple, peach (all wax)	Grape bunch (wax), spoon, pencil

LEVEL III: MATCHING BY ASSOCIATED FUNCTION

On this level, we are interested in establishing categorization and conceptualization based on associated functions of objects that are basically different in form and physical features. This is the function tested in the Illinois Test of Psycholinguistic Abilities (Kirk, McCarthy, and Kirk, 1968) subtest for visual association, in which pictures are used and the child is asked to indicate (select) the appropriate item from a picture card to respond to "What goes with this?"

We suggest beginning with one target object and two from the selection assortment. The clinician should demonstrate the selection and matching procedure and then, by pantomime, direct the child to proceed.

Following are some suggested tasks for association by function:

Item to Be Matched	Items for Selection
Cup	Spoon, pencil
Nail	Hammer
Needle	Spool of thread (or piece of black thread)

Paper	Pencil or dark crayon
Lock	Nail, key, comb
Shoe (unlaced)	Lace, spoon
Purse	Coin, nail
Bowl	Soup spoon, pencil
Paper (orange or red)	Scissors, nail

This step may be repeated with additional items added to the selection box.

If the child begins to indicate some comprehension of spoken language at this stage, the instruction may be given verbally; for example, "Show me which one goes with this."

Items such as those listed may also be used to have the child demonstrate actual use. However, threading a needle and lacing a shoe should not be included in these demonstrations. These tasks exceed what can be expected in the way of visual-motor coordination. After teacher or clinician demonstration, however, the child may be encouraged to stir a spoon in a cup, put a coin in a purse, indicate the use of a soup spoon in a bowl, and mark a paper with a pencil or crayon.

VISUAL REPRESENTATION (PICTURES)

The use of three-dimensional objects chosen so that they are within the child's experience imposes obvious restraints and limitations on the tasks involved in establishing categorical matching. The use of pictures widens the selection and raises the level of representational functioning. At first, the pictures should be in realistic color and should be life size. The target picture (picture to be matched) should be on a card with a framed border. The selection card should contain two pictures for the first tasks and no more than three items, widely separated, for the later tasks. The first selections should be pictures of items that were used in the object matchings. Later selections may include any picture representations of animate or inanimate items in the child's environment.

After the child has demonstrated ability to match full-size pictures, ones of reduced size (half to quarter size) should be introduced. The first assortment should include realistic color. These should be followed by black-and-white pictures, and finally by line drawings. If the child has difficulty at any of these stages, intermediate steps, in which items from one level can be matched with items from the next, can be introduced—for example, a picture to a three-dimensional object, a reduced-size color picture to a full-size picture, a black-and-white picture to a color picture, or a line drawing to a black-and-white picture. As review, and to avoid any tendency for the child to become stimulus-bound in his or her matching behavior, the child should be given opportunities for practice along the lines just suggested.

Following are some samples that can be used for picture matching and association. A slot board may be used with most children for the exercises that follow. The target item or items are placed on the highest slot level and the selection items on the lowest level.

Identical Pictures

Target Picture	Items for Selection
Orange	Orange, block of wood
Apple	Apple, comb
Pencil	Pencil, pea pod
Spoon	Spoon, pencil, carrot
Cup	Cup, knife, comb
Comb	Comb, spoon, pencil
Button	Button, key, block
Saucer	Saucer, comb, orange
Key	Key, nail, pencil
Glass (drinking)	Glass, cup, apple

Like Pictures

The items just listed or other common object pictures may be used, but with variations in size, color, and decoration. However, avoid using pictures that are too highly decorated or busy.

A variation of like pictures may be introduced that show animate beings in different postures—for example, a cat sitting and a cat lying asleep, a dog standing (walking position) and a dog in begging position, a child full face and a child in profile, a boy walking and a boy hopping on one leg.

Categorical Matching

Target Picture	Selection Assortment
Cup	Saucer, block, pencil
Apple	Peach, spoon, crayon
Shoe	Stocking, apple
Cup, saucer	Bowl, comb, key
Pencil, pen	Crayon, spoon, banana

Apple, orange

Paper, envelope

Potato, carrot

Peach, knife, key

Pencil, spoon, saucer

Ear of corn, pencil, ball

Matching by Function

The task now is to associate items that complement one another in terms of use. Essentially, if verbalized, it would be to answer the question "Which one do you use with *this?*" *This,* of course, is the target item.

Target Item	Selection for Matching
Lock	Key, comb
Cup	Spoon, apple
Shoe	Sock, block
Hand	Glove or mitten, potato
Nail	Hammer, cup, shoe
Glass (drinking)	Pitcher with fluid, stocking, block
Shoe	Lace, glove, crayon
Needle	Thread or spool of thread, block, shoe
Paper	Scissors, crayon, cup
Toothbrush	Toothpaste tube, button, key

A variation of categorical matching is to train the child to discern and select the odd item, the one that does not belong, in a presented series. Thus, the items just listed may now be presented in a slot board that includes those indicated as the target items and those from the selection assortment—for example, apple, orange, peach, block; shoe, sock, hammer, glove; comb, hair brush, glass; cup, nail, saucer, spoon, and so forth. The clinician must be careful to vary the placement of the odd item in the series so that the child will not make a decision on the basis of position.

Matching of geometric forms may now be introduced, using the basic forms of a circle, square, triangle, rectangle, pentagon and hexagon. A first step in this matching, to permit easy handling, may be to use three-dimensional figures about one-quarter-inch thick. If the child has difficulty in manual manipulation, further matchings should continue with three-dimensional forms. If the child has no manipulative difficulty, sturdy cardboard cutouts may be used. In training, the child should learn to match any like form, regardless of material, to another like form, with variations introduced in size and color of form. Finally, matching should be made with pictures of forms on cards or on pages of a manual, with pointing rather than placing as the method.

Categorical training may take place with geometric forms by having the child match two or three target objects from an assortment in a box. If the child finds this confusing, then the clinician may hand the child one form at a time from an inventory under the clinician's control.

Form boards are used to train the child to a different mode of visual perception. The child must now see the relationship between the receptacle or well-space for a form and the three-dimensional object. We suggest beginning with a single-target form board and two quite different forms, such as a circle and a square. Then introduce a rectangle (circle plus rectangle from selection) and the other forms one at a time for matching against a circle. A further step is to use the same sequence of forms for matching against a different target object—for example, a square. A final step, which many of the children may not achieve, would be matching a pentagon or a hexagon with a pentagon and a hexagon in the selection assortment. In any of the form board tasks it is acceptable for the child to employ pointing rather than placement to indicate the matching.

If the child has difficulty in initial matching, the form board well-space should be outlined in red or black to provide a clear frame for the target form.

SEQUENCING

The task in sequencing is for the child to decide "What comes next?" when presented with an array of visual events with an established order. Such an order might be wooden cubes with alternating top surfaces of red–white–red–white–red or with pictures on the top surfaces of orange apple–red apple–orange apple–red apple, and so on. Another procedure, which is employed in the Leiter scale, is to match blocks to a visual strip display. This may be used as a first step and as a demonstration teaching approach. However, the ultimate objective is to have the child finish a sequence based on a rule or principle that he or she evolves, rather than on a match-to-sample basis.

Plastic chips should replace blocks for children who are able to manipulate them. We suggest using chips, or sturdy cardboard squares, with pictures of objects, animals, and persons (girl, boy, man, woman; baby, mother, etc.), for the early sequencing tasks. Later sequencing may include use of the geometric forms: circle, square, triangle, pentagon, hexagon, and cross. Alternations should at first be for a pattern such as ○ □ ○ □ ○ . . . followed by a pattern such as ○ ○ □ □ ○ ○ □ □ ○ ○ □ □ . . . . The items to complete the pattern should be limited at first to only those that are appropriate. In later tasks, the selection items may include one or two that would not be appropriate, such as fruit chips in a people sequence, or people chips in a geometric series.

SEQUENCING AND RECALL

This level of sequencing requires the child to observe an arrangement of stimulus items and to reproduce the arrangement based on recall. The child must now perceive that there is a pattern or arrangement of events and reproduce it based on memory or inner perception. If a principle is involved (e.g., alternation), the task calls for the child to apply the principle to the available materials.

The materials used in sequencing may include any of those used in the matching tasks that will maintain their position once put in place. We recommend the use of materials that are interesting and meaningful to the child, rather than abstract or nonsense forms. The reproduction of a three- or four-item series is a reasonable objective. First selection of sequences should include only those items that were used in the presented patterns. Later selections may include one or two inappropriate items, so that the child may exercise discriminative ability. If the child becomes confused by the inclusion of nonbelonging items in the selection assortment, these items should be removed.

Visual Sequential Memory is included as a test item in the ITPA battery (Kirk et al., 1968). Chips are used in the ITPA. The stimulus item (sequence) is a card with an arrangement of forms, which is exposed to the child for 5 seconds. After the exposure period, the stimulus card is removed, and the child is expected to replicate the exposed sequence by arranging chips on a tray in a corresponding order.

VISUAL-AUDITORY ASSOCIATION

Up to this point in our program for the nonverbal child, we have bypassed the auditory modality to establish visual perceptual and representational behavior. Through our procedures and materials, we intend to provide the child with opportunities to develop strategies for coping (for behaving appropriately) in situations that are within his or her sensory and perceptual capacities. Our objective at this stage of training for visual-auditory associations is to involve the child in listening, to induce and, if necessary, seduce the child in the processing of auditory events so that he or she can make sense out of sound. This is especially important for the child who has turned off sound and has ceased trying to listen even to the nonhuman (nonspeech) sounds that he or she has the capacity to process.

The next major step in the prelanguage training program is to establish associations between a characteristic sound and the object that is involved in its production. Visual-auditory associations may include animate as well as inanimate objects, which, when acted upon, make consistent and identifiable noises.

Animate Noise Producers

Fortunately, many toy animals are now available that can be manipulated to produce sounds (noises) that are close approximations to the real animal sounds. At first, the representational animate objects should be limited to sound (noise) producers—human speech not included—in the child's environment. Such a selection might include a cat, a dog, a bird, and a baby doll. An expanded inventory, depending upon the individual child and his or her particular extended environment, might include a cow, a lamb, zoo animals, a rooster, a bee, and so forth. The criteria for selection are the actuality of experience for the child and the natural noise made by the object.

In establishing the association, the clinician should demonstrate how the noise is produced by the manipulation of a toy object. After the demonstration, the child is then helped to do the manipulation, preferably by direct imitation of the clinician. Then the routine is repeated with a second object. When the noise-producing manipulation is established, the child is presented with two noise producers and is directed to match (point to) the noise produced on tape or by a toy manipulated out of sight by the clinician. Three and finally four animate noisemakers may be used in later matchings.

Nonanimate Noise Producers

Doors bang, bells clang, telephones ring, vacuum cleaners whir, horns toot, drums beat, and so on. Actually, these objects need to be acted upon to make their characteristic noises. Here, too, toy manufacturers have made available materials that can be readily employed in clinical training. With procedures modified as necessary along the lines described for animate noisemakers, associations can be established between the toy object and its own kind of noise. For most children, the success in selecting the object for producing the appropriate noise should be enough reinforcement to keep the visual-auditory association game going.

Picture Representation and Auditory Association

As soon as the child has demonstrated the ability to make the appropriate associations between objects and their characteristic noises, pictures should be introduced as substitutes for the objects. The use of pictures widens the scope of possible noisemakers, which might now include food mixers, airplanes, trucks, hammers, and other environmental noisemakers. These noises can be recorded and played on tape. The child's task now becomes pointing to one of two, and then one of three or four, pictures for appropriate selection.

Sequential Matching

At this stage, the object is to train the child to listen to a series of noises and, first, manipulate the objects and, later, point to the pictures that correspond to the order of the presented noises. The first series should be for two noises produced on tape, with clinician manipulation of the noise producer out of the child's sight. The selection of noise producers is placed on a table in front of the child. After the child has learned to produce a two-noise sequence, the series should be increased to three and finally to four. Immediate material rewards, preferably quickly edible ones, are recommended for each success.

Onomatopoetic Word Association: First Words

In a strict sense, there are very few, if any, words that actually represent the sounds or noises made by the objects associated with them. A number of words, however, come close enough to the natural sounds or noises to provide a small inventory of first words that have no more than four phonemes, including continuant voiced consonants, which are ordinarily produced with a fair amount of energy. These features make the words dramatic and easily audible. Presumably, also, the phonetic nature of the words should make them easily processible by a child who is beginning to listen.[4]

Our first lexicon for visual-auditory associations includes the words *meow, woof, boom, bang, moo, oink,* and *wha-wha,* the last being for a baby's crying. (We assume that there is no need to indicate appropriate associations for the other onomatopoetic terms.) We suggest that each of these words be produced twice for the child, on tape or through object manipulation, as stimulus events for the child's response. As in earlier procedures, the first association may be made with the toy object, and later associations may be established by associations with pictures.

SPONTANEOUS SOUND PRODUCTION

In any stage of auditory matching, spontaneous attempts by the child to make the noise of the stimulus object should be recognized and encouraged. Especially deserving of reward should be the child's oral efforts at noise imitation. The clinician should accept and reinforce any approximation of the stimulus sound. However wide of the mark the approximation may be, spontaneous noise imitation indicates that the child has tuned in to sound and is processing rather than ignoring the audible events in the environment.

SUMMARY

The suggested program for training the nonverbal child is intended as a guide, not as a prescriptive series of steps to be rigidly followed by a clinician. In a one-to-one relationship, or even in a small-group setting, the clinician–teacher is soon able to know how much, as well as how fast and how often, a child needs to be involved in each of the subprograms described. Although three-dimensional objects have motivational and interest value, many children are able to move rather quickly from them to picture representations. Such progress brings the child closer to representational behavior than would long involvement with objects.

The objective for the child is to establish visual perception, on the assumption that the visual modality will be more effective than the auditory. Through such perceptual functioning, the child is also expected to learn

---

[4]We suggest a review, at this point, of our discussion on the functions of the auditory cortex in Chapter 4, on brain mechanisms and language functioning.

strategies for coping, for knowing what he or she may be able to do in relation to visual events. Though it is not specifically stated, we also believe that the child acquires a form of inner language, a way of talking to himself or herself without words, so that he or she can relate and transform experiences into a set of rudimentary visual symbols. In effect, we have suggested a program and procedures that reverse the normal order of the acquisition of language, which presumably proceeds from sounds, words, spoken language, and aural-oral symbolization to written language for literate persons. Our basic philosophic principle is that the establishment of a representational system and inner language as bases for symbol behavior should not be postponed until conventional language is established. Ultimately, we believe that symbol behavior in general, including behavior that is dependent on aural-oral functioning, will be more advanced and will progress to a higher level if we begin with the capacities a child has and train to his or her comparative strengths. We consider training first to overcome weakness in auditory perceptual functioning in the hope that, through such therapy the child will begin to make sense out of sound, to be wasteful of early effort and productive of frustration. All too often we may enhance the likelihood that the child, already turned off from human speech, may completely withdraw from the world of auditory events and be regarded as autistic. We believe that our philosophy and our program for the nonverbal child reduces this possibility.

The program outlined in this chapter is not prescriptive in specific content or in order. The program as a whole is intended as a guide for the clinician, who alone can determine the stage or level of functioning—where to go from where a given child is. Based on such a decision, the clinician decides, perhaps only tentatively, on the initial level and on when and how to progress from that stage or level to the next.

Based on responses to this program guide, we have found that some clinicians prefer the following stages or levels in establishing representational understanding as a first major (prelingual) stage for training in representational (symbol) behavior:

1. Identical object matching.
2. Identical picture matching.
3. Matching of identical objects to pictures.
4. Matching of similar objects.
5. Matching of similar pictures.
6. Associated object grouping.
7. Associated picture grouping.
8. Object categories.
9. Picture categories.
10. Which one is different (objects and pictures)?

The following chapter will present a program for linguistically retarded children who are in the first stages of oral linguistic proficiency. The program will emphasize established lexical and syntactic competencies that are consonant with cognitive abilities.

REFERENCES AND SUGGESTED READINGS

Bruner, J. S. "On Cognitive Growth II," in J. S. Bruner, R. R. Olver, P. M. Greenfield, et al. (eds.), *Studies in Cognitive Growth*. New York: Wiley, 1967.

Ginsburg, H., and Opper, S. *Piaget's Theory of Intellectual Development*. Englewood Cliffs, N.J.: Prentice-Hall, 1969.

Johnson, D. J., and Myklebust, H. R. *Learning Disabilities*. New York: Grune and Stratton, 1967.

Kirk, S. A., McCarthy, J. J., and Kirk, W. D. *Illinois Test of Psycholinguistic Abilities*, Rev. ed. Urbana: University of Illinois Press, 1968.

Piaget, J., and Inhelder, B. *The Psychology of the Child*. New York: Basic Books, 1969.

chapter 9

Semantic-Syntactic Approaches for Establishing and Developing Language in Aphasic and Dysphasic Children

The previous chapter presented a program to establish representational behavior for severely linguistically retarded (aphasic) children. The approach is intended to establish representational behavior as a prelude to linguistic understanding and expression. A preliminary first lexicon of onomatopoetic words was suggested as a bridge between nonverbal sounds and linguistic representations.

In this chapter, the plan is to take the child over the bridge into linguistic territory. Our primary concern will be with congenitally aphasic children, some of whom may still be at the single-word stage. Others may be less severely delayed but considerably retarded compared with their age peers. A small percentage of the children, for reasons that may not be readily discerned, may be capable of acquiring language but continue to be perceptually defensive against spoken language.

For practical purposes we will assume that we will be dealing with children who are at least 3 years of age and who, based on formal or informal assessment procedures, are significantly inferior in language comprehension and production but are not mentally retarded, impaired in hearing, or autistic.

What is obvious in aphasic and dysphasic children is that they are linguistically retarded. What is not always readily apparent is that the congenitally aphasic's primary deficit is for the decoding of language at the rate and quantity at which chronological- and mental-age peers have no difficulty. In the complete absence of decoding, there is no linguistic content to encode. With lesser degrees of decoding impairment (dysphasia), there may be levels and quantities of content that can be decoded. Encodings, however, are likely to reveal limitations in vocabulary and, to an even greater extent, in appropriate syntax in multiple-word productions. These limitations are not based on severe articulation impairments, such as we find in the orally apraxic child. This child, if not turned off by language, may have normal language comprehension.

BASIC ASSUMPTIONS TO JUSTIFY DIRECT INTERVENTION

1. The child has passed the normal critical period of language acquisition and has failed to show appreciable increments in verbal behavior. Table 2.1 on maturational milestones in Chapter 2, "Normal Language Development," shows that the period between 24 and 36 months is one during which most children have a great acceleration in vocabulary growth as well as in the establishment of syntax. Because of these normal accomplishments we consider 36 months the upper age limit of the critical period for language acquisition.[1]

2. The child is not progressing from single-word utterances to phrases of two or more words. This achievement is normally expected within 3 or 4 months after the onset of speech. In regard to correlates of maturational milestones, two-word utterances begin to occur when the child takes his or her first unaided steps and begins to show evidence of hand preference. In relation to other aspects of language acquisition, two-word utterances may be expected when a child has a lexical inventory of about 50 words.

A more rigorous test of delay in language acquisition occurs when children, through training or natural acquisition, have established a lexical inventory of 50 words or more, but fail to combine words into utterances of their own. They then may be lacking in creative ability for self-formulation. With training, some children may be taught two- or three-word utterances. However, they are still linguistically retarded if their word strings do not include any of their own creation. In brief, children may be regarded as linguistically retarded if their acquisitions are limited to formulations they are specifically taught.

3. The child is able to discriminate speech sounds and speech-sound sequences of at least three phonemes. If not, then training toward that end is in order.

4. The child does not have oral apraxia or dysarthria and is capable of producing, by imitation, at least a consonant-vowel-consonant sequence. If

[1]See our discussion of the critical period for language in Chapter 1. The concept of critical period implies "a timed unfolding of a certain type of behavior, with a corresponding biologically based period of sensitivity to, or need for, normal supporting stimulation" (Kohlberg, 1968, p. 1044).

there is evidence of such motor involvements, then the approaches suggested in Chapter 10 should apply.

5. The way a child uses language should express the individual child and her or his cognitive responses to the environment. It follows that for a child to use a linguistic construction with intended meaning, the child must first understand what the construction means.[2]

Our concern, as indicated earlier, will be with the most severely linguistically retarded children. For reasons that will soon be considered, these children require therapeutic intervention to help them to establish language behavior.

THE ROLE OF THE CLINICIAN

Normal children, as well as those who are somewhat delayed in language development, do not learn language by learning a vocabulary and a set of rules to go along with the words. Normal children, through active involvement in situations that include language, somehow arrive at the rules from significant experiences. These experiences include persons and objects that are relevant to needs and events in which children can gainfully engage and interact with other important persons.

The other important persons may be parents, older siblings, teachers, clinicians, or even peer-age, older, or younger children with proficient language. We shall assume, however, that in the case of the aphasic child, exposure to other important persons has not been productive, so that clinical instruction to help the child to establish useful language is now in order. What, then, is the role of the clinician? Bloom and Lahey (1978) suggest that the clinician (speech pathologist) is responsible for planning a treatment program and for advising others who have daily, ongoing interactions with a child on how to provide appropriate linguistic content and forms relevant to meaningful situations. The view in this book is that, in most instances, the clinician or teacher must also have primary responsibility and take an active role in the child's language training. Because the congenitally aphasic child is often beyond the critical age for normal language acquisition—that is, acquisition by exposure to speakers with little or no direct teaching—direct intervention is now required. We agree with Reid and Hresko (1981), who state:

> The growth of language depends on the intensity and quality of the *interaction* between the person guiding the intervention and the child. The person who intervenes must direct, develop, and monitor the interaction, maintaining its focus and direction while incorporating those aspects of

[2]We are aware that it is possible to train (condition) mentally retarded, linguistically deficient children to use a linguistic construction appropriately according to a given situation and to receive a response that is satisfactory. Such training, Guess, Baer and Sailor (1978) found, does not require or establish comprehension. However, because we are not concerned here with mentally retarded children, we strongly urge that, in all instances, comprehension must either precede or accompany teaching for linguistic production.

language to be stressed for the particular child. ... The cognitive-psycholinguistic view of language assumes that language cannot be taught in a didactic manner, but rather that language intervention depends upon the development of opportunities for the child to discover and internalize appropriate adult forms of language. In a variety of settings (both at home and in the school), the child is expected to *extract* the appropriate language structures. (p. 222)

The clinician, then, is both a stimulator and a teacher. Wherever and whenever possible, parents, and possibly teachers, if the child also attends a school, should participate in the instruction, with ongoing advice from the clinician.

Our most optimistic goal as clincians is to help the child discover and internalize adult language forms. Such constructions, however, may have intermediate and more modest forms, which are used by normal children as they progress to adult forms. As clinicians-teachers for severely linguistically retarded children, we will find it necessary to present more tokens of a construction type than normal children need for generalization. We are also likely to find that it helps to speed the generalization process by making obvious statements to suggest the rule that governs a construction.

Clinicians need to be guided by the pace of the child but not bound by it. As indicated earlier in our discussion of the parent or caretaker's role in verbal interchanges with the young child (see Chapter 2), the structure (form) and content should not be so far beyond the child as to be out of reach, yet far enough (or close enough) to make the reaching attainable and worth the effort.

RATIONALE FOR THIS APPROACH

Professional Teaching or Family Training

It must be evident to the reader that we have placed considerable emphasis on appreciating normal language development and normal cognitive maturation as a basis for understanding the problems of severely linguistically retarded children. This position seems to be in keeping with that of Miller and Yoder (1974), and we may therefore be able to take a developmental approach in our direct language teaching of the children with whom this book is concerned. Who, then, will do the teaching?

Tentatively, we can answer that question by saying that, ideally, parent or parent surrogates should do the teaching. However, children who are so severely retarded as to be considered congenitally aphasic, as well as those with lesser amounts of language retardation who are designated as dysphasic, have already failed to learn at the hands of older speakers in their home environments. If the children have older siblings who have adequate language proficiencies, we can find no fault with the parent or parent surrogates unless the familial picture has changed. If, on the other hand, the linguistically retarded child is the oldest sibling, the familial picture may have changed for the worse.

Obviously, with an only child, there is no basis for comparison. These observations are speculations that in all too many instances do not affect the course of treatment for the children with whom this book is concerned.

Our clinical experience indicates that, in many instances, a much more realistic situation is the absence of a parent or parent surrogate and of any other primary caretaker who is well informed or who has the time and the inclination to undertake the role of language teacher or language stimulator. When this is so, it is not in the best interest of the child to place the burden of language instruction on the family—at least not until counseling or some positive change in the family picture indicates that direct family involvement may be assumed. As a general principle, we agree with Guess, Baer, and Sailor (1978) and MacDonald and Blott (1974) that language instruction should be carried out in the best social contexts available to the child. Furthermore, whenever there are members of the child's family who are available and willing as well as capable of being instructed to provide the necessary language training, the family should be included to the maximum possible degree. However, when sophisticated clinical judgment suggests that any given time the family is or may be a negative influence, the responsibility for language training must go to the agency to whom the child has been referred. This observation in no way implies that the family should never become involved. Whenever circumstances so indicate, and as soon as possible, caretakers should be taught to share and ultimately to take over the largest possible portion of the training. As a start, opportunities should be provided for observation and follow-up discussion about what the clinician has tried to accomplish in a training session. A subsequent role may be that of teacher aide, with even greater responsibility shifted to the observer-caretaker. This is an ideal goal, but it may not be a realistic one.

Spradlin and Siegel (1982) sum up the issues and problems in language training that is conducted in natural, versus clinical, environments. A key problem in structured programs, especially when they are carried out in clinical settings, is how to promote generalization so that the child can apply the taught and presumably learned linguistic information and skills in a wide variety of appropriate situations. Ideally, the solution is to "embed the teaching in the natural environment and, perhaps, to use the parent as the teacher." As indicated earlier, we share with Spradlin and Siegel (1982) the following awareness:

> For some families . . . this may not be a feasible arrangement, because of the nature of the child's problem, the characteristics of the environment, or some interaction. It may then be most appropriate to teach the child in a clinical or laboratory environment and to use a formal language training program. When such programs are implemented, there is often a problem in extending or generalizing the child's newly acquired skills. Careful consideration of the manner in which stimuli are presented, the kinds of responses that are required, and the way in which reinforcement is dispensed may help to solve the difficulty in moving from laboratory to natural setting.

Syntactic-Semantic Training: The Setting

The setting for direct language training should be as natural as can be found or devised. It is not limited to the clinician's room or the teacher's classroom. The setting should be the most effective environment where the teaching can take place—if at all possible, at home for language content that is related to the home, at the playground for relevant language, and so on. If this can be observed, and to the extent that it can be observed, it increases the likelihood that meanings will be generated from the combination of linguistic (verbal) semantics and situational semantics.

The syntactic-semantic approach, which will be presented as the basic procedure, will incorporate motivational content (what is important for the child to know and be able to say) with form (how to say what the child needs to say to make his effort effective). We continue to recommend and offer a syntactic approach rather than exposure to listening to language, as if we were dealing with an infant with full potential for normal language acquisition, because we are dealing with a special population for whom presumably this has not worked. Most of the children who come to us for training will be past the age for the critical period for spontaneous language acquisition. During the period when normal children make their greatest strides in language proficiencies, these children have experienced failure. Therefore, formal and direct language instruction is in order.

Basic to our rationale for direct syntactic training as well as other aspects of formal and direct teaching is that we are dealing with children who are obviously different in their potentials for language learning. The difference, manifest in severe language delay and language deviancies, has its etiology in neurological deviancy. Linguistic acquisitions that are perceived and become apparent to normal childen are not perceived by the congenitally aphasic and by the other groups of children discussed here, with the exception of the oral apraxic. Menyuk (1981) in comparing the requirements for second language learning by adolescents and adults, following along the lines of Krashen (1975), suggests:

> The requirements of the adult second-language learner may be analogous to the requirements of some handicapped children learning a first language and may lead to the same results; that is, a nonnativelike competence in syntax, semantics, and phonology. If these requirements for language are necessities, not only is what is learned about language different but also the conditions for learning are different for normally developing children acquiring a first language, adult learners of a second language, and handicapped children.

The formal (direct and different) intruction that we recommend helps to isolate the features, rules, and lexical items that the child needs to learn. Fortunately, responses to feature isolation provide opportunities for external and direct feedback and reinforcement. We believe that congenitally aphasic children, as well as the others with whom we are concerned, benefit from the highlighting and isolation of criterial language features.

THE FIRST LEXICON

The first words should enable linguistically retarded children to label (name) persons, things, and events, to make demands according to their needs, to assert themselves as persons, and to negate what they do not want. First words should be tools that make things happen, or put an end to their occurrence. First words should bring persons and things in view and available for the child. The words should also be able to get these things out of view when they are not needed, at least for the moment.

Bloom and Lahey (1978) and Lahey and Bloom (1977) suggest other criteria for determining the selection of verbal items for a first lexicon. These criteria include the relations of content and form interactions as input. We shall review these suggestions as well as those offered by Holland (1975). In addition, we shall apply the findings of Morehead and Ingram (1973) on the development of base syntax in normal and linguistically deviant children.

Lahey and Bloom (1977) observed three basic principles that relate to content and form in the selection of the first words (lexicon) to be taught to linguistically retarded children.

1. The selected forms were based on "the ease with which the content they code can be demonstrated in the nonlinguistic context" (p. 341). Practically, this means that a word that can be demonstrated as a real object or event has priority over a word that is only shown in picture form. If the word to be taught is either *eat* or *cookie,* it is preferable to present a child with a *cookie to eat* rather than a picture of a child eating a cookie. Similarly, giving a child a *ball to throw* is better than showing a picture of a child *throwing a ball.* However, a child may be shown a picture of an object or an act and told the appropriate word (label). If possible, the child should be encouraged to fit the deed to the word and so encode the word linguistically and behaviorally.

2. Selections reflected the potential usefulness of the forms in likely communicated situations for the child. The application of this principle for selection of a lexicon requires that the teacher-clinician know the child well enough to choose terms that are readily usable, terms that can be used frequently in daily living and so can enhance communication. Such words may also improve the quality of life for the child and thus become reinforcers for what they are being taught as well as motivators for learning still more.

3. The selected lexicon was organized "according to the regularities in the interaction between linguistic forms and the semantic content that such forms encode" (Lahey and Bloom, 1977, p. 341). Practically, this means that children must be taught the forms that will help them to encode their ideas most effectively, first in single-word productions and later in multiple-word utterances that include acceptable syntax. At this time, substantive words, action words, and relationship words are taught. There will be more about these words in the discussion of syntactic forms.

There are other practical considerations regarding the selection of a first lexical inventory. Ease of pronunciation for a given child is one such practical consideration. If there is a choice of synonymous terms, the one a child can pronounce should have priority over one that incorporates sounds or sound blends the child does not yet have under control. Single-syllable words or duplicated monosyllables, such as *mama* and *dada,* are among the first learned by virtually all children and so should be among the first for those who are linguistically retarded. In establishing a lexicon, we agree with Bloom and Lahey (1978) that words with wide phonetic contrasts, such as *kitty* and *baby,* are better included within a single lesson than are words close in phonetic features, such as *cup* and *pup* or *make* and *bake.*

Holland (1975) describes a psycholinguistic language therapy program that includes a core lexicon. She states: "Diagnostic categories of language disorders are ignored . . . because I am convinced that the context and content described are relevant to al language disorders."

Holland presents a rationale for each of 35 terms for a recommended core lexicon.[3] She states: "To assure that no preferential rank ordering is implied, words are listed in a helter-skelter fashion without regard to grammatical function." The terms are as follows:

me (or I)	name of favorite food
you	name of least favorite food
child's own name	very angry word
names of signiificant others	allgone
kiss	name of loved activity
hate	up
gimme	down
scared	there
wash	that
more	hi
go	my (mine)
no	your
ycs	

In addition, Holland recommends the following words as "possibly more representative of clinically appropriate language environments than of core lexical words. They grew out of linguistic combination possibilities primarily, and clinical good sense secondarily."

[3]For the rationale for these terms, see Holland (1975, pp. 520–521).

big and little   doll (or stuffed cuddly toy)

ball, block, car   clinician's name

beads

A SYNTACTIC APPROACH TO LANGUAGE THERAPY

Experience with severely linguistically delayed and deviant children has made it clear that they require a larger base lexicon and need to spend considerably more time at each syntactic level (more tokens of each type of construction) to be ready to move to new forms and constructions. Perhaps, because of this observation, clinicians may be tempted to assume that linguistically deviant children learn no linguistic constructions that they are not directly taught. Fortunately, this is not so. These children may be slower at generalizing and generating, slower to apply rules that they know, than are linguistically normal children. The slowness may be a product of insecurity and anxiety, of apprehension about taking a chance in the linguistic game. Even more than other children who are mildly or even moderately delayed, these children need periodical informal assessments, language sampling, and formal testing. Such assessments will help to inform, confirm, and sometimes even surprise the clinician as to the progress of the child. If all is going well, the clinician may learn that the child has somehow acquired new language constructions that were not directly taught. In any event, through reassessment, the clinician will be able to determine where the child is and needs to go, what next needs to be directly taught to continue progress in the language game.

Crystal, Fletcher, and Garman (1976) emphasize that an effective syntactic remediation program must in the interest of the child and must provide the teacher (clinician) with knowledge about (1) the structures the child has acquired (and with what degree of mastery) and (2) the structures that have not been acquired but that would be appropriate and ordinarily expected at the child's stage of development. According to Crystal et al. (1976), the teacher (clinician) "has to make himself aware of the entire range of structures that ought to be developing at any given stage, so that he knows clearly *what* he has *not* taught as well as what he has" (p. 21). This position is acceptable, provided, as indicated earlier, that the teacher-clinician also makes it a point to learn what the child does not need to be directly taught because that child has somehow learned how to learn (acquire) some language by exposure and without direct teaching.

Implicit in the foregoing is that we plan to present a syntactic approach to teaching severely and moderately linguistically retarded children to be more proficient users (comprehenders and producers) of language. Nothing in this approach is in any way incompatible with other procedures that are identified as experiential, pragmatic, or environmental. We are in complete accord with Bloom and Lahey (1978) on the essential nature of language intervention:

Language intervention involves modifying a child's environment in a manner that will enhance the ability to induce the interactions among language content/form/use. Certain of these modifications are specific to the contexts in which the goals of language for a particular child will be facilitated; other modifications are more general in that they may apply to many contexts or need to be considered prior to or concurrent with planning specific contextual modifications. Such considerations include (1) reducing the influence of any factors that may be maintaining difficulty with language learning; (2) the context in which language will be facilitated; (3) the child's response behaviors—the techniques of eliciting and maintaining these behaviors, the sense modality to be used, and relative emphasis on comprehension versus production. (p. 553)

BASE SYNTAX RELATED TO MEAN LENGTH OF UTTERANCE

Morehead and Ingram (1973) studied young, normal children and a group that was severely linguistically delayed (language disordered) and compared the two groups on mean length of utterance (MLU) rather than on age or other usual criteria. One of their relevant conclusions was that the differences between normal and linguistically delayed children were quantitative rather than qualitative and were primarily related to time of onset of language and rate of development, rather than to types of rules that govern the syntax of their utterances. A projection of this observation is that it should be possible to anticipate the kinds of syntactic structures the delayed children would acquire. The projection here is that knowledge of normal acquisitions (developmental order) may be used as a guide for therapeutic intervention. Syntactic structures that are absent or rarely used by the delayed children but are needed for understanding and production to enhance normality of communication are targets for intervention. Because most severely linguistically delayed children are at a single-word stage, intervention can begin with those constructions that are first produced by normal children. Other guides include the obligatory morphemes (Brown, 1973) and the first recommended lexicons of Holland (1975) and Lahey and Bloom (1977). However, the emerging linguistic and social needs of the individual child are certainly both the initial and the ultimate factors in selecting the constructions that should be taught.

LEVEL I: MEAN LENGTH OF UTTERANCE, 2.0 TO 2.5 MORPHEMES

Average utterance range is 2 to 2.5 words, most of which are a single morpheme.

1. Agent-action (noun + verb)
   The sample constructions include a noun plus an action word (verb).[4]

---

[4]The clinician will present the adult form (e.g., *baby cries*), but at this level will accept *baby cry* from the child. As a general practice, the clinician should first present the adult (full) construction form but not insist that the child produce the form. If it becomes evident that the child does not understand the adult or full form (see later constructions), then the samples should be reduced to the early, normally produced child construction.

baby cry	boy jump	mommy kiss
baby eat	girl eat	mommy wash
dog run	bird sing	boy fall
kitty run	daddy throw	car go
Tommy wash	daddy drink	boy kick

2. Action-Agent (verb + noun)

The sample construction forms consist of a verb (an action word) and a noun (something or somebody) related to the action.

eat banana	hold stick	throw stick
eat cookie	hold ball	see kitty
throw ball	pull wagon	hold baby
kick ball	kiss mommy	hit ball
wash baby	wash doggy	give cookie

At this level, it is not mandatory for the child to include the article (*the,a*) in his or her productions. However, the child should be exposed to them, at least in initial presentations, so the clinician should include the appropriate (adult) form, such as *eat the banana* or *hit the ball*. If the clinician is acting out the construction, the full form should be spoken as the words suitable to the action. At this stage, there should be no correction if the child reduces the construction by deleting the article.

3. Attribute (adjectives) + noun

Whether color should be used as an attribute should be first determined and, if important for the child, separately taught before including it in sample constructions. These samples include the primary colors, *red, yellow,* and *blue.*

big ball	pretty doll	tall man
small ball	red wagon	short man
big dog	yellow wagon	red box
small dog	blue wagon	blue box
big tree	happy girl	yellow box
small tree	happy puppy	happy boy

4. Agent (possessor) + Object (noun)[5]

The adult form would be *Tom's book.* See the earlier note for the presentation of the adult form of construction and the acceptance of a child's reduced form.

[5]In keeping with earlier suggestions, the full (marked) possessive form should be presented, but the unmarked child form is accepted.

boy ball	Mary kitty	Mary candy
Tom ball	Bobby kitty	girl book
baby cookie	baby shoe	boy book
girl wagon	mommy shoe	baby cup
boy wagon	daddy hat	mommy hat

5. Words used singly or in combination with action words or nouns to indicate wishes.

These include words denoting continuation (recurrence) of an event, cessation of an event, negation, state of affairs. For older linguistically delayed children, these words may be too infantile and should not be taught.

No, stop (for rejection or putting a stop to an action)

no drink	stop jump
no eat	stop push
no ball	stop run
no kitty	stop throw

More (for recurrence)

more cookie	more pull
more milk	more jump
more throw	more drink

All gone

all gone cookie	all gone ball
all gone milk	all gone doggy

6. Noun + verb as statement of a situation (predicate adjective)
The adult form would be *wagon is red;* the child form is *wagon red.*

car blue	girl big	box big
car red	girl small	box small
tree big	stick big	truck yellow
tree small	stick small	box yellow

7. *This* and *that* to identify an object or note its existence
These forms include *this, that* + predicate noun, as in *this ball (this is a ball)* or *that wagon (that is a wagon).*

this man	that man
this boy	that boy

this kitty	that kitty
this puppy	that puppy
this girl	that girl
this wagon	that wagon

8. Noun + locative (*here, there*)

boy here	Tom here	apple here
boy there	Tom there	apple there
man here	bird here	flower here
man there	bird there	flower there

9. Verb (action word) + locative (e.g., *throw here, throw there*)

run here	walk here
run there	walk there
jump here	kick here
jump there	kick there

10. *In* and *on* as contrasting prepositions for containment (*in*) and support (*on*)

in box	in car	on car (top of car)
on box	in pot	on floor
in truck	in cup	on shelf
on table	in wagon	on chair

11. Expansions of previous constructions
    a. Verb + preposition + noun

sit in wagon	give to boy	sit on box
sit in car	throw to Tom	put on table
put in cup	look in bag	put on box

b. Preposition + adjective (attribute) + noun (e.g., *in (the) big wagon*)

in big truck	in big cup	on big box
in yellow box	in small cup	on small box
in big bowl	on red box	in big house

c. Preposition + possessive noun + noun (e.g., *in Tom's wagon, in Tom wagon*)

in boy truck	in daddy car	in Tom house
in girl truck	in mommy car	in Bobby box
in Mary wagon	on Bobby box	in Mary pocket

12. Pronouns: *me, my, I, you, it*
    a. Action word (verb) + *me* (pronoun)

feed me	hug me	carry me
hold me	kiss me	wash me

   b. *I* + action word (verb)

I eat	I kick	I drink
I run	I throw	I wash

   c. Action word + *it* (pronoun as recipient of action)

hold it	throw it	push it
carry it	drink it	pull it

   d. Pronoun *it* as agent + action (verb)

it eat(s)	it fall(s)	it jump(s)
it run(s)	it fly (flies)	it wash(es)

   e. *it, you, here, there* as locative

it here	it there
you here	you there

   f. *You* + action word

you drink	you walk	you wash
you throw	you help	you fall

   g. *My* (possessive) + noun (person or thing associated with possession)

my cup	my kitty	my bunny
my book	my wagon	my doggy
my mommy	my daddy	my cookie

   h. Expansion: *my* + attribute (adjective) + noun

my red wagon	my big ball	my heavy box
my yellow box	my big cup	my dirty dress

13. Greeting (*Hi*) or introduction (*see, look*) + thing or person to be greeted or noted

hi boy	hi man	hi kitty	hi mommy
hi doggy	hi girl	hi daddy	hi birdie
see boy	see doggy	see birdie	look man
see Betty	see men	see wagon	look dog

14. *Bye* or *bye-bye* as social gesture (informal *good-bye*)

Most often, *bye* or *bye-bye* is used as a response to another person who has initiated the social gesture associated with departure. Children also use this construction to verbalize an action that is taking place (something or somebody leaving or about to leave). *Bye* (*bye-bye*) may also be used to instigate an action—"to speed the parting guest."

bye man	bye mommy	bye birdie
bye lady	bye doggy	bye kitty

15. Action word (verb) + verb particle

fall down	pick up	put down
go down	go in	throw down

15a. Expansion: noun or pronoun + verb particle

boy go down	man go in	doll fall down
girl go down	lady go in	Tom fall down
it fall down	it go in	you pick up
I go in	I fall down	I pick up
it run (runs) away	I jump up	
it go (goes) away	I jump down	
it jump (jumps) down	it jump (jumps) up	

Expansions and Combinations of Previously Established Constructions

16. Action word + *in* + *it*; *on* + *it*

jump in it	go in it	walk in it
jump on it	go on it	walk on it
look in it	put in it	put on it

17. Action word (verb) + *in* + attribute (adjective) + noun

go in (the) big house	look in (the) blue box
jump on (the) yellow box	look in (the) big book
put in (the) red wagon	look in (the) big bag

18. Action word (verb) + *in* + noun-possessive

look in Mary's book   put in mommy's box
ride in Tom('s) wagon   look in Bobby('s) truck
ride in daddy('s) car   go in boy('s) house

19. Verb + *my* (possessive) + noun (object possessed)

look in my book   ride in my wagon   sit on my box

put in my bag   put in my box   look in my basket

20. Action word + *in* + locative (*here, there*)

see in here   run in here   throw in here

see in there   run in there   throw in there

21. *Want* (*wanna*) + object

wanna (want) milk   wanna (want) cup

wanna (want) doll   wanna (want) box

wanna (want) water   wanna (want) doggy

At this point it is time to stop and take inventory of what the child has retained and incorporated into his or her language proficiencies. What does the child comprehend and what is the child producing that is the complement of comprehension? We may find, in fact, that there are a few constructions that the child is using without evidence of comprehension, constructions that may be triggered off and, at least on the surface are appropriate for the situation. If this is so, then teaching for comprehension is in order. We may also find that the child, perhaps because he or she is now tuning in to spoken language, has acquired forms we have not taught. So much the better! A language sample should again help us to know when we need to go from where we find the child to be. Perhaps all or most of what is assigned to level II will need to be taught or perhaps only a few constructions call for direct teaching. In any event, it is better to assess than to guess.

It may also help to give us some idea of what we have tried to achieve in behalf of the child by comparing his or her accomplishments with some of the guidelines for our program. For the sake of convenience Table 9.1 reproduces the list of the "Fourteen Obligatory English Morphemes" (Brown, 1973) We will refer to Lahey and Bloom's (1977) Organization of "A First Lexicon," and Morehead and Ingram's "Minor Lexical Categories" (1973) as sources. It will also help to review the suggestions of Holland (1975) for a core lexicon. We hope that it will become apparent that our recommended syntactic constructions have been in accord with most of the recommendations that served as guidelines and that they will continue to serve in the subsequent levels.

**Table 9.1   FOURTEEN OBLIGATORY ENGLISH MORPHEMES (SUFFIXES AND FUNC-
TION WORDS) AND THEIR LIKELY ORDER OF ACQUISITION BY CHILDREN**

Morpheme form	Likely intended meaning	Example
1. Present progressive: *-ing*	Ongoing action	Joe is eat*ing* lunch
2. Preposition: *in*	Containment	The cookie is *in* the box.
3. Preposition: *on*	Support	The cookie is *on* the box.
4. Plural: *-s*	Number (more than one)	The bird*s* flew away.
5. Past irregular: e.g., *went, ran*	The event took place earlier (before the time of the speaker's utterance)	The boy *went* away. The boy *ran* away.
6 Possessive: *-'s*	Possession	The girl*'s* dress is red.
7. Uncontracted form of the verb *to be* (copula): e.g., *are, was*	Plural number; past tense (earlier in time)	These *are* cookies. It *was* a cat. It *was* on the tree.
8. Articles: *the, a*	Definite and indefinite article	Bob has *the* stick. Bob has *a* stick.
9. Past regular: *-ed*	Event happened earlier in time	Tom jump*ed* (over) the fence.
10. Third person regular: *-s*	Third person, present action	He walk*s* fast.
11. Third person irregular: e.g., *has, does*	Present state (situation; ongoing action (third person)	He *has* a ball. She *does* the cooking.
12. Uncontracted auxiliary of *be:* e.g., *is, were*	Ongoing action; past action	Bob *is* eating. They *were* fishing.
13. Contracted form of *to be:* e.g., *-'s, -'re*	State of being (existence)	It*'s* a kitty. We*'re* at home.
14. Contracted auxiliary of *be:* e.g., *-s, -'re*	Time, ongoing action	He*'s* going. They*'re* eating lunch.

Sources: Based on Brown (1973, p. 271) and adapted from Clark and Clark (1977, p. 345).

LEVEL II: AVERAGE UTTERANCE RANGE, 2.5 TO 3.0 OR MORE MORPHEMES

At the outstart of this level, children may continue to use constructions that lack the syntactical markers or other features of adult forms. However, they should be increasingly exposed to the adult form. Some, in fact, may begin to use syntactic markers at this level, at least as related to mean length of utterance (MLU); others may not use such syntactic features until they are at the next level. An outstanding advance in language usage is the beginning of the use of questions that include *wh* words. Other minor lexical items will be introduced, generally in keeping with the findings of Morehead and Ingram (Morehead and Ingram, 1973).

Basic Constructions

1. Agent—action noun (object)

girl hold (holds) doll	girl kick (kicks) ball
boy hold (holds) doll	boy kick (kicks) ball
baby eat (eats) cookie	girl wash (washes) doggy
boy throw (throws) ball	kitty wash (washes) face
girl throw (throws) ball	boy catch (catches) ball

2. Action word + attribute + noun

kick red ball	kick big ball
throw red ball	kick small ball
see big man	catch yellow ball
hold small box	hold baby doll

3. *This* and *that* as demonstratives in constructions, such as *this is a man* (adult form), *this man* (child form)
   Children may use such constructions as *this a baby* and *that a baby* before using the full adult form, *this is a baby*. Either is acceptable (*this baby* or *this is a baby*) but we recommend exposure to the full adult form.

this baby (this is a baby)	that birdie (that is a birdie)
this kitty	that kitty
this car	that car
this doggy	that doggy
this lady	that lady

4. *This, that* + attribute of demonstrative (predicate adjective)

this yellow (this is yellow)	that yellow
this big (this is big)	that big
this small (this is small)	that small
this pretty (this is pretty)	that pretty

5. *On* (as support) + attribute + noun

on big box	on yellow roof
on small chair	on big chair
on red carpet	on yellow table

6. Expansion: agent (noun) + action word + *on* + attribute + object

   girl put on red carpet

   boy put on big box

   Mary put on round table

   kitty sit on small chair

   Mary sit on white pony

7. Expansion: agent (noun) + action word + *in* (containment) + object

   Tom put in red box

   Mary put in big box

   Tom put in yellow wagon

   baby sleep in small bed

8. Articles: *a* (as singular, one of several objects) in contrast with *the* (as a
   contrast-specific indicator between objects)
   a. Article *a* + noun

a hat	a flower
a kitty	a box
a ball	a lady

   b. Article *the* + noun

the lady	the doggy	the boy
the kitty	the cookie	the girl
the ball	the chair	the man

   c. Action word + article *a* + noun in contrast with use of *the*

eat a cookie	eat the cookie
hold a ball	hold the ball
throw a ball	throw the ball
kick a ball	kick the ball

   d. Agent (noun) + action (verb) + article + noun

baby eat a cookie	boy pull a wagon
mama hold the baby	Mary hold a rope
boy kick the ball	Tom eat a banana
girl throw the ball	Bob catch the ball

e. Article (*a* or *the*) + attribute + noun

a big box	the big boy
a small box	the small boy
a yellow wagon	the yellow wagon
a red house	the red house
a green ball	the green ball

9. Plural marker (regular *-s*) in contrast with singular

bell	bells	boy	boys
cookie	cookies	girl	girls
cat	cats	hat	hats
bird	birds	book	books
stick	sticks	table	tables

10. Action word + noun (singular and plural)

throw ball	throw balls	hold book	hold books
eat cookie	eat cookies	see lady	see ladies
see bird	see birds	hold flower	hold flowers
see bunny	see bunnies	feed bunny	feed bunnies

11. Agent-action + article + noun (singular and plural)

girl hold(s) a flower	girl hold(s) the flowers
man hold(s) a book	man hold(s) the books
baby hold(s) rattle	babies hold(s) the rattles
Tom see(s) a car	Tom see(s) the cars

12. Verb *-ing* (ongoing action)

baby eating	cat washing
Tom running	bird flying
Mary jumping	lady walking
man swimming	man fishing

13. Agent + verb *-ing* + noun

baby eating cookie	lady driving car
girl hitting ball	boy riding bicycle
boy kicking can	mama holding baby

14. Expansions and combinations of previously established constructions
    a. Agent + action + *in* + *a* or *the* + noun

Tom sit on a box	boy look in the window
Mary look in the house	lady sit on a chair
Tom jump on a carpet	baby sit in a wagon
fish swim in the water	man sit in the car

    b. Verb + preposition (*in* or *on*) + possessor + noun

put in Mary('s) wagon	ride in boy('s) wagon
ride in lady('s) car	sit on Tom('s) box
look in Mary('s) box	come in Bobby('s) house

15. Agent + action + pronoun *it*

boy catch it	man throw it
Tom throw it	lady hold it
girl kick it	man see it

16. Agent + action + *me*

baby kiss me	mama hug me
man hold me	daddy see me

17. Pronoun *I* + action word + noun

I throw (the) ball	I eat (a) cookie
I hold (the) flower	I see (a) kitty

18. *You* + verb + noun[6]

you drink (the) milk	you hold (the) doll
you catch (the) ball	you kick (the) ball
you hit (the) ball	you kiss (the) baby

19. Verb + *my* + noun

hold my book	smell my flower
kick my ball	eat my cookie
hold my stick	read my book

---

[6]The pronoun *you* is included by Morehead and Ingram (1973) as a Level III item. We introduce *you* here as a contrast to *I*.

20. Verb *-ing* + plural noun

eating grapes	making mudpies
building blocks	holding sticks
eating cookies	pulling wagons

21. Expansions incorporating features previously taught
    a. Noun (singular and plural) + verb *-ing* + noun (object)

boy eating cookie	boy pushing wagon
boy eating cookies	boy pushing wagons
boys eating cookies	boys pushing wagons
girl riding bicycles	boy feeding dog
girls riding bicycles	boys feeding dogs

   b. Verb *-ing* + article (*a* or *the* as contrasts) + noun

eating a banana	eating the banana
eating a plum	eating the plum
pushing a wagon	pushing the wagon
holding a stick	holding the stick
kicking a ball	kicking the ball

   c. Noun + verb *-ing* + article + noun

boy eating a banana	boy eating the banana
lady eating a plum	lady eating the plum
girl pushing a wagon	girl pushing the wagon
girl holding a stick	girl holding the stick
man kicking a ball	man kicking the ball

   d. Noun plural + verb *-ing* + article + noun

boys eating a pie	mamas holding the babies
girls eating the plums	boys pulling the wagon
girls holding a rope	boys pulling the wagons

Questions

The first questions of English-speaking children are usually distinguished from statements by the use of a rising intonation; that is, the word order is the same as that of a declarative sentence (e.g., "I can eat cookie?"), but the intonation

changes from a falling final inflection to a rising one. The reordering of words
to produce "May I eat cookie?" is an advanced accomplishment. By the third
year, most children begin to ask questions that include an interrogative word—
that is, to construct *wh* questions. The usual order is *where, what, whose, who,*
followed by *why, how,* and *when.* However, as Bloom and Lahey (1978)
observe: "It appears that children learn to ask particular kinds of questions
only after they learn to respond to questions of the same kind, and they do not
learn to ask and answer questions in general" (p. 188).

In the early use of *wh* questions, children tend to confuse some of the *wh*
words, such as *where* and *when, why* and *what.* De Villiers and de Villiers
(1979) explain this confusion, as well as the correct understanding and, hence,
production of other *wh* constructions, by the following observation:

> Children begin by answering *what, who,* and *where* questions quite well,
> since this is the kind of information—agents, objects, and locations—that
> their own sentences can express. However, they do not yet understand the
> notions of manner, causation, purpose, or time, and they are apt to answer
> questions that relate to those notions as if they were familiar questions. (p.
> 63)

De Villiers and de Villiers also provide examples of wrong answers to
some *wh* questions:

> Q. When are you having lunch?   A. In the kitchen.
> Q. Why are you eating that?   A. It's an apple.

Morehead and Ingram (1973) found a relative absence of questions in the
language sample of their deviant (severely linguistically retarded) group of
children. They conjecture that the paucity of questions "could reflect either a
general sampling problem inherent in children with productive liabilities or a
general sociolinguistic posture which is antithetical to seeking information by
linguistic code." Furthermore, the note: "It would be difficult to assume that
question transformations are psychologically more difficult than many of the
transformations acquired by the deviant group."

The assumption that severely linguistically retarded children can be
directly taught verbal constructions based on model sentences is not readily
tenable for *wh* questions. Normally, an adult-presented question to a child is
intended to produce a response in the form of an act or a verbal statement,
positive or negative; thus, "What do you want?" when asked by an adult is
intended to elicit behavior to indicate what the child wants. The child may point
to something as an answer to the question or state "I want———."

The matter of eliciting *wh* question constructions from the linguistically
retarded demands ingenuity and creative techniques on the part of the clinician
or teacher. A technique that we have found reliably productive is to structure a
situation that involves the child in an interchange of roles with the clinician.
Specifically, the clinician asks a question intended to elicit an overt response

from the child; thus, "Do you want a cookie?" is likely to evoke "Yes," and the child is given the cookie. When it becomes clear that the child understands the question, the clinician changes places as well as roles with the child, who is duly instructed: "Ask me to tell you what I want."[7]

Puppets may be manipulated either to act out or to utter the questions and answers as identification models for the child. Considerable ingenuity will be needed for the clinician or teacher to create meaningful and likely situations that go beyond a "What do you want?" question–answer interchange. Appropriate pictures may stimulate answers to questions such as "What will the boy (girl, man, woman) do?" Following are some sample question constructions in adult and acceptable child forms for children at Level II, based on mean length of utterance. In succeeding levels, we will present other *wh* question constructions.

Where

1. *Where's that?* (adult form); *Where that?* (acceptable child form). Use to elicit an answer in the form of a preposition plus a locative noun, (e.g., *Where's that? In (the) wagon.*).
2. *Where is the man going?* (adult form); *Where man go?* (acceptable child form). Use as in 1 to elicit answers in forms that include a preposition plus a noun (e.g., *to the house.*).
3. *Where does the boy run?* (adult form); *Where boy run?* (acceptable child form). Use with a variety of activities to elicit a location (place) answer. This may be in the form of a preposition plus a noun, as in *to the playground,* or just a noun, as *playground.*

What

1. *What is (what's) that?* (adult form); *What that?* (acceptable child's form). The *What is that (what's that)?* form should be used with a series of objects or pictures to elicit an identification term (e.g., ball, boy, chair, kitty, doggy, man, and so on).
2. *What does the man do?* (adult form); *What man do?* (acceptable child's form). Use this form with a variety of subjects (e.g., girl, man, dog, cat) engaged in various activities, such as jump, hit, eat, climb, push, pull, and so forth.
3. *What does the boy hold?* (adult form); *What boy hold?* (acceptable child form). Use this form with various verbs (e.g., drink, eat, push, hold, carry) to elicit an appropriate nominal term.
4. *What is the girl's name?* (adult form); *What girl name?* (acceptable child form). Use this form to elicit a variety of names.
5. *What does the baby want?* (adult form); *What baby want?* (acceptable child form).

---

[7]Many linguistically deviant (pseudoverbal) children with primary (infantile) autism typically respond to questions by a repetition (echoing) of the presented construction.

LEVEL III: MEAN LENGTH OF UTTERANCE, 3.0 TO 4.0 OR MORE MORPHEMES

Basic Constructions

1. Continue with agent (noun) + action (verb) + noun

Articles and prepositions are supplied in presentation but are not required in child's formulation. However, do acknowledge by special approval if articles or propositions are included. The noun-verb-noun construction was introduced earlier for Level I. It is reintroduced here because it is so basic a construction and provides a formulation for expansions to be presented later. An actual presentation might be *The boy eats a pear*.

man open (opens) door	man hit (hits) ball
lady open (opens) box	girl pull (pulls) wagon
dog eat (eats) bone	boy catch (catches) ball
mama hold (holds) baby	man throw (throws) stick

2. Verb-noun-preposition (*in* or *on*) + noun.

These constructions may be used to contrast *in* for containment and *on* for support. They should be presented initially in full adult form (e.g., *Put the spoon in the cup*) and then reduced, if necessary, to child form if it becomes apparent that the adult form produces errors.

put ball in wagon	hit ball on ground
put stick in box	put stick on box
sit doll in chair	throw ball in air
put spoon in cup	put cup on dish

3. Modal (auxiliary) verb + noun

Many, perhaps most, children are more likely to hear the colloquial form *gonna* rather than *going to* in these constructions. From the point of view of presenting tokens of types of constructions prevalent in a child's environment, and, thereby establishing comprehension as well as production, the colloquial form is acceptable. Practically, if the clinician ascertains that *gonna* is the form the child is most likely to hear, it should become the first form for introducing the modal (auxiliary) verb construction.

going (to) eat apple	going (to) drink juice
going (to) pick flowers	going (to) read book
going (to) pull wagon	going (to) feed baby
going (to) throw ball	going (to) push wagon

4. Noun + verb + noun + preposition (required) + noun

Present in full adult form to include article (*a* or *the*) as well as preposition; accept reduced form from the child, but require or at least encourage inclusion of the preposition.

boy put box in wagon	Bob put spoon in cup
girl put doll in box	mommy put baby in car
girl throw ball in air	girl put cake on plate
Tom put kitty in wagon	Mary put doll in bed

5. Noun + form *is* (copula) of verb *to be* + predicate noun

Tom is boy	mommy is woman
Susan is girl	lady is woman
kitty is animal	dog is animal

6. Demonstrative (*this, that*) + *is* + noun

this is Tom	that is Mary
this is lady	that is girl
this is boy	that is kitty
this is wagon	that is car

7. Noun + locative (*here, there*)

Tom is here	mommy is there
dog is here	Bobby is there
lady is here	kitty is there
girl is here	boy is there

8. Noun + *in, on* (containment, support) + noun

dog is in wagon	man is on bicycle
ball is in hand	book is on table
girl is in house	kitty is on roof
lady is in car	cup is on table

9. Noun + *is* + predicate adjective (e.g., *dog is big, baby is small*, or contracted forms, *dog's big, baby's small*)

lady is pretty	ball is yellow
man is tall	dolly is small
wagon is red	girl is happy
bunny is soft	stone is hard

10. Demonstrative pronoun + *is* (copula) + attribute + noun

This is a big cookie.	That is a tall man.
This is a small kitty.	That is a big stick.
This is a yellow wagon.	That is a red apple.

11. Expansions featuring preposition and/or article plus inflectional ending *-s* as a plural marker

put a ball in the wagon	put a cookie on the dish
put the balls in the wagon	put the cookies on the dish
put the balls in the wagons	put the cookies on the dishes
boy sits on the box	girl picks up a stick
boys sit on the box	girls pick up a stick
boys sit on the boxes	girls pick up the sticks

12. Modal (*going to, gonna*) + plural marker *-s*

going to (gonna) push the wagon	going to (gonna) make a tower
going to (gonna) push the wagons	going to (gonna) make the towers
going to (gonna) kick the ball	going to (gonna) open the box
going to (gonna) kick the balls	going to (gonna) open the boxes

13. *Is* or auxiliary + ongoing action

man is walking	dog is jumping
boy is eating	baby is sleeping
girl is swimming	lady is sitting

13a. Expansion: *is* or auxiliary + ongoing action + noun as object of action

girl is catching the ball	man is driving the car
boy is feeding the dog	lady is riding the bicycle

13b. Expansion to include articles (*a* and *the*)

If the addition of these function words produces confusion in comprehension or production, then drop 13b.

A girl is catching the ball.	A lady is riding the bicycle.
A boy is feeding the dog.	A mommy is feeding the baby.
A man is driving the car.	A dog is holding the stick.

13c. Articles *a* and *the* in full sentences

Put a cookie on the dish.   Put a block on a box.
Put the cookies on the dish.   Put the blocks on the box.

Throw a stick in the air.   Put a doll in a wagon.
Throw the stick in the air.   Put the dolls in the wagon.

14. Conjunction *and;* expansion to include definite article *the*

baby and mommy   See the baby and the mommy.

boy and dog   See the boy and the dog.

cup and dish   kick the ball and the box

block and wagon   hold the ball and the stick

15. Preposition *to* + noun (place); verb + preposition + noun

to (the) store   Ride to (the) store.

to (the) playground   Walk to (the) playground.

to (the) house   Run to (the) house.

to (the) garden   Go to (the) garden.

16. Noun + verb (action) + preposition *to* + noun

man drive to store   dog jump to boy

boy run to playground   kitty run to girl

lady walk to house   boy go to wagon

17. Pronouns (third person) *he, she, they* + present state or action

He throw (throws) ball.   He throw (throws) a ball.
She drink (drinks) milk.   She drink (drinks) the milk.
They catch sticks.   They catch the sticks.
He play (plays) piano.   He play (plays) the piano.

17a. Pronouns *he, she, they* + *her, him, them*

he hold her   hc hold them

she push him   she hold them

he kiss her   he pull them

she kiss him   she pull them

he see her   she chase them

she see him   he chase them

18. Pronoun (third person singular) + *is* (copula) + preposition *in, on* + noun (locative)

She is in (the) garden.	He is in (the) wagon.
He is in (the) car.	He is on (the) bicycle.
She is in (the) house.	She is on (the) box.
He is in (the) playground.	He is on (the) carpet.

19. Pronoun (third person singular) + *is* (copula) + *here, there*

She is here.	She is there.
He is here.	He is there.

20. Pronoun + modal auxiliary + verb + *noun*

As indicated earlier, the modal may be presented as *going to* or *gonna*, as determined by the prevalence of the form in the child's environment.

He (is) going to (gonna) push wagon.	He (is) going to ride bike.
She (is) going to eat (the) cookie.	She (is) going to throw (the) ball.
He (is) going to open (the) box.	He (is) going to pull (the) wagon.
He (is) going to drive (the) car.	She (is) going to feed (the) baby.

21. Pronoun + action word + noun + preposition *in, to* + noun (statement of an action)

The full form should be tried but then reduced if there is evidence of confusion in comprehension or production.

He put (puts) the box in (the) wagon.
She put (puts) the baby in (the) carriage.
She throw (throws) the stick in (the) air.
He give (gives) the ball to (the) girl.
She carry (carries) cake to (the) table.
He pull (pulls) dog in (the) wagon.

22. Plural pronoun (*they*) + modal auxiliary (*going to, gonna*) + verb + noun

It is likely that the full but contracted forms, *they're going to* or *they're gonna*, are a later-level achievement. They might be tried here and maintained, or dropped, depending on evidence of comprehension or confusion.

They going to (gonna) bake cookies.
They going to (gonna) push wagon.

They going to (gonna) fly kites.

The going to (gonna) ride bicycles.

23. Plural pronoun (*they*) + verb + preposition *to, in* + noun

They pull (the) wagon to (the) store.

They carry (the) kitty in (the) basket.

They throw (the) balls in (the) air.

24. Expansions incorporating modal auxiliary form

Mother going to (gonna) go to (the) store.

Girl going to (gonna) go to (the) playground.

Boy going to (gonna) run to (the) house.

Lady going to (gonna) look at (the) flowers.

Girl going to (gonna) play in (the) house.

25. Noun + present progressive (ongoing action) + preposition + noun

Man is walking to (the) car.

Lady is standing at (the) bus stop.

Boy is running to (the) house.

Girl is eating at (the) table.

Dog is running to (the) man.

26. Pronouns *she, he, they* + present progressive

He is eating.   She is eating.

He is running.   She is running.

He is sleeping.   She is jumping.

They are hopping.   They are swimming.

They are reading.   They are cooking.

27. Pronouns *she, he, they* + verb (present tense)

She pulls (the) wagon.   He feeds (the) kitty.

He holds (the) dog.   She feeds (the) baby.

He throws (the) stick.   He reads (a) book.

They pull (the) wagon.   They push (the) wagon.

They eat (the) cookies.   They read (the) books.

28. Questions

    Introduce questions that may be answered by "Yes" or "No" as transformation of declarative sentences with *is* as initial word.

a. Noun + *is* (copula) + noun (predicate noun)

Declarative Statement	Question Transformation
Daddy is (a) man.	Is daddy (a) man?
Susie is (a) girl.	Is Susie (a) girl?
Tom is (a) boy.	Is Tom (a) boy?
Fluffy is (a) kitty.	Is Fluffy (a) kitty?

b. Noun + *is* (copula) + preposition + noun (locative)

Statement	Question
Kitty is in box.	Is kitty in box?
Block is in wagon.	Is block in wagon?
Man is in car.	Is man in car?
Lady is in house.	Is lady in house?

c. Noun + *is* (copula) + progressive verb

Statement	Question
Dog is running.	Is dog running?
Kitty is meowing.	Is kitty meowing?
Girl is jumping.	Is girl jumping?
Man is eating.	Is man eating?

29. *O.K.?* as a tag question (e.g., *I pull the wagon, O.K.?*)

Introduce the tag question with a demonstrated action for which the expected and usually appropriate answer is "Yes." Follow this by the question addressed to the child as a request for permission to do something. The child is in control of the situation by his or her decision to answer either "Yes" or "No."

I push wagon, O.K.?
I eat (the) cookie, O.K.?
I sit on (the) box, O.K.?
I kick the ball, O.K.?

30. *Wh* questions

Review *where* and *what* in Level II. Expand the form to an adult construction. Note that the contracted form (*what's* for *what is*, *where's* for *where is*) is acceptable.

Where is the boy?	Where's the boy?
Where is the kitty?	Where's the kitty?

Where is the cookie?   Where's the cookie?

What is the girl doing?   What's the girl doing?
What is the man reading?   What's the man reading?
What is the baby drinking?   What's the baby drinking?

31. Preposition *with*

   Bob go (goes) to party with Susan.

   John go (goes) to store with Tom.

   Jane go (goes) to market with mother.

   Bill go (goes) to playground with daddy.

   Mary go (goes) to airport with mother.

32. Expansion including pronoun *them*

   Give the cookies to them.

   The dog runs with them.

   Bob pulls the wagon with them.

   Mary jumps rope with them.

   Daddy drives the car with them.

33. Auxiliary modal: *has to* (*hasta*) and *have to* (*hafta*)
   In a strict sense, *has to* and *have to* are not modals, as are *do, must, shall,
will, can,* and *must.* However, *has to* and *have to* and their colloquial forms,
hasta and *hafta,* serve functionally as modals and are usually acquired at Level
III.

   I have to (hafta) eat.

   You have to (hafta) leave.

   She has to (hasta) play.

   The dog has to (hasta) jump.

   The baby has to (hasta) sleep.

   The kitty has to (hasta) wash.

LEVEL IV: MEAN LENGTH OF UTTERANCE, 4.0 TO 5.0 OR MORE MORPHEMES

At this level, utterances of normal children are close to full adult forms. Some
children still may not include grammatical markers. The constructions should
now be presented to include such grammatical features, as well as articles and
prepositions that have previously been taught and those that will be introduced. However, do not reject a response that omits a verb marker.

Basic Constructions

1. Noun + verb (present tense) + noun and article *the*

   The boy throws the ball.   The girl holds the rope.
   The cat drinks the milk.   The man catches the ball.
   Tom reads the book.   Bob rides the horse.
   The lady drives the car.   Susan closes the door.

2. Expansion to include preposition + article *a*

   The boy puts a box in the wagon.
   The girl puts a doll in the carriage.
   Tom throws a stick in the air.
   The dog digs a hole in the ground.
   Bob pulls a wagon in the garden.

3. Noun + verb (present tense) + attribute + noun and article

   Bob hits the red ball.
   The girl wears a red dress.
   The dog eats a big bone.
   The man drives the yellow car.
   Susan feeds the white kitty.
   Bill eats the big apple.

4. Noun + modal *going to* (*gonna*) + verb + noun

   Mary going to (gonna) eat a banana.
   The lady going to (gonna) drive the car.
   The mother going to (gonna) feed the baby.
   The boy going to (gonna) dig a hole.
   The girl going to (gonna) read the book.
   The dog going to (gonna) jump the fence.

5. Article + adjective + noun + verb (present tense)

   The small kitty washes.   The happy boy laughs.
   The tall man walks.   The big boy runs.
   The black kitty meows.   The little baby sleeps.

6. *at* + article + noun; noun + preposition *at* + noun (locative)

at the playground	at the house
at the party	at the store
at the school	at the market
boy at the playground	mommy at the house
girl at the party	man at the store
girl at the school	lady at the market

7. Expansion to include copula *is* an article

The boy is at the playground.	The mother is at the house.
The girl is at the party.	The man is at the store.
The teacher is at the school.	The lady is at the airport.

8. Expansion to include noun + verb (copula) + adjective + noun

Susan is a pretty girl.	That is a pretty girl.
John is a strong boy.	That is a strong boy.
A kitty is a small cat.	That is a small cat.

9. Pronouns *his, her, their* to indicate possession (attributive adjective before a noun)

This is Mary('s) wagon.	That is Susan('s) book.
This is her wagon.	That is her book.
This is Tom('s) dog.	This is Sam('s) ball.
This is his dog.	This is his ball.
This is mother('s) car.	Fluff is Mary('s) kitty.
This is her car.	Fluff is her kitty.
This is their box.	
This is their dog.	
This is their house.	

10. *Him, her, them* as objects of action

The stick hit Tom.	Bill pushes Bob.
The stick hit him.	He pushes Bob.
It hit him.	He pushes him.
The ball hit Mary.	Mary sees daddy and mommy.
The ball hit her.	She sees daddy and mommy.
It hit her.	She sees them.

11. Pronouns *you, I, we*

You and I play.   You and I run.
We play.   We run.

You and I jump.   You and I eat.
We jump.   We eat.
You and I drink.   You and I hop.
We drink.   We hop.

12. Noun + verb + pronoun (*me, you, us*)

Daddy holds me.   Tom pushes me.
Daddy holds you.   Tom pushes you.
Daddy holds us.   Tom pushes us.

Mary sees me.   Mommy touches me.
Mary sees you.   Mommy touches you.
Mary sees us.   Mommy touches us.

13. Pronouns *I, you, we* + verb + noun

You and I play ball.   You and I read books.
We play ball.   We read books.

You and I jump rope.   You and I push the wagon.
We jump rope.   We push the wagon.

14. Copula verb constructions
    a. Noun + *is, are* as part of present progressive

The dog is barking.   The lady is singing.
The dogs are barking.   The ladies are singing.

The girl is walking.   The cat is climbing.
The girls are walking.   The cats are climbing.

The baby is sleeping.   The boy is swinging.
The babies are sleeping.   The boys are swinging.

The man is driving.   The dog is eating.
The men are driving.   The dogs are eating.

    b. Demonstrative (*this, these*) + copula + noun phrase

This is a hat.   This is a wagon.
These are hats.   These are wagons.

This is a cup.   This is a spoon.
These are cups.   These are spoons.

This is a flower   This is a top.
These are flowers   These are tops.

   c. Noun + copula + predicate adjective and appropriate article (*a* or *the*)

      A baby is little.   The wagon is red.
      A ball is round.   The box is yellow.
      A kitty is small.   The men are strong.
      A horse is big.   The trees are tall.

   d. Pronouns (*you, I*) + copula (full and contracted forms) + article + predicate adjective or predicate noun

      I am (I'm) hungry.   You are (you're) hungry.
      I am (I'm) strong.   You are (you're) strong.
      I am (I'm) thirsty.   You are (you're) thirsty.
      I am (I'm) happy.   You are (you're) happy.
      I am (I'm) a girl (boy).   You are (you're) a girl (boy).

   e. Pronoun + copula (full and contracted forms) + present progressive

      I am (I'm) laughing.   You are (you're) laughing.
      I am (I'm) swimming.   You are (you're) swimming.
      I am (I'm) playing.   You are (you're) playing.
      I am (I'm) jumping.   You are (you're) jumping.

15. Grammatical markers
   a. Verb, present tense (*-s*)

      The baby sleeps.   The bird sings.
      The cat meows.   The bee stings.
      The dog barks.   The man walks.
      The boy runs.   The lady drives

   b. Noun or pronoun + verb (present tense) + noun.

      John eats an apple.   He eats an apple.
      Bob climbs a tree.   He climbs a tree.
      Mother drives a car.   She drives a car.
      Tom pulls a wagon.   He pulls a wagon.

   c. Possessive marker *-'s; his, her*
     (1) Demonstrative + copula verb + noun (possessive marker); *his, her*

      That is Mary's mother.   That is Tom's stick.
      That is her mother.   That is his stick.

That is Bob's wagon.	That is Susan's friend.
That is his wagon.	That is her friend.
That is Fred's box.	That is Ellen's book.
That is his box.	That is her book.

(2) Pronoun + verb + noun with possessive marker

I see the boy's wagon.	He sees the boy's wagon.
I see the girl's book.	He sees the girl's book.
I see the man's car.	He sees the man's car.
I see the girl's kite.	He sees the girl's kite.

You see the baby's mother.

You see the girl's friend.

You see the boy's wagon.

16. Functional modals: *have to* and *has to* (*hafta* and *hasta*)
   a. Noun phrase + modal + verb

The boy has to (hasta) drink.	The dog has to (hasta) run.
The boys have to (hafta) drink.	The dogs have to (hafta) run.
The baby has to (hasta) eat.	The girl has to (hasta) read.
The babies have to (hafta) eat.	The girls have to (hafta) read.

   b. Expansion to include final noun phrase

The girl has to (hasta) go home.

The girls have to (hafta) go home.

The mother has to (hasta) feed the babies.

The mothers have to (hafta) feed the babies.

The boy has to (hasta) go to school.

The boys have to (hafta) go to school.

17. Modal auxiliaries: *can, may, will, would*

I can run.	Tom can push.
We can jump.	Ellen can kick the ball.
Mary can run.	Mother can drive the car.
Matt can swim.	Daddy can cook the food.

Bob may leave.   Mother may read a book.
Susan may go home.   Ellen may come late.
Tom may go with Susan.   Dick may feed his cat.

May I leave?
May Tom push the wagon?
May Betty sit in the wagon?

We will play ball.   Susan will jump rope.
Tom will go home.   They will run and hop.
Mother will drive the car.   I will read my book.

I would like to go.   Susan would not like to go.
He would like to drive.   She would not like to drive.
Betty would like to jump rope.   Tom would not like to jump rope.
We would like to play ball.   They would not like to play ball.

Question Constructions

Review Level II discussion for techniques for eliciting questions.

1. Review *yes* and *no* questions of Level III with inverted *is*
   At the present level, require the use of the appropriate article for producing a full (adult) sentence.

Ellen is a girl.   Is Ellen a girl?

The boy is in the wagon.   Is the boy in the wagon?

The man is swimming.   Is the man swimming?

The boys are fishing.   Are the boys fishing?

2. *What* used in constructions that call for expanded grammatical responses.
   The clinician will probably need to employ modeling and role-playing in creative situations to elicit responses to questions.

What is (what's) that?   What is the baby drinking?

What is (what's) the man   What is the dog chasing?
  doing?

What is the lady driving?   What is the man hitting?

What is the girl reading?   What is the boy catching?

3. *Where*, including contracted form of *where is* as *where's*

Where is (where's) the lady   Where is Tom? (Where's Tom?)
  going?   Where does the dog run?

Where is (where's) that? .   Where does the bird fly?

4. Inverted questions with modal *will*

Statement	Question
Ted will run.	Will Ted run?
Susan will read.	Will Susan read?
The dog will jump.	Will the dog jump?
The boy will pull Ellen.	Will the boy pull Ellen?
The lady will go home.	Will the lady go home?
The boy will feed the cat.	Will the boy feed the cat?

5. *Why* in expanded constructions

Statement	Question
The boy pushes the girl and she cries.	Why is the girl crying?
The kitty is thirsty and drinks.	Why is the kitty drinking?
The father spanks the boy and the boy cries.	Why is the boy crying?
The dog is hungry and eats.	Why is the dog eating?

6. *How* questions

These forms will probably require an accompanying action or the use of a picture to illustrate the activity.

How do you jump?	How do you fish?
How do you climb?	How do you throw?

7. *Whose*

Whose cookie is this?	Whose book is this?
Whose hat is this?	Whose apples are these?
Whose wagon is it?	Whose car is this?

8. *Which*

Which boy is Tom?	Which man is driving?
Which girl is jumping?	Which boy is washing?
Which lady is singing?	Which child is talking?

9. Preposition *for* and *yes* or *no* question form

Is the book for Susan?	Yes, the book is for Susan.
Is the cookie for Tom?	Yes, the cookie is for Tom?

Is the milk for the baby?	Yes, the milk is for the baby.
Is the food for the kitty?	No, the food is for the dog.
Is the flower for the boy?	No, the flower is for the girl.

LEVEL V: MEAN LENGTH OF UTTERANCE, 5.0 TO 6.0 OR MORE MORPHEMES

1. Continue modal constructions (negatives): *won't, can't, didn't, don't*

Do is a rather interesting auxiliary that most children begin to use correctly between ages 2 and 3. Ervin-Tripp (1977) observes: "*Do* doesn't do anything in terms of semantics. It's a carrier for tense and number or can be left out, as when we say colloquially 'You want some tomato juice?'" (p. 11). Ervin-Tripp also notes: "It's hard for foreigners to learn the use of the word because it does no semantic work. It's pure syntax." In the following constructions, *do* carries the negative affix for the verb.

a. Noun phrase + modal + verb

The dog won't jump.	The girl can't climb.
The baby can't walk.	The baby can't run.
The lady didn't leave.	The boy didn't jump.
The apple doesn't fall.	The apples don't fall.
The boy doesn't run.	The boys don't run.

b. Noun phrase + modal (negative) + verb + noun phrase

The baby won't eat the cereal.	The boys won't fly the kites.
The baby can't eat the nuts.	The girl can't drive the car.
The baby didn't drink the juice.	The man didn't pull the wagon.

2. Function words (prepositions) to express spatial relationships: *up, out, over, under, near, off*

The cat is up the tree.	The plant is out the window.
The man is up the ladder.	The bird is out of the nest.
The kite is up the sky.	Ellen is out of the garden.
The cloud is over the house.	The box is under the desk.
The airplane is over the field.	The basket is under the table.
The kitty is near the cat.	The pillow is off the bed.
The house is near the garden.	The cup is off the shelf.

3. *Down* as contrasted with *up*, and expansions to include noun phrase + verb + preposition + noun phrase

The boy climbs up the ladder.	The smoke goes up to the sky.
The boy slides down the slide.	The rain falls down to the ground.
The bird flies up to the sky.	The boys run up the hill.
The bird flies down to the nest.	The boys run down the hill.
The kite flies up to the clouds.	The cat climbs up the tree.
The kite falls down to the ground.	The cat climbs down the tree.

4. Copula *was* (past action) in contrast with *is* (ongoing action)

The dog is swimming.	The baby is sleeping.
The dog was swimming.	The baby was sleeping.
The lady is sewing.	Daddy is driving.
The lady was sewing.	Daddy was driving.
Tom is happy.	The kitty is drinking.
Tom was happy.	The kitty was drinking.

5. Past tense regular (*-ed*) in contrast with present (*-s*)

The boy skates.	The boy climbs.	Mary smiles.
The boys skated.	The boy climbed.	Mary smiled.
The cat meows.	The baby laughs.	Rover barks.
The cat meowed.	The baby laughed.	Rover barked.
The girl hops.	Ellen skips.	The mother talks.
The girl hopped.	Ellen skipped.	The mother talked.

6. Irregular past tense

As an indication of an ability to generalize, children tend to regularize verb affixes to transform present to past. Thus, lawfully, they may construct *eated, runned, holded, standed,* and so forth, as past tense forms. Linguistically retarded children usually require direct teaching to learn the exceptions to the rule for the past.

Bob eats a cookie.	Mary goes home.
Bob ate a cookie.	Mary went home.
Susan holds the rope.	Ellen breaks the stick.
Susan held the rope.	Ellen broke the stick.

7. Possessive pronouns *their* and *our, his, her*

This is his ball.	This is her dog.
This is our ball.	This is our dog.
This,is his book.	This is his house.
This is our book.	This is our house.
This is her doll.	This is his box.
This is our doll.	These are their boxes.
These are their cookies.	These are their flowers.
These are their pencils.	These are their hats.

8. Restrictive relative clause; noun phrase + clause that identifies or modifies the immediately preceding noun

Bob sees the bird that is flying.

Betty sees the wagon that's painted yellow.

The girls drink the juice that is cold.

The man fixes the wheel that is broken.

The cat feeds the kitty that is hungry.

We will go to the park that is near.

Constructions for *wh* Questions   Also review question constructions presented in previous levels.

1. Questions with negative modals, *won't* and *can't*

Won't the dog jump?	Can't Susan hop?
Won't the cat eat?	Can't you eat the candy?
Won't the baby sleep?	Can't you read the book?
Won't the boy run?	Can't you go to the park?

2. *Who* + *is* + verb

Who is laughing?	Who is driving?
Who is talking?	Who is yelling?
Who is running?	Who is kissing?

3. Expansion: *who* + *is* + verb + noun phrase

Who is eating candy?	Who is chasing the dog?
Who is drinking juice?	Who is hitting the ball?
Who is riding the bike?	Who is driving the car?

4. Expansion: *who* + *is* + verb + prepositional phrase

    Who is running to the park?
    Who is sitting at the table?
    Who is sleeping in the nest?
    Who is standing near the tree?

5. *When*

When will we go?	When do we play?
When do we eat?	When will we read the book?
When will the baby sleep?	When will the cat meow?
When will the boys swim?	When will the baby talk?
When do we hear the stories?	When will Mary come home?
When will our daddy come?	When will we play in the garden?

Constructions Beyond Level V

Almost all of the model constructions presented in this chapter are under control—that is, understood and used—by normal children when they are about 3 years of age. Linguistically retarded children, depending on the degree of retardation, may be age 8, 9, or older before they have learned these constructions. Of course, there is still much more to be learned by linguistically retarded children as well as by linguistically normal children. For example, even at age 10 many normal, bright children still have to learn the sometimes subtle differences in using *ask, tell, allow,* and *promise* in sentences that begin with one of these words followed by *him to go,* as in "Ask him to go," "Tell him to go," and so forth (Chomsky, 1969). Differences in the use of *may* and *might, could* and *should,* may not be clear. Also to be learned are how to coordinate clauses and how to subordinate them, how and when to employ or avoid constructions that begin with "If I were . . . ," and much more about the ways human beings have with words and words have with human beings. Clark and Clark (1977) consider some of the things normal children learn of their language and the strategies they seem to employ in their learning in their chapter "Meaning in the Child's Language."

    There is no end to this kind of learning, the acquisition of meanings according to use in situational and verbal contexts. For all children, there is a continual process of decoding meaning from language in situational use. Though not always with the same degree of proficiency, there is also an ongoing process of encoding of language for meaningful communicative purposes. Clark and Clark (1977) note: "As children find out more about how each word is used, they refine their hypotheses and strategies until their meanings coincide with the adult ones. This process can take years to complete" (p. 513). Indeed, we believe that the process is never complete.

    It is obvious that we cannot possibly teach any child all that a child needs to know and learns of the language or languages of his or her special culture. Normal children require relatively little direct language teaching. The linguistically retarded require considerably more of our time and attention to learn what they need to know about language. Nevertheless, we should not assume, however delayed or deviant the children may be linguistically, that we can possibly teach them all they need to know or are capable of learning about language. Fortunately, when most linguistically retarded children reach Level V, they have become sufficiently sensitive to language and to the ways of words so that, for the most part, they can be left on their own. Some of them will continue to need direct instruction, however. Our clinical experience has shown that they, more than most children, may have difficulty in learning to read. Some may have word-finding problems, in that a word they want and usually know becomes elusive. Others may be slow in putting words together in acceptable syntactic constructions.

What we have offered in this and the preceding chapter are approaches for getting children who are severely linguistically retarded started and moving toward their potential as verbal beings. We should anticipate that many of these identified children will continue to need clinical instruction throughout their school years. There is reason for guarded optimism that most of the children who begin their verbal careers as linguistically retarded can, with instruction, catch up and overcome most of their delays by the time they are adolescents.

REFERENCES AND SUGGESTED READINGS

Bloom, L., and Lahey, M. *Language Development and Language Disorders*. New York: Wiley, 1978.

Brown, R. *A First Language: The Early Stages*. Cambridge, Mass.: Harvard University Press, 1973.

Chomsky, N. *The Acquisition of Syntax in Children from 5 to 10*. Cambridge, Mass.: M.I.T. Press, 1969.

Clark, H. H., and Clark, E. V. *Psychology and Language*. New York: Harcourt Brace Jovanovich, 1977.

Crystal, D., Fletcher, P., and Garman, M. *The Grammatical Analysis of Language Disability*. New York: Elsevier, 1976.

deVilliers, P. A., and deVilliers, J. G. *Early Language*. Cambridge, Mass.: Harvard University Press, 1979.

Ervin-Tripp, S. M. "Language Development," in *Master Lectures on Developmental Psychology*. Washington, D.C.: American Psychological Association, 1977.

Guess, D., Baer, D., and Sailor, W. "A Remedial-Behavioral Approach to Teaching Speech Deficient Children," *Human Communication*, 3, 1978, 55–69.

Holland, A. "Language Therapy for Children: Some Thoughts on Content and Form," *Journal of Speech and Hearing Disorders*, 40, 1975, 514–523.

Kohlberg, L. "Early Education: A Cognitive-Developmental View," *Child Development*, 39(4), 1968, 1013–1062.

Krashen, S. "The Critical Period for Language Acquisition and Its Possible Bases," *Annals of the New York Academy of Medicine*, 263, 1975, 201–224.

Lahey, M., and Bloom, L. "Planning a First Lexicon: Which Words to Teach First," *Journal of Speech and Hearing Disorders,* 42(3), 1977, 340–350.

Lasky, E. Z. and Klopp, K. "Parent-Child Interaction in Normal and Language Disordered Children," *Journal of Speech and Hearing Disorders,* 47,(1) 1982, 7–18.

MacDonald, J. D. and Blott, J. P. "Environmental Language Intervention," *Journal of Speech and Hearing Disorders,* 39(3), 1974, 244–256.

Menyuk, P. *Language and Motivation.* Cambridge, Mass.: M.I.T. Press, 1977.

Miller, J. F. and Yoder, D. E. "An Ontogenetic Language Teaching Program for Retarded Children," in R. L. Sckiefelbusch, and L. L. Lloyd (eds.), *Language Perspectives—Acquisition Retardation, and Intervention.* Baltimore: University Park Press, 1974.

Morehead, D. M., and Ingram, D. "The Development of Base Syntax in Normal and Linguistically Deviant Children," *Journal of Speech and Hearing Research,* 16, 1973, 330–352.

Reid, D. K., and Hresko, W. P. *A Cognitive Approach to Learning Disabilities.* New York: McGraw-Hill, 1981.

Spradlin, J. E., and Siegel, G. H. "Language Training in Natural and Clinical Environments," *Journal of Speech and Hearing Disorders,* 47, 1982, 2–6.

Tyack, D., and Gottesleben, R. *Language Sampling: Analysis and Training.* Palo Alto, Calif.: Consulting Psychologists Press, 1974.

chapter 10

Congenital Motor Impairment for Speech Production

APRAXIA FOR SPEECH (Articulatory Apraxia)

In acquired disorders of speech and language, it is usually possible to identify the pathology that underlies the new impairment or impairments in verbal behavior. If we are concerned with an older child, an adolescent, or an adult, we are provided with a considerable developmental history up to the time of the pathology and change in functioning. Such a history permits us to make diagnoses in keeping with established facts and knowledge about cause or causes related to the impairment. With congenital problems, no extensive body of information is available. We have to call on the early medical and developmental history to learn or conjecture what was not produced that we normally would expect to be produced. Thus, in dealing with a child who has congenital apraxia for speech, we are concerned with a failure or impairment of a complex oral behavior to be established, rather than with the breakdown of previously established behavior. Nevertheless, the following description of the *acquired* impairment (Darley, Aronson and Brown, 1975) will help us appreciate what the behavior is that we identify as congenital apraxia for speech (articulatory apraxia):

> As they speak, they struggle to position their articulators correctly. They visibly and audibly grope as they struggle to produce correct articulatory postures and to accomplish a sequence of these postures in forming words. Their articulation is frequently off target. They often recognize that they are off target and effortly try to correct the error. Their errors recur, nonetheless, but they are not always the same; the errors on a series of trials are highly variable. (p. 250)

It is important to distinguish between articulatory apraxia and dysarthria. In general, *apraxia* implies an impairment in motor planning for an intended sequence of movements. In apraxias for speech, the impairment is in a planned sequence of movements of the organs of articulation. Dysarthrias are also articulatory impairments associated with neuropathologies, but not necessarily of central (cerebral) origin. In *dysarthria,* the intended movements may be made, but with overt evidence of weakness, slowness, and lack of precision. The phonological consequences create difficulties in comprehension. However, the type of error or distortion in dysarthria is characteristically consistent. In contrast, apraxic errors characteristically reveal variability and inconsistency of production.

CONGENITAL APRAXIA AND CONGENITAL APHASIA

Some congenitally aphasic children may also have articulatory apraxia. If and when they do, such children will have primary difficulty in decoding spoken language as well as impairments in producing whatever language they are able to decode and attempt to encode for response by a listener. However, congenital articulatory apraxia may exist as a separate (discrete) impairment. When it does, the child is able to process and decode (comprehend) spoken language but cannot readily plan the appropriate sequence of articulatory movements to produce an oral message.

We will define apraxia for speech (articulatory apraxia) as impairment in the ability to produce a sequence of voluntary and intended movements involving the muscles of the mouth (tongue, lips, palate, cheeks), pharynx, and larynx on the basis of cerebral pathology. Automatic movements of the same muscles can be performed, although there is considerable clinical developmental evidence that movements of the oral mechanism may also show impairment during the first year or two of life.

Some children with apraxia for speech are occasionally identified, probably erroneously, as motor or expressive asphasics. McGinnis (1963), for example, includes them in her basic classifications as belong to Class I—motor or expressive aphasia—and describes such children as (1) having intelligence within normal limits, (2) having normal hearing and understanding of language, (3) impaired in their ability to imitate words, and (4) impaired or limited in their ability to imitate speech sounds.

These children are more appropriately designated as suffering from congenital articulatory apraxia. If the impairment is less than very severe, then the term *dyspraxia* should be used.

Hardy (1978), in describing the child with congenital articulatory apraxia, emphasizes:

In particular those phonemes that require complex articulatory movements are seldom heard. Hence the articulatory problem is characterized by frequent omissions and distortions of sounds. . . .

> In addition, the child will have an extremely difficult time changing
> articulatory patterns ... disability in performing nonspeech movements of
> the articulators may or may not be present, but the articulation problems of
> children with developmental speech apraxia is typically quite severe. (pp.
> 236–237)

Yoss and Darley (1974) in comparing adult and congenital apraxic children,
note: "An accompanying oral apraxic component is usually seen in children."

THE APRAXIC CHILD

The child with congenital oral (articulatory) apraxia, as indicated earlier, does
understand language (speech) and may indicate such understanding by behavior that does not require an oral (verbal) response. In an approximate sense,
the oral apraxic child is much like young children between 12 and 18 months of
age who are beginning to understand a considerable amount of the language of
their environment, but who have little productive language of their own. The
important difference between the young normal child who is acquiring language and the child with congenital oral apraxia, however, is that the former
acquires productive language while the latter continues to be impaired. As they
grow older, oral apraxic children become frustrated by their productive
limitations. In some instances the frustration begins to overshadow its underlying cause, and such children may be viewed and designated as emotionally
disturbed.

The term *articulatory dyspraxia* is perhaps better and more specific to our
problem than *oral dyspraxia*. Morley and Fox (1969) suggest that articulatory
dyspraxia may be present when no other oral disability can be detected.
Articulatory dyspraxia (apraxia, if severe) is restricted to the child's ability to
organize and produce the appropriate movements for the production of certain
phonemes or sequences of phonemes, and is likely to include phonemes related
to consonant sounds requiring movements of the lips or movements of the
tongue tip or tongue blade. According to Morley and Fox (1969):

> The child who has such a disability, in achieving the complex motor
> coordination required, ... may have a reduced phonemic vocabulary, may
> omit those distinctive features which are for him most difficult, and may
> substitute those which he can produce more easily, or he may omit difficult
> phonemes entirely. (p. 157)

Background and Developmental History

In our earlier discussion of the child with oral apraxia, we cited a number of
factors that, despite many developmental similarities, nevertheless distinguish
such a child from the normal speaking child. We shall now briefly review some
of the similarities and differences that distinguish the child who acquires speech
normally and spontaneously from the child with oral (articulatory) apraxia.

Responsiveness to Environmental Sounds   The developmental history of the child with oral apraxia reveals that he or she is normally responsive to the sounds of the environment—mechanical, animal, and human. The child's orienting movements and postural changes—anticipatory modifications of motor set—are consonant with the ongoing auditory events in his or her milieu. In brief, the child's overt behavior reveals generally acceptable and appropriate auditory discrimination and auditory perception. By the end of the first year or the beginning of the second, the child, if stimulated and given the opportunity, is usually able to play baby games—clapping hands on cue and perhaps pointing to parts of the body, as well as interacting with an adult in "peek-a-boo" activity. In all, except that such a child is not also a verbal imitator and does not engage in echolalic activity, parents have little cause for concern that he or she will not be speaking by 15 to 18 months.

Parental concern may be expressed when, at 18 months or later, the child continues to be productively nonverbal, despite obvious gains in speech comprehension. Even then, especially if the child's family history includes some late talking by siblings or other members of the family constellation, the parents may well have been reassured by a pediatrician or a language clinician that all will be well and that the child will probably be talking in a short while. Concern tends to increase when the prediction is not realized by age 2½ or 3, especially when the family constellation provides no evidence of late onset or retarded language development.

Early Oral Activity   In some instances, the mother is able to recall that, as an infant, the child presented problems in feeding. Frequent regurgitation, difficulty in accepting food that required chewing, rejection of semisolid and bulk foods, and lazy chewing are recalled. The child may have continued on liquid and soft foods at an age long after siblings had accepted and enjoyed chewy foods. At age 5 or 6, the child is happier with liquids than with chopped foods that require even a minimum of chewing.

Early vocal play is often notably absent or is present only in token form. Babbling might be recalled, but lalling (self-sound imitation) and echolalic play are often notably absent. Although the child is neither silent nor an excessive crier, as in some cases of infantile autism, there is comparatively little sound play as might be expected from a child with normal hearing.

Articulatory Activity   Examination of the peripheral speech mechanism often reveals that the child is impaired in executing movements with specific parts of the oral mechanism. Such activities as imitating tongue pointing, lip licking, and tongue wagging (lateral movements) present difficulties. These activities may show improvement if the child is able to imitate them in front of a mirror, especially if the movements can be performed slowly with opportunity for visual cueing. Difficulties tend to increase if rapid movement is expected, or if a series of movements—for example, tongue followed by lip activity—is required. Difficulties are also likely to be manifest if actual sound production (articulatory behavior) is required. Thus, a child may be able to pantomime slowly the movements for *pee-kee* or *lee-nee* but will have difficulty in the actual production of the sounds that are a normal product of such lip and tongue activities.

Sequential Activity   The articulatory apraxic child's predominant difficulty is an impairment in the production of the sequence of movements essential for a unit of utterances. The degree of impairment varies considerably from child to child. With individual exceptions, severity appears to be negatively related to age; that is, younger children (ages 3 to 4), even with allowances made for normal differences in articulatory proficiency, are generally more impaired than older children (ages above 4). In the most severe form, the child may not have sufficient control of the organs of articulation to imitate an isolated movement of the tongue or lips. In other instances, the child may imitate an isolated movement but have difficulty in executing a series of two or more movements, even though each can be produced separately. Performance tends to break down when the rate of activity is accelerated. Thus, though a child may be able to imitate and maintain a sequence such as *ba–da–ga,* the product may, if the model for imitation is presented more rapidly than at first, become *ba–ga* (omission), *ba–ba–da* (perseveration and omission), or *ba–ba–ga,* or may be compressed into *bada* or presented with transposition, as *da–ba* or *ga–ba–da,* and so forth.

   Failures to maintain sequential order are not likely to be associated with any underlying difficulties in auditory perception or auditory sequencing. Most children with oral apraxia who are also of normal intelligence are likely to do as well as their age peers in tests for auditory discrimination, such as Wepman's, or in any informal matching-to-sample tests of sequences of auditory events, including those for speech sounds, provided that memory span is not taxed beyond expected limits for the age of the child.

   By age 3 or 4, when most children are well on their way to becoming syntactically proficient and have a productive vocabulary of 1000 words or more, the child with articulatory apraxia may be struggling to produce intelligible utterances of two or three phonemes. The child is likely to be most proficient with combinations of readily visible labial (lip) plus vowel sounds. Thus, he or she may be successful with *m, n, b,* or *p* plus a vowel and so may produce *ma* and *moo* correctly. He or she may have most vowel sounds under fairly good control. Therefore, if the child attempts an utterance with such sounds and if the intonation contour is appropriate, as it is fortunately likely to be, the utterance may suggest the speech attempts of a child who is just beginning to combine words into a two-word utterance. In effect, the child will sound infantile. Nonvisible sounds and attempts at sequences of five or six phonemes may reveal distortions and sound transpositions, again suggesting the efforts of a child of between 15 and 18 months or a slower child of about 2 years. Syntactical (grammatical) markers, of course, are almost always absent.

Aphasia and Oral Apraxia

As indicated earlier, it is possible for a child to have both articulatory apraxia and congenital aphasia. In such a case, the child will suffer from failure to make adequate sense out of speech sounds and will also be impaired in the production of the limited amount of language he or she does understand. In the absence of intake, there will be little motivation for output except for emotional expression. The aphasic and articulatory apraxic child is essentially perceptually deaf for speech and impaired in motor capacity for communicating what he or she understands of nonspeech environmental auditory events. In essence, the child is reduced to living in a visual world. If we recognize this as a reality situation and train the child on a visual-visual basis, then some representational appreciation and some language behavior can be established to serve as a basis for future training in auditory speech perception and oral language production.

Related Evidence of Dyspraxia

Clinical histories reveal that many articulatory apraxic children present findings that suggest some degree of overall dyspraxia. Some of the children are conspicuously awkward, and their early developmental histories include late walking (past 2 years of age) and a severe lack of manual dexterity. Handedness and other indications of laterality preference may not yet be established at age 4 or 5. Essentially, some of these children may best be designated as ambinonlateral, slow, and awkward in all forms of motor expression. A clinical impression about some of the children is that they seem capable of stumbling over a chalk line. McGinnis (1963) describes a child with motor aphasia and normal intelligence in a manner that is almost typical of a majority of the children we designate as orally apraxic:

> There was delay in all physical development. He was nearly two years old before he began to walk, and then needed physical therapy to improve control of his feet and leg muscles. The parents reported that he made an attempt to say "daddy" at the age of two, but at five he had made no gain in acquiring intelligible speech. He made few attempts to talk, even though his hearing and comprehension of speech were good. (p. 36)

Expressive Impairments of the Congenitally Aphasic Child

The congenitally aphasic child without dyspraxic involvements may have no functional language or, depending on the degree of severity and the child's age, may have a vocabulary limited to a few words that may be used appropriately, with specific meanings communicated and enhanced through the use of gesture. Some children may develop a fairly elaborate gesture system, with vocalization employed essentially as an attention-getting device to engage another person in a communicative interchange. As the child begins to acquire speech, later and more slowly than age peers, productive language is likely to consist largely of nouns and verbs, or words that serve verb or whole sentence functions. He or she appears, in effect, to be fixed at the single- or two-word-utterance stage in language acquisition for a considerably longer period of time than the normal child. As in the normal child, receptive language development is considerably greater than productive language. Unlike the normal child, however, the child with congenital aphasia has a greater disproportion of language he or she understands to language he or she can produce.

Syntax develops slowly, even with direct training. Thus, the aphasic child builds up a much larger inventory of single-word utterances before progressing to two-word asyntactic formulations. Two-word utterances may continue to be asyntactic (an absence of functional words and inflectional markers) long after the normal child has begun to use conventional sentences. When aphasic children attempt syntactic formulations, they sometimes appear to be suffering from anomia, apparently hunting for the word needed for the utterance to be conventional and acceptable. The appearance of anomic difficulty is really an indication that the child is striving, however belatedly, to express himself or herself in a sentence unit, that he or she is working out a complete verbal formulation and is no longer satisfied with asyntactic utterance. In this stage, the child's utterances may suggest the repetitions and hesitations of the normal dysfluencies of the 3-year-old, or even the excessive dysfluencies of the primary stutterer.

Therapeutic approaches for the congenitally aphasic child are considered in Chapters 8 and 9.

THERAPY FOR ARTICULATORY APRAXIA

The objective in the treatment of the child with articulatory apraxia is to establish the ability to produce a sequence of voluntary oral movements essential for intelligible utterance. The corollary of this objective is to extinguish (discourage) random oral movements, which produce the effect of jargon or gibberish as well as some of the perseverative articulatory products that sometimes seem to burst at and overwhelm a would-be listener. A related goal is to discourage a child who has control of a few appropriate, short utterances from surrounding and incorporating them into a larger flow of jargon.

Complicating Problems

In some instances, children with articulatory apraxia may turn off listening in order to avoid the need for responding. In effect, they may withdraw from persons and situations that normally call for oral (verbal) responses. In instances when the problem is compounded by auditory aphasia, we must deal with this impairing intake component and provide an outlet for expression. One approach is to teach a syntactic signing system for productive purposes while establishing intake language along the lines recommended for severely linguistically retarded children.

For children who have turned off or turned away from speakers and speaking situations, efforts at seduction are in order. It should help to begin with the approaches recommended in Chapter 8, "Establishing and Developing Language in Severely Linguistically Handicapped Children," and moving on to those in Chapter 9. As a measure of insurance that we are not overlooking any related intake or receptivity problem, phonological functioning should be assessed. If results so indicate, the recommendations for the treatment of children with phonological deficiencies (Chapter 7) should be instituted.

Establishing Intelligible Speech

Our realistic therapeutic objective for children with articulatory apraxia is to establish intelligible speech. This implies that it may be necessary to settle for considerably less than the level of articulatory proficiency we expect from all but a very small percentage of children with normal hearing and normal intelligence. Overall speech production may need to be at a slower rate than for age peers. Some sound blends may be simplified for an indefinite time to a single phoneme; for example, the clusters *sps* or *sks* may be beyond the reach of the child's articulators. However, for most children with articulatory apraxia, intelligible speech is an obtainable objective. For a very few it is not, however, and we have no other recourse but to teach a signing system as the effective output means of expression. For the more fortunate large majority of children with articulatory apraxia who can learn to control their oral articulators in order to plan and execute a sequence of movements, we recommend the following approaches.

Establishing Sounds in Isolation

If we consider the articulatory apraxic child as one whose impairment is in articulatory production, not in auditory perception or speech comprehension, we may then take advantage of the capacities implied in this designation in our therapeutic efforts. The capacities are for normal auditory and visual intake, and thus for the sequencing of speech events. We may assume that visual stimulation is associated with the auditory, and this, in turn, with articulation. Since even a single sound is a product of a synergy (series) of related movements, the basis for sequencing is established even when we are dealing with an isolated sound or, preferably, a consonant followed by a vowel. We recommend the following general approach in the initial phonetic-phonemic training.[1]

[1]McGinnis (1963) describes a series of initial training steps under the heading "development of the elements of speech." These are exercises for gross tongue movements and tongue position (tongue protrusion, tongue pointing, tongue clicking) that may be performed in an individual or group situation. McGinnis, it should be noted, recommends that a mirror should not be used in training a child to imitate gross muscle patterns. "Unless there is extreme difficulty in tongue control the child should be able to imitate tongue movements from the pattern given by the teacher" (p. 135). Other procedures are described by McGinnis for training an apraxic child. The essentials of the motokinesthetic (Young and Hawk, 1955) are also appropriate for the establishment of isolated speech sounds and for sound sequences.

1. With clinician and child facing a mirror, the clinician slowly pantomimes the articulation for [pɑ]. The child is directed to imitate the movements. If the child does not succeed after several trials, the movements should be broken up (separated) into distinct [p] . . . [ɑ]. When this is achieved, the interval between the separate movements should be reduced until the combination [pɑ] is produced as a continuous articulatory effort. If the two-phoneme sequence or two-phoneme succession is not possible, then the child should be trained to imitate a single, isolated sound. If mirror imitation does not result in successful imitation, then the clinician should feel free to place the articulators in position by manual manipulation, using a tongue depressor (spatula) or a rounded probe stick or manipulating the child's fingers to the appropriate articulatory position. As soon as possible, however, the visual stimulus alone, and then visual recall, should constitute the basis for imitation. Ultimately, of course, the auditory stimulus should replace all of the other stimuli. In some instances, it may be helpful to photograph the child's face in appropriate articulatory states. Then the child is, in fact as well as in effect, imitating himself or herself. Videotape playbacks, if available, provide an ideal though somewhat expensive apparatus and medium for early training.

The first isolated sounds should be /m/, the sound /p/ or /b/. We would then recommend /k/, /g/, and /n/, in that order, followed by /t/ and /d/ and /l/ and /r/. The sibilant sounds, /s/, /z/, /ʃ/, and /ʒ/, should follow, and finally /θ/ and /ð/. However, if the child produces /θ/ or /ð/ as a substitution (approximation) for one of the other sounds, we would establish the child's product on a voluntary and appropriate basis by training him or her to imitate these sounds.[2]

2. Repeat as step 1, but this time without a mirror and with the child facing the clinician.

3. Direct the child to produce the movements with eyes closed, so that visual memory becomes the basis for recall.

4. Introduce vocalization so that the child now hears and sees the activity producing the contexts [pɑ] and [bɑ]. If necessary, separate the phonemes, as in step 1.

If the child fails to appreciate vocalization, or fails to produce voice when necessary, the child's hand may be placed on the clinician's face or throat, and then on his or her own, when the voiced sound needs to be made. As soon as possible, however, the manual contact should be replaced by a written symbol for the voiced phoneme—for example, a checkmark over a sound that should be voiced.

5. Reverse the order of the phonemes to produce the combination [ɑp]. Repeat whatever steps are necessary to arrive at the combination.

When the child succeeds with a two-phoneme combination beginning with a consonant-vowel (CV), the next objective is to establish a consonant–vowel–consonant (CVC) combination. We suggest that the first three-phoneme context consist of the same consonant, preferably a bilabial, in the

---

[2]The suggested order of consonants approximates that of the normal child's phonemic acquisition.

initial and final positions, for example, [pɑp]. Following this, the vowel should be varied so that the child ultimately establishes control over combinations that include each of the vowels in the medial position. As each combination is achieved, the child should be given a card with the symbols orthographically represented (e.g., *peep, pip, pep, pap, poop, pup,* etc.). In training, we recommend establishing the combinations with the greatest differences in articulatory position for the vowels, *peep* vs. *pop,* and then working toward the smaller vowel differences, *peep* vs. *pip, poop* vs. *pawp.* Do not hesitate to use in-front-of-the-mirror imitation if this helps the child. However, the clinician should encourage the child to recall and rely on visual memory to produce the articulatory movements necessary for the production of the stimulus combinations. Be generous with both verbal praise and material rewards (the candy reward approach). Such rewards (reinforcements) should be given at first with every successful or nearly successful (reasonable facsimile) imitation. In later stages, material rewards may be given for a series of successful efforts.

When three-phoneme (CVC) combinations are established with readily visible combinations—bilabial, labiodental, and alveolar consonants—combinations with velar consonants should be introduced. We recommend repeating the five steps previously detailed to establish [kɑ], [gɑ], [ɑk], and [ɑg]. The combination vowel + ng [ŋ] is a later aspiration. Following this, we would again train for CVC combinations, including the velar consonants in medial position, and then for VCV combinations with the same initial and final vowel. After this major achievement, the consonants and vowel combinations may be varied in position, taking care not to introduce any unnatural or nonexisting combinations—for example, no [ppɑ] as a syllabic utterance. On the other hand, we would introduce repeated two-syllable combinations, such as *ma ma, da da, pa pa, ba ba, moo moo,* and the like. Fortunately, these are real words in English and so can provide the reinforcement that comes, as it does to the normal young child, of being able to say something.

It is likely that the clinician will have to learn the technique of slower-than-normal utterance so that the chld will have a model to imitate consistent with his or her developing abilities. Whenever necessary, the child should be directed to separate the sound combinations to ensure accurate articulatory movement. However, as soon as possible, the sequence of continuous movement should become the objective. If the synergy breaks down because of a rate too fast for the child, then a slower rate should be tried. A slow but accurate effort is generally more desirable than a more rapid one that impairs correct sequential articulation.

After the child has built up an inventory of words, nonsense or real, based on consonant-vowel combinations, he or she should be introduced to units that include consonant blends (e.g., *pl, bl, kl, gl, tr, dr, gr, fl, st, sn, mz, nz, dz, nd*) and other frequent consonant-consonant sequences that occur within a syllable and between syllables in spoken language.[3]

---

[3]Our reference is to a phonetic syllable—the sequence of sounds produced on a breath impulse—not to orthographic spelling rule syllabication; for example, the word *asking* is articulated as *as king,* not as *ask ing.*

Sentence Practice

On the basis of the child's inventory of sound combinations under control, short sentences should be constructed and presented to the child with appropriate intonation. At first, these sentences should maximize the use of words with sound and syllable reduplication and alternating consonant-vowel sequences, such as "I want a (wanna) cookie," "I want a cake," and "I want a candy." These sentences, it might be noted, also make use of the repeated carrier phrase "I want," which provides the basis for the generation of many sentences that the child may produce as his or her own verbal formulations.

The following list of words may be used for sentence building:[4]

I	mama	baby	and	in	candy
me	mommy	boy	to	on	bunny
my	papa	girl	of	book	kitty
you	daddy	the	for	cooky	cat
we	up	down	under	over	high
is	was	moon	run	ran	low
has	have	wash	washing	am	read
write	book	ball	kick	catch	draw
paper	cut	will	go	going	went
what	why	this	that	these	those
hand(s)	feet	mouth	talk	sing	yell
come	here	there	coming	see	seeing
now	soon	quick	please	later	may
hop	skip	dance	jump	play	walk

This, of course, is only a sample list of one- and two-syllable words, with none having more than five phonemes. Many hundreds of sentences can be generated from this list. The list is heavily weighted with words that are picturable. This makes it possible for the sentences to depict specific actions, which may be drawn for the child with the sentence written beneath the picture.

Morley and Fox (1969) recommend the use of rhyme words and rhyming phrases, built on the child's established inventory of words, as a device, and we concur in this suggestion. The use of rhymes provides an interesting and motivating exercise for the child and also directs the child's attention to auditory discrimination and perception. Thus, word pairs such as *boy-toy, pat-*

---

[4]See also Holland (1975) and Lahey and Bloom (1977) for suggestions on words for a basic lexicon.

cat, hat-bat, go-toe, run-fun, and the like, may be used. Short sentences employing rhyme words, such as

I pat the cat.	My bunny is funny.
The boy has a toy.	We swing and sing.
To run is fun.	The girl has a curl.
Candy is dandy.	I go up with the pup.

and short couplets, such as

I am a boy. I play with a toy.	Susan has a kitty Who is very pretty.
The moon is high, Up in the sky,	He had a fall When he kicked the ball.

may be devised, based on the child's inventory. It is important that sentence length be limited to the child's capacity for recall. However, after presenting a longer unit than the child can recall, the clinician may present part of the context and direct the child to provide the rhyme word, or the second half of each line. The game of rhyming may also be played by having the child present a line for the clinician to rhyme. The child may also be encouraged to make up rhymes with nonsense words. This provides practice in articulation as well as auditory training.

SUMMARY

We have outlined procedures for the child with congenital articulatory apraxia or, less severely, dyspraxia. Such a child is usually one whose hearing is normal and whose early understanding of speech shows no impairment, but who cannot order and control his or her organs of articulation to produce the necessary sequence of sounds to manage intelligible speech. The procedures described emphasize the use of the visual modality as a basis for imitating speech sounds, beginning with the isolated phoneme and progressing to short sentences. The practice materials and the order of the sounds follow the articulatory acquisitions of the normal child. Concepts of distinctive feature contrasts for articulatory training are incorporated in the practice materials.

REFERENCES AND SUGGESTED READINGS

Darley, F. L., Aronson, A. E., and Brown, J. R. *Motor Disorders of Speech.* Philadelphia: Saunders, 1975.

Hardy, J. C. "Neurologically Based Disorders," in J. Curtis (ed.), *Processes and Disorders of Communication.* New York: Harper and Row, 1978.

Holland, A. "Language Therapy for Children: Some Thoughts on Content and Form," *Journal of Speech and Hearing Disorders,* 40, 1975, 514–523.

Lahey, M., and Bloom, L. "Planning a First Lexicon: Which Words to Teach First," *Journal of Speech and Hearing Disorders,* 42(3), 1977, 340–350.

McGinnis, M. E. *Aphasic Children.* Washington, D. C.: Alexander Graham Bell Association, 1963.

Morley, M. E., and Fox, J. "Disorders of Articulation: Theory and Therapy," *British Journal of Disorders of Communication,* 4(2), 1969, 151–165.

Yoss, K., and Darley, F. L. "Developmental Apraxia of Speech in Children with Defective Articulation," *Journal of Speech and Hearing Research,* 17, 1974, 399–416.

Young, E. H., and Hawk, S. S. *Moto-Kinesthetic Speech Training.* Stanford, Calif.: Stanford University Press, 1955.

chapter *11*

Acquired Aphasia in Children

DEFINITIONS AND PRELIMINARY OBSERVATIONS

In Chapter 5 the term *acquired childhood aphasia* was used to designate the condition of children who had established language normally and had subsequently suffered impairment as a result of cerebral pathology caused by accident or disease. *Acquired dysphasia* was suggested as the appropriate term for residual deficits following a period of recovery.

The nature of the language impairment and the recovery process—what is in fact impaired and what remains as deficits—is different for children with acquired aphasia, for those with congenital aphasia, and for adults with acquired aphasia. As a preliminary statement, it might be said that many of the differences in acquired childhood aphasia are related to the stage and overall proficiency of the child. What a child may be able to recover quickly in language functioning and what the child may have difficulty in establishing may vary considerably, according to the age of the child and so, presumably, according to level of language development if the child is normal, and according to the child's linguistic proficiency if the child is either linguistically slow or possibly precocious. We are more likely to find greater linguistic variability in 3-year-old children than among 12-year-olds. What may be a retrieval (recovery) for a 12-year-old may be initial language acquisition for a younger child. Cromer (1978) emphasizes this point in his observation: "In developmental or even early acquired aphasia the child has been prevented from the initial acquisition of a complete language system" (p. 87).

CAUSES

Acquired aphasia in children, as indicated earlier, is caused by cerebral pathology associated with accident or disease. As a general observation, a child may become aphasic—that is, suffer from impairments of previously established language functions—as a result of pathology of the brain, especially of the hemisphere that is dominant for language. As with adults, the damage is almost always in the left hemisphere for right-handed children. Also, as with adults, the cerebral damage may be in either hemisphere for most left-handed children. Acquired aphasia in children may also be associated with lesions in the right hemisphere, especially in children below age 5 (Krashen, 1973). A possible explanation for this observation is that young children (below age 5) may not yet have lateralized cerebral dominance for language; hence, damage to either hemisphere may temporarily produce some language disruption. However, Satz and Bullard-Bates (1981) note that acquired aphasia in children is more often associated with bilateral cerebral pathology than is the situation in adults.[1]

Although the onset of initial aphasic involvements is higher in children than in adults, the outlook and course of recovery is different and, fortunately, better for most children. As a summary observation, Satz and Bullard-Bates (1981) note: "In fact, the pattern of childhood aphasia departs significantly from the adult form in terms of incidence, type, and prognosis" (p. 401).

As already noted, the patterns of acquired childhood aphasia also depart significantly from that of congenital aphasia. The following discussion will consider these patterns.

PATTERNS OF EARLY LANGUAGE IMPAIRMENTS

Marked reduction in fluency, often to the point of virtual mutism, is a frequently observed feature of early acquired aphasic involvement in children. (Satz and Bullard-Bates, 1981; Chase, 1972; Alajouanine and Lhermitte, 1965). Based on his own observations and a review of the literature, Hécaen (1976) notes that a positive feature of acquired aphasia in children is "the frequency of mutism, of loss of initiation of speech or more generally of the inability to communicate." Furthermore, Hécaen notes that, in the early stages, "Disorders of auditory verbal comprehension appeared in more than a third of the cases. ... However, this relative frequency is a feature only of the acute period ... often there is a rapid and complete disappearance of such disorders." In contrast, he states: "Disturbances of naming have a still greater frequency and tend to persist, the lexical poverty being noted at later stages and even mentioned explicitly in school reports."

Articulatory disorders (dysarthrias) are frequently present in early stages

[1]Based on a review of the literature and their own observation, Satz and Bullard-Bates (1981), generalize: "The risk of aphasia with right brain injury, while higher in children than in adults, is still much lower than the risk of aphasia following left-sided injury, regardless of age" (p. 410).

and sometimes present persistent symptoms. Hécaen (1976) reports that 12 of 15 cases in his longitudinal study had articulatory impairments; in 4 cases the impairments were persistent.

Nonspeech Impairments

Among the associated neuropsychological impairments, acalculia (arithmetic deficit) is high on the list and is frequently reported by observers of children with acquired aphasia. Hécaen (1976) found acalculia to be present in 11 of 15 cases of childhood aphasia associated with left cerebral lesion. Table 11.1, from Hécaen (1976), presents the frequency of aphasic symptoms in 15 cases associated with left cerebral lesions that were studied over a period of 14 years. The children in the study ranged in age from 3½ to 15 years.

Written Language Impairments

Disturbances in reading and writing are found in a majority of children with acquired aphasia. Hécaen (1976) reported such deficits to be present in his study. He found reading disorders in 9 of 15 cases and writing impairments in 13 of the children. Persistent deficits were found in reading for 3 children and for writing in 7. Alajouanine and Lhermitte (1965) reported that disturbances for written language often were more persistent than those for speech.

Alajouanine and Lhermitte (1965) found that age was a factor related to type of symptom in the 33 children, ages 6 to 15, who were the subjects of their study. Obviously, reading and writing were not impaired in the youngest of their subjects. However, of those who had learned to read and to write in the subject population up to age 10, there were frequent disturbances for written language (impaired comprehension) as well as difficulties in comprehension for spoken language. Hécaen (1976) concluded that "it is important to stress

Table 11.1 FREQUENCY OF DIFFERENT APHASIC SYMPTOMS IN 15 CASES DUE TO LEFT HEMISPHERE LESIONS

	Number of cases	Percentage	Evolution
Mutism	9	60	from 5 days to 3 months
Articulatory disorders	12	80	persistent in 4 cases
Auditory verbal comprehension disorders	6	40	persistent in 1 case
Naming disorders	7	46	persistent in 3 cases
Paraphasia	1	7	disappearance
Reading disorders	9	60	persistent in 3 cases
Writing disorders	13	86	persistent in 7 cases

Source: Hécaen, H. "Acquired Aphasia in Children and the Ontogenesis of Hemispheric Specialization in Children," *Brain and Language,* 3, 1976, 114–134.

the persistence, at times permanently, of mild verbal deficits, particularly in writing."

Satz and Bullard-Bates (1981) reviewed studies of the clinical picture of speech and language disorders in children with acquired aphasia. They caution that there is no fixed pattern of symptoms and that there is considerable variability in reported features and patterns of aphasic manifestations. They emphasize: "The linguistic differences, if real, could be due to a number of factors including lesion site, etiology, age of lesion, lesion size, type of lesion (acute versus chronic), time of language assessment postonset, and the linguistic age of the child" (p. 415).

Cognitive and Educational Deficits

Estimates of cognitive deficits in young children are necessarily based on assumptions of the intellectual potential that was manifest either in language development or in educational achievement. In some instances there may be actual objective measurements based on psychometric evaluations related to appropriate school placement. The published literature does not regularly provide such information. Unless there is evidence to believe otherwise, we will assume normal intellectual potential in the population of children reported in the literature. As a general finding, most of the studies report a striking contrast between the usually good and rapid recovery of speech functions and the retardations and deficits in educational (school) achievements and cognitive status.

The findings of Alajouanine and Lhermitte (1965) are typical of studies on the recovery patterns of children with acquired aphasia. Alajouanine and Lhermitte studied 32 children, ages 6 to 15, with acquired aphasia. After one year or more, 24 of the 32 children had regained normal or close-to-normal speech, "but none made further normal school progress." Along the same line, Byers and McLean (1962) report a contrast between speech recovery and cognitive functioning. In their investigation, Byers and McLean did a follow-up study of 10 children, ages 3 to 15, most of whom had incurred vascular lesions producing hemiplegias and aphasia. At periods of 1 to 4 years after onset, all of the children had made good (spontaneous) recovery of speech. In contrast, 7 of the 10 showed moderate to severe impairment on tests of verbal and nonverbal cognitive function.

Basser (1962) studied two groups of hemiplegic children, 15 with left cerebral lesions and 15 with right cerebral lesions. He reported that speech disturbances were overcome in less than 2 years after onset of impairments. However, regardless of the site of the lesion, most of the children were found to have suffered intellectual deficits and tested in the retarded range. Assessment of intellectual functioning was limited to the vocabulary and block-design tests of the Merrill-Palmer and Terman-Merrill inventories.

Lenneberg (1967) reviewed the literature on acquired aphasia in children from 1942–1946 and reported on cases he himself had seen and studied. His results are consistent with the others reported.

Satz and Bullard-Bates (1981), after an extensive review of the published literature, conclude that "even in cases of recovery from aphasia, serious cognitive and academic sequelae were found" (p. 421).

Auditory Agnosia

Cooper and Ferry (1978) describe a syndrome of auditory agnosia (failure to understand spoken language) and seizure activity associated with acquired aphasia in children. Their paper presents a comprehensive review of the literature since 1957 and a detailed report of their own cases. In all, 43 cases are reported in the age range of 2 to 13 years. At the outset, a wide variety of speech and language disorders is noted by all of the investigators. Most of the studies reported initial poor comprehension of spoken language, some to the point that the children appeared oblivious to verbal commands "to such a degree that deafness was suspected." Cooper and Ferry generalize that most of the children who had seizures associated with auditory agnosia "are left with some degree of dysphasia that may range from auditory verbal agnosia and no functional verbal communication to less severe difficulties in certain academic areas, such as reading and spelling. Because of the residual deficits, many of the children required special education."

Summary: Cognitive Deficits

A review of the literature clearly indicates that many children with acquired aphasia are left with residual cognitive deficits, even after their language recovery. The deficits are present following damage to either the left or the right cerebral hemisphere. We suggest two possible explanations for this finding. First, in children, the contribution of the right hemisphere to early normal cognitive development is significant and important, although the nature of the contribution is only beginning to be understood. Second, both cerebral hemispheres are involved in early language acquisition and in normal cognitive development. Disturbing either hemisphere has serious negative implications for the other. As a supplement to these observations or speculations, we add a third—that ordinary language functioning, as expressed in ordinary (conversational) speech, is a weak indicator of an individual's higher levels and potentials for language functioning and related cognitive development. The loss of millions and perhaps billions of cortical cells as a result of injury or pathology is not likely to occur without potential losses in higher levels of language usage and cognition. To some degree, the reduced potential is indicated by the negative academic histories of children with acquired aphasia.

Other aspects of language and cognition that may be retarded in development or chronically impaired to some degree in children with acquired aphasia include abilities that normally continue to develop up to and through adolescence and into adult years. Such abilities include the appreciation of wit, humor, irony, analogy (metaphor), and speaker intentions when subtleties or the possibility of more than one meaning are inherent in the message. To these may be added the potential ability to use language as an instrument of imagination and projection (thinking). The possible, but not invariant, limitations or reduced abilities are in keeping with the observations of Chase (1972), Alajouanine and Lhermitte (1965), and Bay (1962) as well as with those of Satz and Bullard-Bates (1981).

PROGNOSIS AND RECOVERY

There is little question that the prognosis and course of recovery is better for children with acquired aphasia than it is for most aphasic adults. Presumably, this is so because of the capability of either hemisphere to take over the language functions normally served by the other. We have already indicated that this takeover may not be complete, but that it is usually better than the progress made by most right-handed adults. The early literature on acquired aphasia in children tended to emphasize the transient nature of the impairments. From our earlier discussion, it is apparent that although some of the disturbances are of short duration, others, especially those for written language, are more persistent and may even constitute chronic deficits.

The process of recovery is different for young children—those below 4 to 5 years of age—and for children above this age. As indicated earlier, few children below age 5 are likley to have learned to read or write or to have learned arithmetic computations. Lenneberg (1967) generalizes:

> If the aphasia occurs early in life, for example at age four, two processes intermingle so intensely during the recovery period that a rather different [compared with adult] picture emerges. The two processes are the interference phenomena caused by the lesions and the extremely active language learning process that may or may not be inhibited at all by the disease, or may only temporarily have come to an arrest, soon to be reinstated. (p. 146)

For children who incur brain damage and aphasia during the 20- to 36-month age range, the course of recovery takes a different form from that of the 4-year-olds. Lenneberg (1967) observes:

> Cerebral trauma to the two or three year old will render the patient unresponsive, sometimes for weeks at a time; when he becomes cognizant of his environment again, it becomes clear that whatever beginnings he had made in language before the disease is totally lost, but soon he will start again on the road toward language acquisition, traversing all stages of infant vocalization, perhaps at a slightly faster pace . . . until perfect speech is achieved. (pp. 149–150)

This observation is in keeping with that of Basser (1962). Lenneberg (1967) emphasizes that, in the very young, the primary process in recovery is acquisition, "whereas the process of symptom-reduction is not in evidence" (p. 150).

In patients older than 4 and younger than 10, the most likely clinical picture is that of a typical aphasic involvement in older persons, with symptoms gradually and usually quickly subsiding. However, in contrast to aphasic adults, the child may have little difficulty in expanding vocabulary and learning to understand and use complex syntactic constructions.

Lenneberg has a less optimistic observation for children above age 10 and onward to puberty. Although some children in this age range also make rapid and good recoveries, many show residual deficits. In speaking, they may be hesitant, may have word-finding difficulties, or may produce words that are inappropriate for what they intend to say. Lenneberg (1967) also notes: "Emotional tension magnifies the symptoms, making their aphasic nature very obvious" (p. 150).

Our own experience confirms Lenneberg's observations for the preteen-age and early teenage children with acquired aphasia. We are more reserved than Lenneberg, however, about the rapid and excellent progress of children below age 4. We have noted residual deficits for word finding and the use of shorter utterances and simpler syntactic constructions than those of normal age peers in the below age 4 population.

Based on their extensive review of the literature on acquired aphasia in children, Satz and Bullard-Bates (1981) found evidence to support a number of general findings, which we will restate to include the following:

1. After infancy, regardless of age, the likelihood of aphasic language impairment is greater when the lesion is in the left rather than the right cerebral hemisphere.
2. The risk of aphasic involvement associated with right hemisphere damage is rare in right-handed children, "particularly after ages 3–5 years, and perhaps earlier" (Satz and Bullard-Bates, 1981, p. 421).
3. Nonfluency occurs in a majority of cases as part of the early aphasic pattern. Other acquired impairments that may coexist or occur independently include disorders of auditory comprehension, naming difficulties, and reading and writing deficits.
4. Spontaneous recovery, "while dramatic in a majority of children, is by no means invariant. After one year postonset of aphasic impairments, studies showed that 25 to 50% of cases were unremitting" (p. 421).
5. Even in cases of good recovery from aphasic (language) impairments, there are often significant cognitive and educational (academic) difficulties.

TREATMENT

Treatment of the child with acquired aphasia is necessarily a family affair. At the outset, the family members need to be informed that early stages of recovery, however rapid and spontaneous, may not be continuous. Temporary setbacks are likely to occur, especially if the child is fatigued, is frustrated— either from a lack of success in communicating, from not having his or her way, or even from not knowing what way he or she may want—or is upset for any reason. Sometimes the setback is for no discernible reason. Furthermore, especially for young children, an early period of sparse talking, possibly to the point of virtual mutism, may be anticipated.

For most young children—those under age 5—no early direct therapy is indicated other than normal stimulation provided by key members of the environment and more than normal willingness to listen. It would be wise, however, for family members to shorten their utterances and speak somewhat more slowly than might otherwise be their inclination. Speaking should be done in direct view of the child. Wherever possible, and certainly in the earliest days of recovery, visual cueing—speaking about what is physically present— will enhance comprehension. Variability in the child's ready comprehension is to be expected, especially if the child is fatigued or upset. Upset behavior and general emotional lability are to be expected. Do not ask the child to explain his or her behavior.

For children in the 5- to 8-year age range, some amount of direct intervention may be indicated. After the first stage of recovery, perhaps by the third or fourth month after onset of the aphasic impairments, a language sample of spontaneous speech or elicited speech in a play situation may be taken to provide information about the child's reestablished language status. If there is evidence of an absence of the words a child needs to be an effective communicator at home and in play settings, or an absence of semantic-syntactic constructions that might be expected on the basis of the child's mean length of utterance, then *situational instruction* may be undertaken. By situational instruction, we mean creating or making use of events and situations that are relevant and meaningful to the child, thus providing opportunities for learning words and word units that the child can readily employ once learned. Such opportunities increase the likelihood that what the child learns or retrieves will be reinforced through use in practical situations. Language functioning will then be naturally reestablished.

Associated language functions—reading, writing, and arithmetic—may show deficits from previously established levels of proficiency. For the most part, such deficits will be limited to the child who is over 6 years of age. If this is so, reteaching is in order. Tutoring may be helpful before the child returns to school. We advise that the tutor be a professional, not a member of the family.

For children in the 8- to 12-year range, some degree of deficit in educational subjects may be expected. It may be helpful to regress the child to a lower than preonset level of achievement and then to reteach the written language subjects. If there is evidence that the child now has difficulty with a phonic or phonetic approach to reading—if this is the way the child was taught initially—we suggest a whole-word and whole-phrase approach to permit the child to look and decide (Eisenson, 1983) when decoding written language. Such an approach is in keeping with what the right cerebral hemisphere is normally better able to do than the left. If the damage is to the left hemisphere, then we should not expect analytical, segmental decoding to be proficient.

Auditory comprehension may be impaired, especially, as indicated ear- lier, for children who had seizures associated with their aphasic involvements.

Therapy should include exposure to a reduced quantity of utterances, simple syntactic constructions, and a slower-than-normal rate of speaking. Visual cueing should be helpful and is especially important in the early stages of treatment. Verbal repetition should be exact, not paraphrased. The use of recorded material that can be played back as often as the child needs it—and alone if the child so prefers—is of considerable help. As a general procedure, we suggest individual professional tutoring before the child returns to school and individualized instruction by a special educator for as long as needed after the child has returned to school.

Cognitive assessment that includes awareness of conditions under which a child performs best as well as poorly will avoid unrealistic expectations and frustrations. If, after repeated reassessments, there is evidence of cognitive deficit, then expectations should be adjusted according to findings. However, we must caution that repeated assessment implies a period of at least a year and possibly two years after the early stages of improvement and at least a year beyond therapeutic intervention. Thus, if there is evidence of reduced cognitive capacity, achievable goals may be established. We strongly suggest that even such goals as these should be considered tentative. No child should be limited by statistics of populations of children without the opportunity to show that he or she is an exception. Success in performance breeds opportunities for further successes, although the increments may be smaller than preaphasic indicators might have implied. For children below age 12, both new learning and reacquisition of impaired language are parts of the continuing process of living with and overcoming the deficits of acquired aphasia.

SUMMARY FINDINGS OF A CASE HISTORY
OF ACQUIRED APHASIA

The following are highlights of the posttraumatic history of M. C., a boy aged 5 years, 1 month, who was seen for psychodiagnostic and language evaluation. M. C. was evaluated approximately 2 years after he had incurred a head injury as a result of an automobile accident. The injury resulted in intraventricular damage and possible brain stem contusion.

Developmental History

M. C. was born after an uneventful pregnancy and a normal delivery. His early health history, except for occasional colds, was not remarkable. His motor development was somewhat accelerated; he sat up at 5 months, stood alone at 7½ months, and walked at 9 months. His speech and language development was well within normal range: first words at 11 months and two-word utterances at 14 months. There was no evidence of abnormal dysfluencies nor any indications of articulation or language problems up to the time of the head injury. M. C. was left-handed, with indications of ambidexterity.

The head injury and brain trauma occurred when M. C. was 3 years, 1 month, of age. When seen, the boy had difficulty in balance and in walking associated with residual right hemiparesis. Visual-field difficulty was suspected. The parents reported that the child had episodes of appearing not to hear or not to understand what was said to him, sometimes accompanied by looking "spaced-out."

Following onset of injury, there was a period of 3 to 4 weeks during which the child neither talked nor responded to spoken language. After the first month postonset, the child made slow but steady progress in speaking, but not reliably in listening and comprehending. Progress continued for about 2 years, until M. C. seemed to have reached a plateau.

Language Assessment

On the basis of formal testing, including Carrow's Test for Auditory Comprehension, Zimmerman's Preschool Language Scale, and a language sample, the child was found to be about 2 years below age expectance for overall language proficiency. He understood simple commands but had some difficulty in following multiple directions. Most *wh* questions elicited a correct response, but he occasionally confused *where* and *when*. Syntactic errors sometimes suggested "pidgin" productions, with confusion of pronouns—for example, *him* and *her* for *he* and *she* and *he* or *she* for *his* or *her*. His articulation revealed a few infantilisms, such as *w/r* and *w/l* substitutions, but his overall articulation was intelligible.

Psychological Evaluation

A range of from 2 to 2.5 years' retardation was found on the basis of nonverbal tests, including the Leiter scale and the performance items of the Wechsler Preschool and Primary Scale. The Beery Visual-Motor Test was used for determining visual-motor functioning. The Peabody Picture Vocabulary Test was employed for determining a language comprehension age. All of the tests indicated retardation. M. C.'s mental age was generally more than 2 years behind age expectancy, with verbal items somewhat higher than nonverbal performance. The Peabody Test produced a receptive quotient of 69. General functioning was at the mildly retarded level.

Academic Achievement

School reports indicated that M. C. was making slow progress. He had shown improvement in auditory comprehension but needed extra time to respond. His overall language skills and communication abilities were estimated to be at about the 3-year-plus level. His articulation was described as "slow, deliberate, and generally intelligible." He was able to name the primary colors and could sort by shape and color. He could cut paper with scissors, string one-inch beads, and complete a six-piece puzzle form. He still had some difficulty holding a pencil in correct position with his left (preferred) hand. In general, he was responding positively to basic eye–hand training and gross motor coordination training for tasks involving balance and positioning of himself in space.

Overall Impressions

M. C. showed numerous definite indications of cognitive and language impairments associated with the brain damage incurred when the boy was 3 years, 1 month old. Although he made significant progress since the onset of his involvements, recent assessments suggest a "plateauing" at a level of about 2 years behind his chronological age and precerebral-insult indications of expectancies.

M. C. is receiving appropriate educational and language training in a special education program. The impression of the psychologist is that the boy is likely to function in the range of the mildly retarded.

Notes on the Case Study

The case of M. C. is not typical of the progress of young children with acquired aphasia. Perhaps no case is really typical. The nature of the child's motor impairments and early indications of bicerebral hemisphere damage made for a guarded prognosis at best. Nevertheless, the child did improve in motor, visual-perceptual, and language areas. Although he appears to have reached a plateau, he has not regressed from his highest postonset achievement level. Continued improvement may therefore be expected. Realistically, a lower-than-normal level of cognitive functioning may also be expected.

REFERENCES AND SUGGESTED READINGS

Alajouanine, T. H., and Lhermitte, F. "Acquired Aphasia in Children," *Brain,* 88, 1965, 653–662.

Basser, L. S. "Hemiplegia of Early Onset and the Faculty of Speech with Special Reference to the Effects of Hemispherectomy," *Brain,* 85, 1962, 427–460.

Bay, E. "Aphasia and Nonverbal Disorders of Language," *Brain,* 85, 1962, 411–426.

Byers, R. K., and McLean, W. T. "Etiology and Course of Certain Hemiplegias with Aphasia in Childhood," *Pediatrics,* 29, 1962, 376–383.

Chase, R. A. "Neurological Aspects of Language Disorders in Children," In J. V. Irwin and M. M. Marge (eds.), *Principles of Childhood Language Disabilities.* New York: Appleton-Century-Crofts, 1972.

Cooper, J. A., and Ferry, P. C. "Acquired Auditory Verbal Agnosia and Seizures in Childhood," *Journal of Speech and Hearing Disorders,* 43, 1978, 176–184.

Cromer, R. "The Basis of Childhood Dysphasia: A Linguistic Approach," in M. A. Wyke (ed.), *Developmental Dysphasia.* New York: Academic Press, 1978.

Eisenson, J. *Reading for Meaning.* Tulsa, Oklahoma: Modern Education Corporation, 1983.

Freud, S. *Infantile Cerebral Paralysis* (L. A. Russin, trans.) Coral Gables, Fla.: University of Miami Press, 1968. (This work by Freud was initially published in 1897.)

Guttman, E. "Aphasia in Children," *Brain,* 65, 1942, 205–219. (This article is a landmark publication on acquired aphasia in children.)

Hécaen, H. "Acquired Aphasia in Children and the Ontogenesis of Hemispheric Functional Specialization," *Brain and Language,* 3, 1976, 114–134.

Krashen, S. D. "Lateralization of Language Learning and the Critical Period," *Language Learning,* 23, 1973, 63–74.

Lenneberg, E. *Biological Foundations of Language.* New York: Wiley, 1967.

McFie, J. "Intellectual Impairment in Children with Localized Post-infantile Cerebral Lesions," *Journal of Neurology, Neurosurgery, and Psychiatry,* 24, 1961, 361–365.

Osler, W. "The Cerebral Palsies of Children," *Medical News,* 2, 1888, 29–35.

Satz, P., and Bullard-Bates, C. "Acquired Aphasia in Children," in M. T. Sarno (ed.), *Acquired Aphasia.* New York: Academic Press, 1981.

Von Dongen, H. R., and Loonen, M. C. "Neurological Factors Related to Prognosis of Acquired Aphasia in Childhood," in Y. Lebrun and R. Hoops (eds.), *Recovery in Aphasics.* Amsterdam: Swets and Zeitlinger, 1979.

chapter *12*

Childhood Autism

ADRIANA L. SCHULER

HISTORY OF THE AUTISTIC SYNDROME

Descriptions of autistic communication, or rather the lack of communication, were first rendered by Leo Kanner (1943) in his insightful case studies of 11 individuals who shared some remarkable features. The striking common behavior observed in these individuals, who were seen over a 20-year period, led Kanner to postulate the syndrome of early infantile autism. The common characteristics observed by Kanner were intense aloneness, an obsessive desire for preservation of sameness, a skillful and even affectionate relationship to objects, an intelligent and pensive physiognomy, and either mutism or the kind of language that does not serve interpersonal communication. What should be emphasized here is the considerable variance that was noted in terms of speech proficiency, prevalence of echolalia responses, and grammatical abilities. Moreover, all individuals described were limited in the communicative interpersonal use of speech. Echolalia, so-called pronoun reversal, metaphoric use of speech, extreme literalness of meanings, and affirmation by repetition were noted as common peculiar language traits. Furthermore, all individuals described by Kanner exhibited some remarkable skills, often involving verbatim recall (for instance, of long sections of the Bible) and memorization of large numbers of tunes and melodies. Despite the fact that language problems are generally viewed as the most prominent feature of the autistic syndrome, some of the individuals described were noted for initial speech precocity, as evidenced by their early enunciations of unusual and elaborate words or phrases. All in all, these individuals presented a picture of rather extreme developmental discontinuity.

CHANGING VIEWS OF THE SYNDROME

In his early writings, Kanner attributed the cluster of autistic traits described to an innate disturbance of affective contact, not unlike the developmental problems that arise from defective sensory mechanisms. However, in keeping with the trends of the time, autism was soon viewed as the tragic result of poor parenting and emotional neglect, whereby the cold or even hostile responses of parents shifted infants away from social interaction into a state of secluded autistic aloneness. Although this interpretation blossomed during the 1950s, definitions of the autistic syndrome became increasingly loose, zeroing in primarily on autistic withdrawal and lack of eye contact, with minimal concern for the idiosyncrasies of language behavior. These psychogenic interpretations of autism changed dramatically in the 1960s. First, language anomalies were reemphasized and were subjected to extensive studies (Cunningham and Dixon, 1961; Wolff and Chess, 1965). Second, a new biological interpretation of autism was offered by Rimland (1964), whose extensive descriptions, discussions, and interpretations of the autistic syndrome favored the notion of an organically based cognitive dysfunctioning, possibly based within a malfunction of the reticular formation. This new orientation set the stage for numerous studies dealing with linguistic and cognitive functioning. More detailed case descriptions, experimental studies, and investigations of the organic bases of autism led to the replacement of the older psychogenic interpretation of autism with a view of autism as an organically based dysfunction of language and cognition, possibly tied to perceptual malfunctioning. Autistic aloneness ceased to be the primary symptom of the syndrome and was now viewed as ancillary to a severe thought and language disorder.

To decrease subjectivity of diagnosis, attempts were made to define the syndrome in more accurate terms, thus allowing for greater consistency in diagnosis and treatment. Among these various efforts, the listing of behavioral traits associated with autism, as put forward by Freeman and Ritvo (1977) has probably been the most widely acclaimed in this country. It has been endorsed by the National Society for Autistic Children and the American Psychiatric Association. According to this definition, autism is viewed as a developmental disability, defined and diagnosed in behavioral terms. The essential features should be manifested prior to 30 months of age, with disturbances in each of the following areas:

1. Disturbances in the rate of appearance of physical, social, and language skills.
2. Abnormal responses to sensations. Any one or a combination of sight, hearing, touch, pain, balance, smell, taste, and the way a child holds his or her body are affected.
3. Speech and language are absent or delayed while specific thinking capabilities may be present. Immature rhythms of speech, limited understanding of ideas and the use of words without attaching the usual meaning to them is common.

4. Abnormal ways of relating to people, objects, and events. Typically, they do not respond appropriately to adults and other children. Objects and toys are not used as normally intended.

Moderate to severe degrees of mental retardation are associated with the syndrome of autism in the majority of cases; the incidence is four to five times per 10,000 births, with the likelihood of males being affected four of five times greater than the chances of females being affected. These incidence figures seem consistent with figures reported in Great Britain and other European countries. However, definitions such as those used in England, put forward by Rutter (1978), reveal a slightly different emphasis. Although early onset is also critical in this definition, the fact that linguistic and social development are out of line with other aspects of development is stressed, along with a preponderance of ritualistic behavior tied to the desire to maintain sameness. The prevalence of self-stimulatory behaviors ("disturbances of responses to sensory stimuli," in Ritvo and Freeman's (1977) terminology), such as repetitive body rocking, is deemphasized here, with social and language impairment playing a more central role.

Since the definitions of autism rely on observations of and inferences about behavior rather than on objective physical tests, considerable room is left for disagreement. Furthermore, the degree of involvement is unspecified. Children who clearly exhibit only one or two of the traits described may end up with the *autistic* label, even when some of their development problems are caused by identified neurological impairment. Consequently, the label is applied to a range of children of much greater diversity than those originally described by Kanner. For purposes of service delivery, this does not create problems, since children who are more accurately described as autisticlike still are in need of similarly intensive educational services. However, for purposes of research and for gaining insights into the nature of the autistic syndrome, it would be helpful to reserve the *autism* label for the more "pure" cases. Therefore, in this chapter, *autistic* will be used in a rather strict sense, referring only to children such as those originally described by Kanner (1943), those with primary problems in the areas of language, social development, and symbolic thought.

SPEECH AND LANGUAGE CHARACTERISTICS: THE EXTENT OF COMMUNICATION PROBLEMS

To gain a full understanding of the nature and extent of autistic speech and language peculiarities, it is necessary to have a careful description of the behaviors involved. This section will show how the adoption of a functional rather than a structural perspective helps resolve some of the heterogeneity and contradictions inherent in the speech and language behaviors associated with the autistic syndrome. Although some autistic individuals never speak a word, the incessant, clearly enunciated speech of others may seem indicative of rather advanced grammatical abilities. The distinction that surfaces here is the one that has traditionally been made between mute and echolalic autistic individuals. According to the literature, about half the children labeled autistic remain mute—that is, never engage in vocalization that approximates adult speech—while the other half engage in so-called echolalia—that is, the meaningless repetition of the speech of others. However, to evaluate communicative proficiency, it is important to take a close look at functional use of speech rather than speech output as such. Both mute and echolalic individuals are limited in their ability to use speech for communicative purposes. This pragmatic failure is particularly striking in those autistic individuals whose speech output illustrates how painfully dissociated speech and language may be. Both muteness and echolalia warrant closer investigation.

Types of Muteness

Regarding muteness, distinctions should be made in terms of communicative intentions and speech approximations. Although these distinctions follow a continuum and do not allow for the identification of discrete subcategories, different types of muteness may yet be identified at the extreme ends of the continuum. Total muteness occurs when both communicative and noncommunicative vocalizations are lacking. No vocalizations are made to express intentions—for example, to get someone's attention, to ask to be tickled, and so forth. Furthermore, vocalizations do not appear as a form of self-stimulation. This type of muteness, however, is not typical of autism. More commonly, some vocalizations do occur, but they seem to serve primarily self-stimulatory purposes. Often, in fact, they are intertwined with other self-stimulatory behaviors; for instance, a child may be twirling leaves and concurrently humming in a sing-song fashion. Vocalizations are used, if at all, only for primitive signalling functions. This prevalence of self-stimulatory rather than functional use may capture the nature of the autistic syndrome, with a pragmatic failure as the overriding factor. The use of rudimentary speech, supplemented by ample use of body language, may be viewed as its opposite. This type of muteness is less common to autism and more typical of speech and language problems that are primarily due to speech production failures; nevertheless, some autistic individuals may demonstrate this type of muteness mixed with the more self-stimulatory forms of sound-making when evidencing further social and communicative growth.

Types of Echolalia

Regarding echolalic behavior in autism (for a more general discussion of echolalia, see Schuler, 1979), distinctions should be made according to communicative intent, accuracy, and clarity of the echoing behaviors involved, and according to the time lapse between the original and the echoed utterance. A distinction is commonly made between so-called delayed and immediate echolalia. The latter refers to repetition of utterances of others as soon as they are spoken, while the former refers to repetition at some later point in time—a lapse that may vary from a couple of minutes to possibly years. Because of this time delay, this type of echolalia is often not recognized as such; instead, linguistic credit is often given because of the apparent proficiency in speech production. Such delayed echolalic pseudolanguage may show varying degrees of communicative intent. At one extreme, the echoing may be of a completely self-stimulatory nature; that is, no changes result in members of the environment subsequent to the act of echoing, and the motivation to echo seems to stem from the sensory stimulation inherent in the echoing behavior. This may best be illustrated by literal but meaningless repetitions of television commercials, which are not directed at anyone but rather indicate a fascination with sound and sound effects.

At the other extreme, delayed echolalia may indicate an intention to influence the behavior of others. A complete set of role-stereotyped phrases may be used to express a variety of meanings strictly tied to specific stimulus context. Thus, memorized "stimulus-response chains" can be observed as constituting a finite grammar, capable of generating only a limited set of messages. For instance, in order to communicate, a child may say, "Do you want a cookie? Say yes," shifting his or her gaze between mother and cookie jar and then raising his or her voice or giving way to a tantrum if the request is not satisfied. Similarly, a child may say, "Be quiet now, be quiet now," in such a fashion that he or she actually becomes more relaxed. Although the functions of delayed echoing have not yet been subjected to systematic studies, some analogous functions may be inferred on the basis of the functional analysis of immediate echolalia. Duchan and Prizant (in press) were able to identify seven different types of immediate echoing on the basis of the functional analysis of videotaped samples of this behavior in the context of accompanying nonverbal behaviors, such as shifts in gaze, body orientation, and activities performed. The one type of echoing identified that did not seem communicative or functional was called "nonfocused." The echoing is rigidly accurate, immediate, and not accompanied by changes in nonverbal behavior. All the other types of echoing identified were accompanied by changes in nonverbal or subsequent verbal behavior—that is *rehearsal* by the subsequent appropriate response, *turn-taking* by an accompanying nonverbal social exchange, *self-regulatory* by concomitant changes in behavior, *declarative* by some demonstrative gesture, and *request* and *confirmation* by the anticipation of someone's response, the latter congruent with Kanner's (1943) notion of "affirmation by repetition" as a substitute for "yes" responses. The clinical implications of these differentiations are of utmost importance, as they suggest how echolalic behavior may be used and shaped into more sophisticated means of communication.

Regarding the clarity and accuracy of echolalia, autistic individuals are often noted for their relatively clear enunciation of echoed speech; the original intonation pattern and the artifacts of vocal delivery, such as the vocal pitch or accent, may even be preserved. This painstaking accuracy or even "parasitic fidelity" (Fay and Schuler, 1980) is generally reversely correlated with the meaningfulness and relevance of the utterance involved. In general, the least literal repetitions of the greatest latency hold the most communicative promise. When echoed speech shows a clearer departure from the original model, the term *mitigated echolalia* is sometimes used (Fay, 1967). Common alterations involve intonational changes, additions of words such as "please," changes in personal pronoun, and so forth. However, it should be realized that some of the alterations noted may be merely a reproduction artifact, often indicative of limited retention skills. To determine whether changes in wording or intonation are indeed intentional, it is necessary to consider the nonverbal parameters of the exchange along with other samples of verbal behavior. Intentional, rule-governed changes are predictable, since they consistently arouse someone's verbal repertoire. Although several autistic individuals have been noted to pass through a mitigation stage before advancing to greater linguistic maturity, it still remains unclear whether interdependency of these phenomena is implied. However, similar phenomena have been observed as part of the normal language acquisition process (Clark, 1974), since children may only partially break down unfamiliar utterances into their component parts (for example, "May I sit my knee?" instead of "May I sit on your knee?"). The occurrence of mitigation should provide a valuable starting point for remediation efforts, as the ability to break down and recompose utterances may be gradually expanded. In fact, language remediation dealing with autistic echolalia should focus on such breakdown and recomposition rather than on repetitive drill.

Summary

In the evaluation of the magnitude and extent of communication problems associated with the autistic syndrome, lack of or limited communicative intent appears to be one of the most striking features. In many cases, autistic children fail to learn that speaking, signing, gesturing, or even vocal grunts or particular intonation patterns may be used to act upon and control their environment. Even when considerable gains are made in phonology and syntax, pragmatic and semantic skills will generally lag behind. Autistic individuals with relatively advanced grammatical abilities tend to be extremely literal in grasping meaning; idioms, puns, irony—that is, play with dual meanings—continue to baffle them. Similarly, signals inherent in nonverbal communication seem to escape them, for they seem unable to figure out the significance of a particular facial expression or tone of voice. Intonational peculiarities may serve as the most profound illustration of pragmatic failure. The effective use of intonation to emphasize or deemphasize a particular part of a message requires the ability to adopt the perspective of the speaker, an ability that is crucial to the act of communication. As will be pointed out in the following section, communication problems reflect not only pragmatic but also cognitive failures, leading to problems of a magnitude that separate autism from other developmental language problems.

DIFFERENTIAL DIAGNOSIS

In the context of this book, the question of differences in language behavior
between children commonly labeled as autistic versus those commonly labeled
as aphasic or severely language impaired deserves careful consideration.[1]
Before becoming involved in an extensive discussion of those differences, we
will first briefly review other developmental language problems that are easily
confused with the autistic syndrome.

Childhood Schizophrenia

As pointed out earlier, children suffering from childhood schizophrenia have
often been confused with autistic or autisticlike children. The first criterion to
be considered is age of onset. The diagnosis of childhood autism is applied only
if the symptoms appear within the first 3 years of life. Although it has been
assumed that autism and childhood schizophrenia are merely early and later
manifestations of the same disease, this has been refuted by Kolvin (1971) and
his colleagues, who found that significant differences could be found in terms of
social class, family history of schizophrenia, evidence of cerebral dysfunction,
symptom patterns, and level of intelligence. For instance, childhood schizophrenia tends to occur more frequently in certain families, and it occurs four
times more often in females than in males, the reverse of the incidence in
childhood autism. Thus, many of the criteria for differentiation rely on case
history and medical background (for a more extensive discussion, see Rutter,
1972). Differentiations on the basis of current language behavior are not so
easily made. Since this matter has not been systematically investigated, some
clinical observations may provide hints. The language behavior of schizophrenic individuals appears more bizarre, tied to hallucinations, more variable, and indicative of more mature linguistic functioning than that
encountered in autistic children. Language behaviors associated with autism
may be explained on developmental grounds, despite some of the apparent
oddities and contradictions involved. In cases of childhood schizophrenia,
language behaviors should have been essentially normal, at least up to age 3,
leaving the roots of language acquisition unaffected.

Elective Mutism

Speech, language, and communication behaviors associated with elective
mutism and other psychological problems differ from those associated with
childhood autism mostly in that they are situational. The child in this case is one
who appears to have chosen not to speak and not to interact in some or almost
all contexts, but who does have the means to speak. Well-developed receptive
and nonverbal communication skills and adequate symbolic development,

---

[1]The term *aphasic* will be used in this chapter to refer to various children whose language
impairments are severe and out of line with other aspects of development. See Chapter 5 for a
detailed consideration of childhood aphasia.

along with adequate speech in some contexts, suggest that the problem is not a developmental linguistic one, but rather one of an emotional, interactive nature. Because of the tendency of these children to be socially aloof and to display gaze avoidance, they are occasionally confused with autistic children. However, adherence to a stricter definition of autism should eradicate such confusions.

Hearing Impairment

Only rarely will children with autism be confused with children with peripheral hearing deficits. Deaf children's advances in the areas of socialization, nonverbal communication, and symbolic development, as evidenced in play behavior, suffice to make these children distinctly different from those suffering from childhood autism. Nevertheless, the apparent sensory deficit associated with autism—that is, the frequent lack of responses to sound—often causes autistic-type children to be suspected of hearing loss. The problem becomes more complicated when children with an apparent centrally based hearing loss are involved. In such cases, hearing loss becomes confounded with other developmental deficiencies and often with some form of retardation. Symbolic development may be impaired, which, combined with the lack of responses to sound, may become apparent in rather high rates of self-stimulatory behavior. Furthermore, the presence of other perceptual problems may be confused with the more pure forms of childhood autism. Refined differential diagnoses would be greatly facilitated by advances in the objective measurement of responses to sound at various points across the auditory pathways. Recent advances in the objective measurement of auditory responses, including those at the level of the brain stem, may shed more light on the presence and type of auditory deficiencies in autistic children, as they differ from other forms of sensory impairment.

Mental Retardation

Particularly because autism is more often than not associated with severe degrees of retardation, it may be difficult to draw the line between autism and more general developmental delay. However, because pure autism is characterized by a dysfunction in social interaction, communication, and symbolic development, with intact motor development, memory, and speech reproduction skills, the distinction is rather easily made (Wing, 1981). In these cases, the combination of echolalia with a lack of communicative speech, poor social development, normal appearance, adequate motor development and memory, and often isolated areas of precocity will be distinctly different from a more generalized pattern of retardation. This is particularly so in cases in which social skills are relatively well preserved. Specifically in terms of language behavior, severely retarded children's communicative intent will often surpass their verbal production skills. Even if echolalia does occur, it often goes undetected because of poor verbal reproduction skills and impaired auditory memory. Furthermore, the pattern of development will adhere more closely to the normal pattern, though with generally slower development. Since mental retardation is such a hetereogeneous category, however, much more needs to be learned about particular patterns of developmental delay. For instance, with regard to language, Curtiss (1981) and Curtiss, Yamada, and Fromkin (1979) found that syntactic development may diverge considerably from overall cognitive development; even semantic development may be disjointed from conceptual development (Cromer, 1981). The study of the interrelations between conceptual development, phonology, syntax, semantics, and pragmatics may eventually help us differentiate between distinct patterns of retardation. If subtypes of retardation could be identified in this manner, rather than on the basis of inferred etiology, it might ultimately help pinpoint various causes of retardation and possibly the prevention thereof.

Childhood Aphasia

In the context of this book, differences between autistic and aphasic children deserve special consideration. Often, children with autistic-type problems are confused with those who tend to be labeled as aphasic. This confusion is not surprising; there are similarities in the severity of the language impairment, the need for intensive and specialized services, and the commonly associated behavioral and emotional problems. Furthermore, both types of children acquire language late, if at all, and some continue to exhibit social and linguistic problems throughout life.

These apparent similarities between the two syndromes have led some investigators to postulate that autism is merely an extreme form of aphasia. A central language deficiency is viewed as the crux of the problem (Churchill, 1978; Rutter, Bartak and Newman, 1971), and the associated emotional and behavioral problems are considered side-products of the primary language deficiency. Closer examination of the language characteristics, however, reveals considerable differences, particularly when language behavior is evaluated in conjunction with communicative and social and cognitive development. Furthermore, attempts to delineate the two syndromes should focus on their purest forms. In the case of autism, this means that only primary autism is considered, not autistic behavior associated with other problems, such as identified neurological impairments, birth defects, and so forth.

From this perspective, differences between childhood autism and childhood aphasia may be found in the following areas.

Nonverbal Communication   Children suffering from the autistic syndrome are less skilled in the use of nonverbal forms of communication. For instance, facial expression, gestures, body posture, and the like, are rarely used to convey a particular message (Ritvo and Freeman, 1977). Communicative intent (De Hirsch, 1967), if present at all, tends to be expressed through more primitive means, revealing a limited awareness of the listener. Frequent temper tantrums, guiding someone else's hand, making eye contact, and stereotyped rituals to make things reoccur may serve to illustrate this point. In contrast, aphasic children are often remarkably apt in getting their messages across; they seem to compensate for their lack of speech by ample use of body language. Similarly, children with aphasia tend to make more rapid gains than do autistic children when an alternative system of communication, such as American sign language, is introduced.

Understanding of Social Relations   Analogous with their lack of nonverbal communication skills, autistic children have a poor grasp of social relationships. In social situations, they have a poor notion of the presence or point of view of the other person. As pointed out in the previous section, their most pervasive problem with language lies within the realm of semantics and pragmatics. As observed by Tager-Flusberg (1981a), the aspects of speech that are language-specific in origin and not closely related to social functioning do not seem to be especially disturbed in verbal autistic children, but those aspects that deal with usage are disturbed. Autistic children seem to have a limited understanding of the functions of speech and have difficulties with the give-and-take of speech in an interactive context (Tager-Flusberg (1981a). Evidence of deviant pragmatic development is reported by Baltaxe (1977), Ball (1978), and Fay and Schuler (1980).

Cognitive and Symbolic Development   Close examination of the level of symbolic development of children with autism reveals that language deficiencies tend to be associated with poor symbolic development. Analysis of the sensorimotor development of mute autistic children (Curcio, 1979) indicates that children who lack intentional communication are also extremely limited in the understanding of means-end relationships. The failure to understand the effects of their own actions and those of others locks such children within the sensorimotor stage of development, because they are unable to grasp the idea of symbolic representation.

Analyses of object-matching skills (Schuler, 1979, 1980; Fay and Schuler, 1980) indicate that autistic individuals are more prone to classify by physical properties, such as size, color, shape, and spatial orientation, rather than by functional attributes, and that lack of functional communication seems correlated with this inability.

Observation of play activities reveals that autistic children do not act upon objects in a symbolic manner, but rather in a repetitive and stereotypical fashion. For instance, they may mouth a toy car endlessly, spin its wheels, load and unload it, bump it into another car or toy, or even make the appropriate sounds when moving it, but they will not move it purposefully. Few examples of relational and functional play were reported in Tager-Flusberg's (1981b) study of 10 autistic children with some language skills. Even if some objects were related in play, the relationship seemed obscure or arbitrary. In contrast, aphasic children exhibit much more advanced levels of play behavior, often indicative of near-normal symbolic development. Similarly, aphasic children are less prone to engage in self-stimulating body movements and are more consistent in their responses to sensory stimuli; therefore, they are less likely to be confused with deaf or blind children.

The differences pertaining to symbolic, communicative, and social development are all interrelated. They imply that the language disturbances exhibited by autistic children are closely intertwined with and probably secondary to social and cognitive problems. This triad of problems involving social interaction, communication, and imagination (for a detailed discussion of this triad, see Wing, 1981) is out of line with other aspects of development. For instance, motor development, memory, and visuospatial discrimination and orientation in autistic children are generally unimpaired or may even be advanced beyond age level. In contrast, aphasic children present language problems of a purer form, not related to social, communicative, and cognitive development. Hence, a comparison between aphasic and autistic children that focuses primarily on language behaviors may fail to illuminate the differences. The more typical autistic traits, such as pronoun reversal, echolalia, and lack of conventional meaning, may not always be sufficiently pronounced as differential factors.

Some additional differentiations can be made between aphasic and autistic children. Social problems associated with aphasia are of a different nature from those associated with autism. Despite the fact that many aphasic children may be socially withdrawn, they are nevertheless socially aware. If social withdrawal occurs, it is more deliberate than in cases of autism. Autistic children fail to engage in social interaction because they do not understand what social interaction is all about. In more behavioral terms, their behavior is not affected by social consequences. Attention from others does not seem to motivate them, or may be even so aversive that they engage in self-destructive behavior, for example, in order to terminate the interaction. In contrast, the aphasic child's social interaction may be limited because of negative social consequences. Similarly, behavioral problems are of a different nature. An aphasic child may communicate through aberrant behavior in a socially aware fashion; for instance, he or she may strike out at someone or choose more premeditated ways of making a point. The autistic child is less inclined to strike out at others; instead, various forms of self-injury are frequently reported. These behaviors, even if they do serve to communicate, still reveal limited awareness of others.

Another distinction pertains to auditory memory. Excessive echolalic behaviors, which are so typical of many autistic individuals, imply good-to-excellent auditory retention skills. In contrast, children with aphasic impairments are often limited in their recall of auditory sequences. In fact, some of their speech and language problems may stem from limitations in short-term memory (Menyuk, 1964, 1969). Failure has also been observed when aphasic children are asked to identify rhythmic sequences, leading Cromer (1978) to use the descriptor "arhythmic." It is interesting that auditory memory limitations fail to account for the types of language problems encountered in autism, despite the fact that auditory memory has been linked with language disabilities and particularly with syntactic skills. Another point of differentiation pertains to visuospatial discrimination abilities. Many autistic individuals do well or even excel in this area. Our own research (Schuler, 1979, 1980, 1981) indicates that this ability may be well developed, even if communication skills are completely lacking. In contrast, many children with aphasic traits have problems perceiving spatial orientation. They perform poorly on tasks that require discriminations between visuospatial stimulus inputs.

The differences discussed are tentative, however; they do not necessarily apply to the populations as a whole and therefore fail to provide reliable diagnostic criteria. More might be learned about the various types of developmental disorders if we were provided with detailed profiles of impairments across various skill areas.

ETIOLOGICAL CONSIDERATIONS

Within the loose boundaries of the existing classification schemes, it is not always possible to draw a sharp line between aphasic and autistic impairments. In fact, cases have been reported that show considerable overlap, necessitating labels such as "aphasic with secondary autistic reaction." Cohen and Caparulo (1976) raised the possibility that some children may be both aphasic and autistic, favoring the notion of a double handicap over those that postulate a continuum. They discuss etiological implications extensively, viewing both conditions as reflections of different neuropathologies—aphasia involving primarily the neocortex, and autism involving older midbrain structures. Such claims regarding the etiology of autism have been made by many other researchers. Damasio and Maurer (1978), for example, presented a neurological account of some of the similarities between autistic children and adults with lesions affecting the mesolimbic cortex, the neostriatum, and parts of the thalamus, including a lack of initiative to communicate. As pointed out by Wing (1981), what needs to be accounted for is the triad of language and social impairments; so far, however, no hypotheses can be supported. Nevertheless, extensive study of the linguistic, social, and cognitive characteristics of autistic children may ultimately help unravel the mystery. The cluster of disturbances and their interrelationships have become increasingly clear during the last few years. The pervasive cognitive and linguistic problems associated with the syndrome of autism are tied to a profound lack of social responsiveness in early life, congruent with Kanner's (1943) early observations. Mechanisms that lead normal infants to seek out human faces and respond to body posture and tone of voice appear markedly deficient in autism. Meanwhile, other skills, including memory and visuospatial orientation and discrimination are remarkably intact. Increasingly refined clinical descriptions of the syndrome and advances in neuropathology may eventually bridge the existing gap in knowledge.

INTERVENTION

Although more traditional psychotherapeutic and language intervention approaches have failed to make much impact on the course of autistic development, the use of operant techniques has often resulted in dramatic behavioral changes, including changes in speech and language. Earlier reports on the use of operant language instruction have dealt primarily with increases in vocalization and with the shaping of single words (Wolf, Risley, and Mees, 1964; Hewett, 1965; Lovaas, Berberich, Perloff, and Schaeffer, 1966), but the scope of intervention efforts has since been considerbly expanded. Reports on operant language instruction have now come to include syntactic and morphological rules (Wheeler and Sulzer, 1970; Stevens-Long and Rasmussen, 1974; Howlin, 1980), and complete operant language programs are used increasingly. For a detailed description of the basic technology involved, the reader is referred to Lovaas (1966, 1977) and Sloane and MacAuley (1968).

Despite the apparent effectiveness of operant language instruction, some serious questions have been raised relative to the real-life validity of the behavioral changes obtained. Evaluation of instructional gains is often limited to the treatment setting; generalization and follow-up data are often missing, and spontaneous use of learned structures and rules in real-life situations is not easily evaluated. Furthermore, outcomes appear to be highly variable. Some children fail to make progress despite intensive intervention efforts. Because background information about the subjects involved is often limited, evaluations are frequently obscured. For instance, levels of intellectual functioning and of proficiency in nonverbal communication are often lacking, despite the confirmed prognostic value of such information. The most critical question— the extent to which language can be taught through operant conditioning— remains unanswered. The results of a detailed investigation of the effectiveness of a large-scale home-based teaching effort may shed some light on this question. In regard to the language component of this intervention, Howlin (1979, 1981) reports that aspects of language that have to do with increased occurrence of socialized speech are particularly affected. Developmental complexity and maturity of language use are much less affected. These changes pertained to relatively simple morphological rules rather than more complex transformational rules. In other words, it appears that intensive home-based intervention is effective in getting children to make increased use of skills that they already possess and to engage to a lesser extent in competing behaviors, such as stereotyped, nonfunctional speech, self-stimulatory behavior, and so on. It would be interesting to know whether the increased social and functional use of language implies pragmatic growth—that is, the use of an increasing number of language functions in a more advanced manner—rather than merely increased fequencies. The data reported fail to clarify this issue. Nevertheless, lack of communicative speech was noted by Kanner (1943) as one of the most striking features of the autistic syndrome. Hence, gains in social, communicative speech and decreases in isolate and repetitive behaviors are of utmost relevance to the management of children with autism. The merits of operant procedures have been well documented, and continued use seems justified.

The limited effectiveness of operant techniques in teaching language concepts may not be an immediate reflection of the inadequacy of the paradigm itself, but rather may reflect the ways in which it has been applied—that is, in a rather rigid and nonfunctional manner, favoring speech imitation and massed practice. Both teaching content and teaching techniques deserve careful reconsideration, as does the emphasis on speech as the sole means of communication. Although these issues overlap, for sake of clarity they will be discussed separately.

Teaching Techniques

Attempts to upgrade instructional efforts should examine the perspectives of innovations within the operant paradigm. Innovations may be applied to components of the stimulus-response paradigm—that is, to stimulus conditions, response characteristics, and consequences applied; these are more extensively discussed elsewhere (Goetz, Schuler, and Sailor, 1979; Schuler, 1980). In this context, a few issues will be raised that are of immediate relevance to everyday clinical practices. First, it should be realized that the pictorial stimuli commonly used for language teaching may not be appropriate in cases of autism that are associated with low levels of symbolic development. Real-life objects of immediate experiential salience would be more relevant. Furthermore, a range of different objects, supplemented by color photographs and pictures, should be used to enhance generalization.

Regarding responses, there is increasing evidence that passive pointing responses are not suitable for nonsymbolic or presymbolic students; their own actions upon objects seem to be crucial to symbolic growth. Thus, responses or referents that involve active manipulation of objects or physical activities of some kind, as in the labeling of actions through verbs, may be most desirable as targets for intervention. Furthermore, words acquired by autistic individuals often refer to static properties of things, rather than to actions and perspectives of people. Such a preponderance of static words should suggest additional caution in teaching passive responses.

A related matter is the relationship between responses and consequences. Rather arbitrary relationships between responses and consequences are often observed (for example, a treat as a consequence for touching a ball), but experimental data suggest that a more natural relationship (for example, "ball" as a request to play ball) may be more conducive to learning. This raises a critical related issue—the need to consider the function of the utterances taught—which will be discussed in more detail in the next section.

A last consideration crucial to everyday clinical practice pertains to the use of so-called massed versus dispersed trials. Often, a same response is trained over and over, without empirical validation of this type of repetitive training. If such responses were taught in a more functional context, a couple of different responses might actually follow each other, producing a sequence of related behaviors and thus facilitating the acquisition of meaning.

Departures from established clinical practices in language teaching may ultimately lead to more effective teaching techniques, adapting the operant format to the teaching of more varied and interchangeable behaviors that are compatible with the true nature of language.

Teaching Content: Pragmatic Considerations

Operant approaches to language training attend more closely to *how* a skill is taught than to *what* is being taught. In fact, some case reports merely demonstrate the effectiveness of operant techniques. Because considerations of which behaviors to teach to whom have received only minimal attention, the limits of the operant paradigm for language instruction may not yet be reached. Improvements could be made, for instance, by providing a closer match between a student's entrance skills and his or her motivation to use language for particular purposes and instructional content. Past teaching efforts reflect a preoccupation with the structures of language, divorced from underlying concepts and, perhaps more important, from the motivation to use the structures for purposes of social interaction. The recent shift in the orientation of psycholinguistic research—that is, the emphasis on pragmatic issues and the interrelationship between cognitive, social, and linguistic development—holds promise for innovative changes in teaching content. Although such a shift has direct implications for the management of all communication disorders, the management of autistic communication disorders merits particular consideration. As pointed out earlier, discrepancies between speech, language, cognitive, and communicative behaviors are often extreme. Speech proficiency often exceeds linguistic and, particularly, communicative abilities, while cognitive abilities do not maintain equality with communicative and linguistic development. Therefore, common instructional practices such as those that serve to increase speech imitation skills tend to be superfluous. Furthermore, comprehension skills are often overestimated, and targeted utterances are often irrelevant to communicative needs. It is unlikely, for instance, that autistic children who fail to be motivated by social attention will spontaneously generate such utterances as "This is a ———," because these words suggest social consequences. Attempts to enhance communication skills should focus on utterances that provide for more relevant consequences, such as an opportunity to engage in a favorite activity, a change in environment, an alleviation of pressure, and so forth. In order to select such relevant speech functions, a careful functional analysis of a student's behavioral repertoire is crucial. Such an analysis might even indicate that certain disruptive behaviors, such as self-injury, perseverative speech, and so forth, serve communicative functions. Through tantrums or self-injurious behavior, for instance, autistic children may communicate their requests to be left alone. If this is so, language instruction may incorporate such requests by providing more appropriate means to accomplish such a function (for a more detailed discussion of these issues, see Schuler and Goetz, 1981), and thus may indirectly serve to decrease behavior problems. In this way, the functional analysis of observed behavior may pinpoint relevant instructional objectives. Also, behavioral problems are often alleviated by minimizing verbal input. Poor speech comprehension is often concealed by fluent speech output, the stereotyped and automatic nature of which may not be apparent at first. Therefore, demands are easily too high, setting a student up for repeated failure because of unrealistic expectations. Again, it is crucial that the various aspects of speech and language behavior are closely examined in relation to each other. In many cases, more basic objectives, such as learning to take turns in a social exchange, may need to be pursued regardless of apparent speech proficiency. Teachers and speech-language-pathologists need to understand that language instruction for autistic children may require a very different approach from, for instance, that for aphasic children or others with language handicaps. Common practices that emphasize speech production and language structure (syntax) may need to be shifted toward the rules of conversation and the logistics of asking questions and of initiating and maintaining conversations. Many autistic students will need specific practice in making phone calls, running errands, reading facial expressions and tones of voice, and so forth. In behavioral terms, the emphasis is being placed on stimulus control rather than on response topography. Obviously, this applies particularly to speaking but primarily echolalic individuals. For the management of nonspeaking or mute individuals, as well as those with persistent nonfunctional echolalia, the use of alternative nonspeech communication systems holds some promise.

Use of Nonspeech Communication Systems

The trend toward using nonspeech communication systems for language instruction of individuals with varying language handicaps has possibly been the most exciting new development in the remediation of language problems during the last decade (for a detailed review, see Schiefelbusch and Hollis, 1979). The increased use of nonspeech systems reflects the growing realization that speech and language are not identical and that language and related thinking processes may be served by a multitude of means. Ironically, the merits of these approaches need to be examined for use with the population whose erratic speech and language behaviors may serve as the best illustration of the extent to which speech and language can be dissociated.

Although the effectiveness of sign language and other nonspeech communication systems has probably been more firmly documented in other populations, increasing efforts have been made to teach various forms of nonspeech communication systems to autistic children. One of the first extensive investigations into the effectiveness of sign language with autistic children was carried out by Creedon (1973). She reported that the use of sign language resulted in gains for all of the 21 children involved; they at least learned to express some basic wants and needs. Several other studies have appeared since, including even a comprehensive manual to direct those who want to teach sign language to individuals with autistic traits (Schaeffer, Kollinzas, Musil, and MacDowell, 1981).

Attempts to use nonspeech communication systems have not been limited to sign language. Premack and Premack (1974), for instance, reported on how the plastic symbol system that they initially designed to teach language to a chimpanzee was used to teach plural markers to an autistic boy. Carrier and Peak (1974) reported on the successful use of an adapted form of this symbol system, called Non Slip (Non Speech Language Initiation Program), with a larger severely and profoundly retarded population, including some autistic individuals; and a more specific data-based study involving children diagnosed as autistic was reported by McLean and McLean (1974).

The precocious writing and spelling abilities that some autistic children exhibit have also been used as a nonspeech communication alternative. A communication board incorporating written-word labels was used by Ratusnik and Ratusnik (1974). LaVigna (1977) taught written-word–object associations to three severely retarded autistic individuals through the use of an errorless discrimination learning paradigm. Our own research (Schuler, 1979a and 1979b) further indicates that written-word labels may be taught successfully to individuals who have been unable to learn to discriminate consistently between spoken words and signs. Other experiments have involved the use of computer consoles (Colby, 1973) to promote communication skills in nonspeaking autistic children. However, despite the apparent promise this medium holds for the autistic population, no systematic studies have been reported on the use of such an approach; the possibilities and limits of this medium need to be determined by future studies. The usefulness of Bliss symbols, communication aids, and communication boards also deserves further investigation. Although largely nonverbal autistic students may not be able to profit much from the symbolic cues inherent in Bliss symbols, communication boards hold some promise because of the spatial nature of the representations involved.

At this point, it is difficult to draw firm conclusions from the various case studies reported because of their preliminary nature, the lack of controls, and the paucity of information pertaining to the entrance skills involved. For instance, descriptions of subjects as nonverbal and as exhibiting severe behavioral problems leave proficiencies in the areas of nonverbal communication and symbolic development unspecified. So far, the results of the use of sign language and other nonspeech communication systems appear to be variable. It is possible that firm conclusions or recommendations relating to the autistic population as a whole will never emerge or be substantiated. What should be realized, however, is that, as a rule, autistic individuals do not excel in nonverbal communication, nor do they spontaneously make up signs and gestures. Because of the paucity of their symbolic and communicative abilities, it would be unrealistic to expect rapid gains. In many cases the use of gesture, body orientation, gaze, facial expression, and the like needs to be explicitly taught. Furthermore, instruction in nonspeech communication needs to proceed in a carefully programmed, systematic manner, and a close match should be sought between student and system characteristics. Furthermore, progress should be continuously evaluated, so that more appropriate approaches can be selected in cases of poor results.

Choosing a Communication System

In the selection of an appropriate communication system, it should be realized that choices may be of a preliminary nature and that one may gradually move up to more complex systems once the notion of communication is grasped in a more limited context. Again, explicit instruction in the use of gesture, body orientation, gaze, and voice may be most suitable both to prepare for as well as to accompany the use of more formal language systems. Such natural gestures are readily understood and will have to clarify communicative efforts otherwise not readily understood by the outside world. In making preliminary decisions regarding the selection of more formal systems, the teacher needs to closely examine student variables as well as system characteristics and, perhaps even more important, the opportunities for communication. Speech obviously remains the system of choice, because the expressive potential and audiences are unlimited. Sign language also allows for virtually unlimited expression, but with a much more limited audience. Fortunately, however, this audience is growing. Other systems, such as plastic symbols, communication boards, and pictorial and written-word systems, allow only a limited number of messages and ideas to be expressed; the only words to be used are those for which pictures, written-word labels, plastic shapes, and so forth, have been constructed in advance. In addition, these word-teaching tools are often not easily portable, leaving the communicator at a loss when the board is out of reach or the written-word cards are misplaced. Furthermore, the usability of a plastic symbol system is very limited when adopted in the real world. Nevertheless, these types of systems are readily put to use; they are relatively easy to teach with because only simple hand movements and varying degrees of visual and spatial discrimination are involved. In fact, the complexity of the discriminations involved should rarely present a stumbling block for the autistic child. The inherent promise of rapid success may greatly alleviate the often severe behavioral problems encountered beginning work with an autistic student. However, the most critical issue in considering the various options available involves the willingness of members of the child's environment—parents, teachers, residential and workshop staff, and so forth—to adopt the system selected.

Regarding the characteristics of various systems, all nonspeech systems bypass the auditory modality. The implications for autism are that this prevents the use of, in some cases, a suspect modality; the excessive use of speech and sound in general may set the stage for behavioral problems in some cases. Also, in cases where the integrity of the auditory modality may be questioned, nonfunctional echolalia persists despite communicative advances through other modes. An important difference between nonspeech and speech communication pertains to the ways in which the information is coded. The discriminations imposed in using speech are all of a temporal nature; the information is transient, since sounds produced are lost within the continuous act of speech production. This does not apply to pictures, plastic symbols, or written words. The information presented is fixed in time and remains visible over time, allowing the user a second look. As pointed out earlier, autistic individuals are often better equipped to deal with information of a spatial nature, which may make the latter systems more accessible. The dual nature of signing is interesting in this respect, since transient hand movements are superimposed upon hand configurations, which are coded in space. Signing may therefore not be so easily grasped by autistic children, who seem to encounter similar problems in comprehending the nonverbal signals inherent in interaction with others. The complexity of the responses involved also needs to be considered in examining the available systems. The use of signs offers a considerable advantage over speech in terms of teaching techniques; signs are readily prompted or molded, allowing us to focus on functional use without the pitfalls of arduous speech-shaping. The teaching of the other systems discussed allows for even more rapid progress, since the hand movements involved are even simpler in nature.

In making the best match between individual students and systems available, the following child variables need to be considered.

Age   Obviously, the higher the age, the slimmer the chances are of developing a comprehensive language system. A limited but functional communication system (geared to the needs of the everyday living situation) may be a more realistic goal.

Communicative Development   The teaching of nonspeech communication systems, such as signing, will proceed more easily if the notion of communication is already established. This may be evidenced by a rich use of gestures, facial expression, and so forth. In such a case, the teaching of signs merely involves the mapping of existing intentions.

Conceptual Development   Poor conceptual development will severely limit the dimensions of the language system to be developed. If a child does not understand the interrelationships between things and events in his or her world, as may be evidenced by poor classification and categorization skills, extreme caution needs to be applied in selecting instructional objectives. For instance, concrete labels for preferred actions and activities will be more suitable than labels for more abstract object attributes. Again, a more limited communication system may be more realistic.

Speech Comprehension   In cases in which speech comprehension is much poorer than conceptual and communicative skills, rapid gains can be expected from the introduction of an alternative nonspeech communication system, deemphasizing the speech component. When speech comprehension far exceeds speech production, a specific speech-production problem is usually indicated. Use of speech paired with signs in such cases not only may further language development, but also may serve to improve speech production.

According to case studies, the use of signed speech seems to enhance speech production in at least a third of the cases reported.

Vocal versus Manual Imitation Skills   If vocal imitation skills are well developed, primary efforts are made to use these skills for the development of functional language. If manual far surpasses vocal imitation, sign language might be a more viable option. In cases in which both vocal and manual imitation skills are poor, other systems might be used that demand less elaborate responses to get the idea of communication across. Concurrent attempts should be made to upgrade imitation skills, allowing for a later switch to a more versatile system.

Visual Discrimination Skills   Although all the nonspeech systems discussed require some visual discrimination skills, the complexity of skills involved varies. For instance, written words are more demanding than pictures, but some autistic children seem to have a facility for the former; therefore, individual differences need to be considered. A great deal of variance has been noted with regard to modality preference as well as so-called stimulus overselectivity are taken into consideration (for a review, see Lovaas, Koegel, and Schreibman (1979). Many autistic children do much better whan information is presented visually, but others may prefer the auditory modality. With regard to stimulus overselectivity, some autistic children become overselective when multiple stimulus input is presented; they attend only to one—and often an idiosyncratic—component of the stimulus complex, apparently ignoring the rest. An everyday illustration of this phenomenon involves the child who "recognizes" a family member only when the relative wears glasses. When this same person doesn't wear the glasses, the child may act as if he or she had never before seen the person. Nevertheless, not all children are that way. Overall, the higher the level of development—particularly of conceptual and linguistic development—the less the likelihood of such overselectivity. In some cases developmental growth may be thwarted, but in other cases it is facilitated through the use of multiple stimulus input. Therefore, it is extremely important to match carefully the child's level of development and learning characteristics with the requirements of the system used and the possibilities for use. In addition, progress should be carefully monitored so that changes in approach can be made to best suit the capabilities of the individual child. Again, progress will most likely be slow, since the language problems of the autistic child are of a broad nature, including communicative and cognitive peculiarities. Nevertheless, even slight changes or minor breakthroughs may be of great help in coping with everyday life. Furthermore, advances made may generate a more profound understanding of autistic language impairments, since the acquisition of language concepts is studied separately from the maturation of speech perception and speech production mechanisms. Consistent success or failure with particular systems or instructional content should further elucidate the extent to which cognitive and linguistic impairments are interwined.

REFERENCES AND SUGGESTED READINGS

Ball, J. "A Pragmatic Analysis of Autistic Children's Language with Respect to Aphasic and Normal Language Development." Unpublished doctoral dissertation, Melbourne University, 1978.

Baltaxe, C. A. M. "Pragmatic Deficits in the Language of Autistic Adolescents," *Journal of Pediatric Psychology,* 2, 1977, 176–180.

Bates, E. *Language and Context: The Acquisition of Pragmatics.* New York: Academic Press, 1976.

Bloom, L. *Language Development: Form and Function in Emerging Grammars.* Cambridge, Mass.: M.I.T. Press, 1970.

Bricker, D. "Imitative Sign Training as a Facilitator of Word-Object Association with Low Functioning Children," *American Journal of Mental Deficiency,* 76, 1972, 509–516.

Caparulo, B. K., and Cohen, D. J. "Cognitive Structures, Language and Emerging Social Competence in Autistic and Aphasic Children," *Journal of the American Academy of Child Psychiatry,* 16, 1977, 630–645.

Carey, S. "The Child as Word Learner," in M. Halle, J. Bresnan, and G. A. Miller (eds.), *Linguistic Theory and Psychological Reality.* Cambridge, Mass.: M.I.T. Press, 1978.

Carrier, J. K. and Peak, T. *A Non-Speech Language Initiation Program.* Lawrence, Kans.: H & H Enterprises, 1975.

Churchill, D. W. *Language of Autistic Children.* Washington: Winston & Sons, 1978.

Clark, R. "Performing Without Competence," *Journal of Child Language,* 1, 1974, 1–10.

Cohen, D. J., Caparulo, B. S., and Shaywitz, B. "Primary Childhood Aphasia and Childhood Autism," *Journal of the Academy of Child Psychiatry,* 15, 1976, 604–644.

Colby, K. M. "The Rationale for Computer-Based Treatment of Language Difficulties in Nonspeaking Autistic Children," *Journal of Autism and Childhood Schizophrenia,* 3, 1973, 254–261.

Creedon, M. P. "Language Development in Nonverbal Autistic Children Using a Simultaneous Communication System." Paper presented at the Society for Research in Child Development Meeting, Philadelphia, 1973.

Cromer, R. F. "The Basis of Childhood Dysphasia: A Linguistic Approach," in M. A. Wyke (ed.), *Developmental Dysphasia.* London and New York: Academic Press, 1978.

Cromer, R. F. "Developmental Language Disorders: Cognitive Processes, Semantics, Pragmatics, Phonology and Syntax," *Journal of Autism and Developmental Disorders,* 2, 1981, 57–75.

Curcio, F. "Sensorimotor Functioning and Communication in Mute Autistic Children," *Journal of Autism and Childhood Schizophrenia,* 8, 1978, 281–292.

Cunningham, M. A., and Dixon, C. "A Study of the Language of an Autistic Child," *Journal of Child Psychology and Psychiatry,* 2, 1961, 193–202.

Curtiss, S. "Dissociations Between Language and Cognition: Cases and Implications," *Journal of Autism and Developmental Disorders,* 2, 1981, 15–31.

Curtiss, S., Yamada, J., and Fromkin, V. "How Independent Is Language? On the Question of Formal Parallels Between Grammar and Action," *UCLA Working Papers in Cognitive Linguistics,* 1, 1979, 131–157.

Damasio, A. R., and Mauer, R. G. "A Neurological Model for Childhood Autism," *Archives of Neurology,* 35, 1978, 777–786.

De Hirsch, K. "Differential Diagnosis Between Aphasic and Schizophrenic Language in Children," *Journal of Speech and Hearing Disorders*, 32, 1967, 3–10.

Duchan, J., and Prizant, B. "A Functional Analysis of Immediate Echolalia in Autistic Children," *Journal of Speech and Hearing Disorders*, in press.

Fay, W. H. "Mitigated Echolalia of Children," *Journal of Speech and Hearing Research*, 10, 1967, 305–310.

Fay, W. H., and Schuler, A. L. *Emerging Language in Autistic Children*. Balitmore: University Park Press, 1980.

Freeman, B. J., and Ritvo, E. R. "Diagnostic and Evaluation Systems." In Budde, J. (ed.), *Advocacy and Autism*, Lawrence, Kansas: University of Kansas Press, 1977.

Goetz, L., Schuler, A. L., and Sailor, W. "Teaching Functional Speech to the Severely Handicapped: Current Issues," *Journal of Autism and Developmental Disorders*, 9, 1979, 325–343.

Hewett, F. M. "Teaching Speech to an Autistic Child Through Operant Conditioning," *American Journal of Orthopsychiatry*, 35, 1965, 927–936.

Howlin, P. "Training Parents to Modify the Language of Their Autistic Children: A Home Based Approach." Unpublished doctoral dissertation, London University, 1979.

Howlin, P. "Language Training with the Severely Retarded, in W. Yule and J. Carr (eds.), *Behavior Modification with the Severely Retarded*. London: Croom Helm, 1980.

Howlin, P. A. "The Effectiveness of Operant Language Training with Autistic Children," *Journal of Autism and Developmental Disorders*, 2, 1981, 89–105.

Kanner, L. "Autistic Disturbances of Affective Contact," *Nervous Child*, 2, 1943, 217–250.

Kolvin, I. "Diagnostic Criteria and Classification of Childhood Psychoses," *British Journal of Psychiatry*, 118, 1971, 381–396.

LaVigna, B. W. "Communication Training in Mute Autistic Adolescents Using the Written Word," *Journal of Autism and Childhood Schizophrenia*, 7, 1977, 135–149.

Lovaas, O. I. *The Autistic Child*. New York: Wiley, 1977.

Lovaas, O. I., Berberich, J. P., Perloff, B. F., and Schaeffer, B. "Acquisition of Imitative Speech by Schizophrenic Children," *Science*, 151, 1966, 705–707.

Lovaas, O. I., Koegel, R. L., and Schreibman, L. "Stimulus Overselectivity in Autism: A Review of Research," *Psychological Bulletin*, 86, 1979, 1231–1254.

MacLean, L. P., and MacLean, J. E. "A Language Training Program for Non-Verbal Autistic Children," *Journal of Speech and Hearing Disorders*, 39, 1974, 186–194.

Menyuk, P. "Comparison of Grammar of Children with Functionally Deviant and Normal Speech," *Journal of Speech and Hearing Research*, 7, 1964, 109–121.

Menyuk, P. *Sentences Children Use*. Cambridge, Mass.: M.I.T. Press, 1969.

Menyuk, P. "Language: What's Wrong and Why," in M. Rutter and E. Schopler (eds.), *Autism: A Reappraisal of Concepts and Treatment*. New York: Plenum Press, 1978.

Premack, D., and Premack, A. "Teaching a Symbol Language to Language Deficient Children," in R. Schiefelbusch and L. L. Lloyd (eds.), *Language Perspectives, Acquisition, Retardation and Intervention*. Baltimore: University Park Press, 1974.

Ratusnik, C. M., and Ratusnik, D. L. "A Comprehensive Communication Approach for a Ten Year Old Nonverbal Autistic Child," *American Journal of Orthopsychiatry*, 44, 1974, 396–403.

Ricks, D. M., and Wing, L. "Language, Communication and the Use of Symbols," in L. Wing (ed.), *Early Childhood Autism*. London: Pergamon Press, 1976.

Rimland, B. *Infantile Autism*. New York: Appleton-Century-Crofts, 1964.

Ritvo, E. R., and Freeman, B. J. "Proposed Definition of the Syndrome of Autism by the National Society for Autistic Children and the American Psychiatric Association DSM III Committee," 1977.

Rutter, M. "Childhood Schizophrenia Reconsidered," *Journal of Autism and Childhood Schizophrenia,* 2, 1972, 315–337.

Rutter, M. "Diagnosis and Definition," in M. Rutter and E. Schopler (eds.), *Autism, a Reappraisal of Concepts and Treatment*. New York and London: Plenum Press, 1978.

Rutter, M., Bartak, L., and Newman, S. "Autism—A Central Disorder of Cognition and Language?" in M. Rutter (ed.), *Infantile Autism: Concepts, Characteristics and Treatment*. Edinburgh and London: Churchill-Livingston, 1971.

Schaeffer, B., Kollinzas, G., Musil, A., and MacDowell, P. *Total Communication*. Matthis, Ill.: Research Press, 1981.

Schiefelbusch, R. L., and Hollis, J. H. *Language Intervention from Ape to Child*. Baltimore: University Park Press, 1979.

Schuler, A. L. "Communicative, Conceptual and Representational Abilities in a Mute Autistic Adolescent: A Serial vs. a Simultaneous Mode of Processing." Unpublished doctoral dissertation, University of California, Santa Barbara, 1979a.

Schuler, A. L. "Echolalia: Clinical Issues and Applications," *Journal of Speech and Hearing Disorders,* 44, 1979b, 411–434.

Schuler, A. L. "Teaching Functional Language to Autistic Children," in B. Wilcox and A. Thompson (eds.), *Critical Issues in Educating Autistic Children and Youth*. Washington, D.C.: U.S. Department of Education Office of Special Education, 1980.

Schuler, A. L., and Baldwin, M. "Non-Speech Communication and Childhood Autism," *Language, Speech and Hearing Services in the Schools,* 12 (4), 1981, 246–257.

Schuler, A. L., and Goetz, L. "The Assessment of Severe Language Disabilities: Linguistic, Communicative and Cognitive Considerations," *Analysis and Intervention of Developmental Disabilities,* 1, 1981, 333–347.

Sloane, H. N., and MacAuley, B. D. *Operant Procedures in Remedial Speech and Language Training*. Boston: Houghton Mifflin, 1968.

Stevens-Long, J., and Rasmussen, M. "The Acquisition of Simple and Compound Sentence Structure in an Autistic Child," *Journal of Applied Behavior Analysis,* 7, 1974, 473–480.

Tager-Flusberg, H. "On the Nature of Linguistic Functioning in Early Infantile Autism," *Journal of Autism and Developmental Disorders,* 2, 1981a, 45–56.

Tager-Flusberg, H. "Pragmatic Development and Its Implications for Social Interaction in Autistic Children." Paper presented at the International Symposium on Autism Research, Boston, 1981b.

Wheeler, A. J., and Sulzer, B. "Operant Training and Generalization of a Verbal Response Form in a Speech Deficient Child," *Journal of Applied Behavior Analysis,* 3, 1970, 139–147.

Wing, L. "Language, Social and Cognitive Impairments in Autism and Severe Mental Retardation," *Journal of Autism and Developmental Disorders,* 2, 1981, 31–44.

Wing, L., Gould, J., Yeates, S. R., and Brierly, L. M. "Symbolic Play in Severely Mentally Retarded and Autistic Children," *Journal of Child Psychology and Psychiatry,* 18, 1977, 167–178.

Wolf, M. M., Risley, T. R., and Mees, H. J. "Applications of Operant Conditioning Procedures to the Behavior Problems of an Autistic Child," *Behavior Research Therapy,* 2, 1964, 305–312.

Wolff, S., and Chess, S. "An Analysis of the Language of Fourteen Schizophrenic Children," *Journal of Child Psychology and Psychiatry,* 6, 1965, 29–41.

appendix

Case History Form: Children with Retarded Language Development

Name _____   Medical record _____

Birth date _____   Date _____

Age at the time of examination _____   Interviewer _____

Address _____   Referring agency _____

_____   _____

Telephone number _____   _____

Father's occupation: Mother's name _____Age _____

_____   Father's name _____Age _____

Mother's occupation: Siblings   Age

1 _____

2 _____

Father's education: 3 _____

4 _____

5 _____

Mother's education: 6 _____

7 _____

Informant:

_____

Reports from other agencies:

_____

_____

_____

_____

I. HISTORY
  A. Statement of the problem
     by informant:

  B. Family background:

  C. Medical:
     1. Pre- and paranatal:

     2. Illnesses:

estimate of child's handicap
attitude toward child
success in communicating with child
estimate of child's attitude toward
    handicap

siblings: problems
socioeconomic status
education
language environment: home,
    elsewhere
history of language disorders
family adjustment
family interests and attitudes
discipline problems

number of pregnancies, miscarriages
stillbirths
health during pregnancy
toxic factors
birth trauma
RH incompatibility
precipitous delivery
prolonged delivery
premature birth
post-term

rubella
anoxia
encephalitis
meningitis
virus infections
respiratory ailments
mumps

                                      high fevers
                                      convulsions
                                      earaches
                                      surgery
                                      measles
                                      allergies
                                      other

D. Development:
   1. Motor:

sitting age
standing age
walking age
climbing
evidence of motor disability
evidence of sensory disability
laterality: left, right, mixed; age
   when established for handedness

   2. Social:

toilet training
self-dressing
eating habits
personal hygiene
sleeping habits
peer relationships
degree of relatedness to
   siblings
   parents
   relatives
   friends
ability to share
play habits
   favorite games
   favorite toys
personal traits
temper tantrums
degree of cooperativeness
ability to establish rapport
degree of physical contact
   with objects
   with persons
degree and type of affect
fears
adjustments to changing situations
ability to attend
distractibility
restlessness
hyperactivity
pulls head, ears
head banging, rocking
demands cleanliness
meticulous
thumb sucking

3. Oral:

prelingual activity
    crying
    laughing
early sound-making history
    babbling
    echolalia
child unusually noisy?
child unusually quiet?
first words—age
how were first words evoked?
types of words?
complexity?
play "noises"
sound imitation
estimate of comprehension
gesture language
How does child express needs?
sucking
swallowing
regurgitation
chewing

4. Educational:

formal schooling
achievement
strengths
weaknesses
special schooling
likes
dislikes

5. Intellectual functioning:

parents' estimate of intelligence
    Mother
    Father
    other

Index of Authors

Index of Subjects